D0949442

DISRUPTIVE BEHAVIOR DISORDERS IN CHILDREN
Treatment-Focused Assessment

DISRUPTIVE BEHAVIOR DISORDERS IN CHILDREN
Treatment-Focused Assessment

MICHAEL J. BREEN
Winneconne Community School District and
University of Wisconsin–Oshkosh

THOMAS S. ALTEPETER
University of Wisconsin–Oshkosh

Foreword by Russell A. Barkley

THE GUILFORD PRESS
New York   London

© 1990 The Guilford Press
A Division of Guilford Publications, Inc.
72 Spring Street, New York, NY 10012

Printed in the United States of America

This book is printed on acid-free paper.

Last digit is print number: 9 8 7 6 5 4 3 2 1

Library of Congress Cataloging-in-Publication Data

Breen, Michael J.
    Disruptive behavior disorders in children: treatment-focused
assessment / Michael J. Breen, Thomas S. Altepeter.
        p.   cm.
    Includes bibliographical references.
    Includes index.
    ISBN 0-89862-439-8
    1. Behavior disorders in children.   2. Behavior disorders in
children—Treatment.   I. Title.
    [DNLM: 1. Behavior Therapy—in infancy & childhood.
2. Child Behavior Disorders—diagnosis.   3. Child Behavior Disorders—therapy.   WS 350. 6 B832d]
RJ506.B44B74   1990
618.92'858—dc20
DNLM/DLC
for Library of Congress   90-3817
                                                              CIP

To our parents, wives, and children:

Robert and Joyce Breen; my wife, Joan; and children, Sara-Beth, Michael, Daniel, Anne-Marie, and the child we loved and lost

—M.J.B.

Arthur and Gloria Altepeter; my wife, Donna; and children, Andy and Maria

—T.S.A.

FOREWORD

To use books rightly, is to go to them for help; to
appeal to them when our own knowledge and power fail;
to be led by them into wide sight and purer conception
than our own, and to receive from them the united
sentence of the judges and councils of all time,
against our solitary and unstable opinions.

—JOHN RUSKIN (1819–1900)

Throughout the history of research in child and developmental psychopathology, one dimension of child behavior repeatedly emerges as the principle component of those problems that result in children being referred for mental health services in Western societies. That dimension is childhood externalizing behavior, what some have called childhood conduct problems or aggresion, and now has officially been labeled the Disruptive Behavior Disorders. This broad band of childhood maladjustment represents behaviors often labeled hyperactive, inattentive, disruptive, aggressive, antisocial, clandestine, delinquent, and even criminal.

Numerous studies attest to the developmental robustness and stability of this behavioral dimension and its significance as a major predictor of later childhood, adolescent, and even young adult social maladjustment, academic underachievement, and psychiatric disturbance. The personal and social costs of these behavioral problems is enormous. A truly effective treatment approach for them that affects the long-term outcome of these children awaits our discovery. Meanwhile, much of what we have in the way of clinical interventions are symptomatic, relatively situation specific, and of little long-lasting benefit once they are terminated. This has resulted in many senior clinical scientists in this field pronouncing this dimension as the behavioral equivalent of the developmental disorders: having an early onset, affecting adjustment across most domains of social functioning, and being relatively chronic such that it affects and hence predicts general adult social outcome.

Recent research suggests that this broad dimension of childhood and adolescent misconduct can be subdivided into hyperactive/inattentive behavior, aggressive or hostile/defiant behavior, and delinquent or antisocial behavior. The most recent version of the official psychiatric nomenclature of the United States, the DSM-III-R, has officially labeled these dimensions Attention–deficit Hyperactivity Disorder, Oppositional Defiant Disorder, and Conduct Disorder, respectively. It is fair to say that more research has been conducted on these disorders, combined, than on any other type of childhood behavioral, developmental, emotional, or learning disorders.

Because these three disorders account for the vast majority of child referrals for mental health services and increasingly for special educational resources as well, there is a tremendous need to extract from this literature that which is of greatest clinical utility in differential diagnosis and treatment planning. Moreover, and in view of the increasing social significations of this cluster of childhood behavioral problems, there has arisen a widespread professional need for a manual that clearly sets forth a methodology for the clinical assessment of this large proportion of the clinic-referred population. This task has been made all the more compelling by the rapid proliferation of numerous formats for clinical interviewing and the plethora of child behavior rating scales aimed at assessing these behaviors for clinical or research purposes. Little guidance exists in the clinical literature to assist the practitioner in deciphering the relative utility of methods in this extensive array of potentially useful clinical instruments, often leaving the impression that one format or rating scale is as good as another. This is hardly the case.

Breen and Altepeter have now provided us with precisely the right guidebook to a sophisticated yet economical approach for the yeoman's work we must do—the assessment of these complex but common childhood disorders. They have nicely summarized the clinical essences of each disorder, providing us with a succinct overview of their nature and associated conditions. But, more importantly, they have waded through the morass of available instruments and formats for us to deduce a well-reasoned, carefully selected set of procedures likely to be of maximum benefit in clinical assessment, diagnosis, and treatment planning. In doing so, they have paid careful attention to both the "artistic" and "humanistic" elements of clinical assessment as well as to the increasingly important scientific and technical components it now demands from the clinician. The result is a concise, up-to-date, and "user-friendly" clinical manual that should prove of great benefit to a variety of disciplines, including clinical psychology and psychiatry, school psychology, developmental/behavioral pediatrics, social work, and special education. It is certainly likely to be one of those very rare books that one keeps on the professional desk rather than the more distant bookshelf as one will refer to it repeatedly throughout the day-to-day stream of child clinical cases in the course of one's practice. Talbot Wilson Chambers (1819-96), the popular American clergyman, once said, "Books are standing counselors and preachers, always at hand, and always disinterested; having this advantage over oral instructors, that they are ready to repeat their lesson as often as we please." More than most, this book will provide such useful daily counsel for a long time to come.

RUSSELL A. BARKLEY, PhD
University of Massachusetts Medical Center

PREFACE

It is widely recognized that children and adolescents characterized as "out of control"—who exhibit a variety of overactive, impulsive, disruptive, and noncompliant behaviors—are among those most commonly referred for professional help by parents and educators. Public and professional interest in children with these behavior problems has increased dramatically during the past two decades. With this increased interest, there has been a proliferation of research examining the etiologies, assessment, diagnosis, and treatment of these disorders. Presently, one is hard-pressed to find a single copy of a child-related professional journal that does not contain several research articles examining issues related to the cluster of childhood disorders currently referred to as Disruptive Behavior Disorders. Due to this focused attention, the empirical knowledge base has grown rapidly in richness and complexity in a relatively short time.

Despite these many positive developments, the translation of this literature into practical, psychometrically sound, treatment-relevant assessment procedures has lagged behind. Indeed, many outdated, inappropriate, and ambiguous assessment and monitoring methods continue to be widely used in research and clinical practice. The need for a more standardized, systematic, and integrated method of assessing children presenting with externalizing behavior problems is clear. The present volume is our attempt to meet this need. In so doing, we offer a hands-on, practical, yet researched-based, treatment-focused assessment protocol for use with children suspected of having one or more of the Disruptive Behavior Disorders. We then provide methods of integrating this information to be used as a foundation for subsequent treatment.

To the degree that we have realized this goal, the volume should prove useful to currently practicing clinicians and clinicians in training, regardless as to discipline. In addition we have suggested that the appropriate treatment and management of many children with Disruptive Behavior Disorders necessarily involves interdisciplinary cooperation. Very often this will involve physicians, clinical and school psychologists, regular and exceptional educators, perhaps social workers, and of course the child's parents. Unfortunately, professionals from these disciplines often have diverse ways of approaching and working with such children. As a result, they often do not "speak the same language," and therefore may have some difficulty working cooperatively across disciplines. Often it is the child and family who suffer, as optimal interdisciplinary treatment is not realized. In preparing this volume, we deliberately have taken an interdisciplinary approach, in order to facilitate better understanding and communication across professions. We hope, then, that practicing clinicians and clinicians in training from each of the relevant professions (pediatrics, child psychiatry, child clinical and school psychology, regular and exceptional education, and social work) will find the text interesting and useful in their work.

We are indebted to Dr. C. Eugene Walker and Dr. Russell A. Barkley for their time and effort in reviewing portions of this text. The enthusiasm and support of Ms. Sharon Panulla at The Guilford Press have been greatly appreciated.

MICHAEL J. BREEN, PhD
THOMAS S. ALTEPETER, PhD

CONTENTS

1

AN OVERVIEW
OF
DISRUPTIVE BEHAVIOR DISORDERS

It is widely recognized that children who are generally characterized as "out of control" and who exhibit a variety of noncompliant, oppositional, disruptive, and aggressive behaviors are among the most commonly referred for professional help by parents and teachers (Herbert, 1978; Kazdin, 1985; Safer & Allen, 1976; Wells & Forehand, 1985). Typical complaints expressed by parents and teachers of these children include noncompliance with primary and secondary authority figures, failure to behave in a manner consistent with common social norms and situation-specific rules (e.g., rules in the home and in the classroom), annoying or aversive interpersonal behaviors (e.g., lying, stealing, frequent yelling, temper tantrums, excessive motor activity, inattention, and impulsivity), and physically aggressive behaviors (e.g., hitting and fighting). Although less common, problems with older children may include serious delinquent behaviors such as persistent lying, truancy, theft, assault, vandalism, rape, and alcohol/drug abuse. Ordinarily, these behavior problems do not occur in isolation, but are exhibited in clusters and repeated over a period of many months or years.

1

Public and professional interest in children with these behavior problems has increased dramatically during the past two decades. With this increased interest, there has been a proliferation of empirical research, particularly concerning issues related to the assessment, diagnosis, and treatment of these disorders (Mash & Terdal, 1988; Rapport, 1987). Barkley (1981) has noted that one type of disruptive behavior problem, Attention-deficit Hyperactivity Disorder (ADHD), has become the childhood disorder most widely studied by professionals. Similarly, a recent review noted in excess of 300 publications between 1976 and 1984 that addressed etiological and/or diagnostic considerations of this disorder (Reatig, 1984). Presently, one is hard-pressed to find a single issue in a child-related professional journal that does not contain several research articles examining some issue related to this general cluster of childhood disorders. Due to this focused attention, the empirical knowledge base relating to the assessment and treatment of Disruptive Behavior Disorders has grown rapidly in richness and complexity in a relatively brief time.

Despite these many positive developments within the field of pediatric psychology and psychiatry, the translation of this rich empirical literature into practical, psychometrically sound, treatment-relevant assessment procedures for the front-line practitioner has lagged badly. Although researchers have recently noted the need for a consistent means of identifying children with Disruptive Behavior Disorders (Barkley, 1988b; McMahon & Forehand, 1988), many outdated, inappropriate, or ambiguous assessment methods continue to be utilized in both research and clinical practice. In a recent review of strategies employed to assess hyperactivity, for example, Prinz, Moore, and Roberts (1986) reported considerable variability across such factors as source of information, behavioral criteria, age, and chronicity. They concluded that there has been far too much variability in the manner in which children have been identified as hyperactive, and they argued that more behavioral specificity is needed. Similarly, we informally reviewed research articles from the 1989 issues of the *Journal of Abnormal Child Psychology* and the *Journal of the American Academy of Child and Adolescent Psychiatry* that were concerned with any one of the three Disruptive Behavior Disorders. Although most focused upon ADHD, a few researchers studied conduct-disordered children. Among the many empirically based articles we reviewed, we did not observe a consistent means by which authors identified their samples, even though all claimed to have identified ADHD or conduct-disordered children. The diversity in selection criteria was surprising. Of those that utilized child behavior rating scales, the degree of deviancy required on a Hyperactivity scale ranged from 1 to 2 standard deviations above the mean. The most comprehensive system of identification noted in any one article included a parent interview, Conners Parent and Teacher Questionnaires, and *Diagnostic and Statistical Manual of Mental Disorders III* (DSM-III) criteria. Others employed, in varying degrees, the

Werry–Weiss–Peters Activity Scale, the Stony Brook Scale, the IOWA Conners Teacher Rating Scale, Barkley's guidelines (Barkley, 1981), the Home Situations Questionnaire, the Rutter Child scales A & B, the Diagnostic Interview Schedule for Children, and DSM-III criteria. Even within the same issue, we found three quite different sample identification methods: (1) DSM-III criteria, the Abbreviated Symptom Questionnaire, and various psychometric measures; (2) DSM-II guidelines, average IQ, no history of significant pathology or neurologic anomaly, and classified as "favorable responders to stimulant treatment"; and (3) teacher-completed SNAP Checklist and the Stony Brook Scale. While some attempt was made to rule out versus rule in behaviors specific to the diagnosis across these studies, researchers identified their samples as having a Disruptive Behavior Disorder from rather different orientations. Inconsistency in defining groups contributes to confusion.

While the degree of inconsistency among methodologies is of concern to those conducting research, it also has clear implications for those providing direct service to these children and their families. Clinicians frequently rely on the literature for support and direction relative to identification and treatment focus. If these sources are themselves inconsistent, it is likely that clinicians would follow in similar fashion. Similarly, despite attempts to improve the reliability and validity of DSM-III and DSM-III-R's diagnostic criteria for these types of disorders, considerable variability in the manner in which these criteria are interpreted and applied by clinicians continues to be identified. Two recent studies highlight the diversity with which clinicians identify children with Disruptive Behavior Disorders.

First, Rosenberg and Beck (1986) sampled child clinical psychologists (American Psychological Association) and school psychologists (National Association of School Psychologists). They provided participants with a list of assessment techniques, including rating scales, standardized tests of intelligence and achievement, drawing tasks, neuropsychological tests, behavioral observations, interviews, and tests for attention and impulsivity. Participants were asked to identify strategies which they would use in evaluating a 7-year-old child of average intelligence suspected of being hyperactive. They were also asked which of these strategies would best support a diagnosis of hyperactivity. It was found that a high percentage of psychologists rely on interview and observation as common strategies. Most alarming, however, was the finding that 80–90% of the psychologists utilized IQ/achievement measures and/or drawing tasks as a primary method of assessment. Almost 50% used projective techniques in assessing hyperactive children. Rating scales were commonly used by 60–70% of the respondents. This survey demonstrates the wide variability of assessment practices currently employed and supports the need for a more standardized, systematic assessment protocol.

The second study was conducted by Copeland, Wolraich, Lindgren, Milich,

& Woolson (1987). Participants were members of the American Academy of Pediatrics. The intent of this study was to gather information regarding assessment and treatment methods used by pediatricians in caring for hyperactive children. In part, their data indicated that most pediatricians (approximately 90%) viewed information presented by parents and teachers as important sources in making a diagnosis of ADHD. However, only about 60% felt rating scales completed by the child's parents and/or teacher were helpful in the diagnostic process. Few reported using DSM criteria in diagnosing these children. Almost 50% of the respondents felt that "soft" neurologic signs were of diagnostic utility in identifying hyperactive children. Of the general pediatric practitioners 77% viewed the child's response to medication, without employing drug-placebo trials, as further evidence for or against the diagnosis of ADHD. These procedures continue to be widely utilized despite the availability of objective, empirically tested assessment procedures that could substantially improve the efficacy of this process (Barkley, Fischer, Newby, & Breen, 1988).

This substantial degree of diagnostic latitude observed within these studies is, we suspect, commonplace in clinical practice. For example, consider the following scenarios (which in our experience have not been uncommon) and how frustrating they must be for parents to experience. Concerned and well-meaning parents are initially told by a teacher that their child's behavior is interfering with his potential to succeed. Parents do some "soul-searching" and also acknowledge that their son's behavior at home is difficult to manage. Behavioral descriptors such as defiant and hyperactive keep surfacing. They decide to seek professional help for their child. Depending upon with whom they consult and how they initially present their situation (and many factors can influence this) they might come into contact with various professionals from several disciplines. From a parental perspective, they may feel "passed around" from one professional to another. Before they are finally satisfied with the services provided (or quit in frustration) they may have consulted many "experts" and: (1) been asked to complete the Connors Hyperactivity Index and participated in a 15-minute office interview, after which they were told that their son is not hyperactive; (2) been told the child is not hyperactive given that he can sit fairly quietly for 10–15 minutes while in the examining room or while watching television; (3) been told the child is hyperactive and oppositional after a brief office visit, given a prescription of methylphenidate, and told to say nothing to his teacher in order to note whether the teacher says anything to the parents relative to changes in the child's behavior; (4) been told he is "all boy" and that he will outgrow such behavior; (5) been told he needs "counseling" due to his poor attitude and emotional problems; and (6) had the child "tested" for hyperactivity, which resulted in being told he had average cognitive and academic skills (even the Freedom From Distractability Factor fell within the norm), but that he was emotionally disturbed and would thus need exceptional education.

We do of course realize that many clinicians offer nothing short of excellent diagnostic and treatment procedures. On the other hand, and by virtue of our interactions with parents and teachers, we have come to understand that some combination of the scenarios just described occurs far too often. If service delivery is to be at a premium and benefit those in need, the basic assessment process needs to be comprehensive in format and geared toward establishing an appropriate treatment program. In order to assess the complexities of child behavior, family dynamics, and parent–child interactions, arrive at a valid and reliable diagnosis, and offer appropriate treatment, a quick review of a child behavior questionnaire and a 15-minute office visit simply will not suffice. The clinician must be able to "rule out versus rule in" other psychiatric disorders that may present with a similar behavioral profile, as well as be in a position to identify circumstances that may contribute to the development and maintenance of the child's behavior problems (e.g., maternal depression, marital discord, or child abuse). Indeed, in order to evaluate, identify, and then treat children with a Disruptive Behavior Disorder, the clinician must be well versed in child psychopathology, follow a comprehensive assessment protocol that is treatment-focused, and have the necessary time to work with the parent, child, and teacher in a manner that will foster the belief that "help" can and will be provided.

In this chapter, we will provide a general overview of the disorders recently organized into the category of Disruptive Behavior Disorders in the *Diagnostic and Statistical Manual of Mental Disorders III-Revised of the American Psychiatric Association* (DSM-III-R; APA, 1987). We will review current definitions, commonly accepted research findings concerning primary and associated features, prevalence, etiology, developmental course and prognosis, and issues related to family characteristics and interaction patterns. Differential diagnostic considerations will also be reviewed briefly. Finally, we will discuss the need for systematic and integrated assessment strategies that incorporate multiple sources of information, are behaviorally oriented, and can be directly tied to subsequent treatment planning.

THE DISRUPTIVE BEHAVIOR DISORDERS

The conclusions consistently reached in comprehensive reviews (Achenbach & Edelbrock, 1978; Quay, 1979) support two major dimensions in child psychopathology, generally referred to as *internalizing* and *externalizing* disorders. Internalizing disorders are characterized by behaviors that are overcontrolled, inhibited, anxious, withdrawn, etc., and include diagnostic categories such as depressive, avoidant, and overanxious disorders. Typically children with these disorders suffer more than others in their environment as a result of their difficulties. The externalizing disorders, on the other hand, are characterized by behaviors that are undercontrolled, noncompliant, defiant, socially disruptive, aggressive, etc., and include DSM-III-R diagnostic categories such as Attention-Deficit Hyperactivity, Conduct, and Oppositional Defiant Disorders. Typically others in the environment, such as parents, siblings, peers, and teachers, suffer more than the children with these behaviors.

There is evidence suggesting that these disorders significantly overlap and, as a result, there is debate in the literature about whether they constitute separate disorders per se (Barkley, 1982; Henker & Whalen, 1989; Hinshaw, 1987; Loney & Milich, 1982; Prinz, Connor, & Wilson, 1981; Quay, 1986; Stewart, Cummings, Singer, & deBlois, 1981; Szatmari, Boyle, & Offord, 1989). For example, Hinshaw (1987) recently provided a thorough analysis of empirically identified similarities and differences between children with Attention-deficit Hyperactivity and Conduct Disorders (the reader is referred to the original article for a more detailed discussion). He reached several interesting conclusions. First, with respect to strict criteria (e.g., common etiology, signs/symptoms, prognosis, and treatment response for individuals within a category) the evidence does not support distinct narrow-band disorders of hyperactivity/attention deficit versus conduct problems/aggression. In particular, there is little evidence of differential biological precursors/etiologies, or of significant differential responses to available treatments. Second, separate but correlated behavioral dimensions have frequently emerged between the two "disorders" in factor analytic studies. Important differences between subgroups of children within these two domains have been identified. For example, antisocial parents and chronic family hostility are highly associated with children with Conduct Disorders, but not in ADHD children. Similarly, in structured situations, such as a classroom, ADHD children are more frequently off-task than conduct-disordered children. Hinshaw noted that the ambiguity of these findings is in part attributable to contaminated research samples (e.g., samples identified as "hyperactive" which were in reality a mixture of hyperactive and conduct-disordered children). Hinshaw concluded that the evidence suggests that the domains of hyperactivity/attention deficit and conduct problems/aggression have significant overlap, yet are partially independent, and recommended continued research addressing the degree of overlap and discriminative criteria between these two disorders. A similar analysis could be undertaken comparing the Conduct and Oppositional Defiant Disorder categories. For example, the primary distinction between the two is one of severity, and the two disorders have considerable behavioral overlap. Thus, the Oppositional Defiant Disorder is essentially a less severe form of Conduct

Disorder, and one could argue that the two do not constitute distinct diagnostic categories.

It is important to acknowledge at the outset that these ambiguities exist, and that there are many important theoretical and practical questions that are in need of further analysis and research. These ambiguities will no doubt continue to be debated, and hopefully more definitive conclusions with more precise diagnostic criteria will result. A detailed analysis of relevant issues regarding these ambiguities is beyond the scope of the present text. Rather, we will be concerned with a practical review and application of the literature as appropriate for the practitioner. We would now like to present a brief overview of each of the Disruptive Behavior Disorders.

ATTENTION-DEFICIT HYPERACTIVITY DISORDER

Historical Overview

Early references to the disorder currently referred to as ADHD date back to the late 1800s (Barkley, 1981; Rutter, 1989; Shaywitz & Shaywitz, 1989). These early reports made reference to the restlessness, impulsivity, difficulties with concentration, and excessive motor activity in mentally retarded or severely neurologically impaired children. These signs were attributed to specific neurologic trauma, such as head injuries (Goldstein, 1936; Meyer, 1904) or diseases, such as central nervous system infection (Bender, 1942; Hohman, 1922) experienced by the children. During the 1930s and 1940s, investigators reasoned that since these behavioral changes were associated with or followed known neurologic trauma or disease, any child exhibiting this cluster of behavioral signs must also have some neurologic impairment (Strauss & Lehtinen, 1947; Werner & Strauss, 1941). This argument gradually gained wide acceptance. Eventually, it became commonplace to assume that children exhibiting hyperactivity suffered from mild diffuse brain damage or neurologic abnormalities, even in the absence of supportive neurologic evidence. Through the 1960s and 1970s this constellation of behavioral signs was often referred to as minimal brain dysfunction (MBD) (Clements & Peters, 1962).

Until recently, predominant conceptualization of this disorder and the corresponding diagnostic label have reflected an assumption of a neurologic anomaly. However, despite widespread acceptance of a neurologic basis for hyperactivity, the weight of evidence did not support the conclusion that hyperactivity was the result of structural damage or abnormalities in the central nervous system. Rutter (1983) indicated that much of the rationale supporting the MBD syndrome was based upon circular reasoning, and the hypothesized neurologic basis for hyperactivity had not been supported by subsequent empirical evidence. In 1977, Rutter had concluded that only a small minority (less than 5%) of hyperactive children have hard biomedical evidence of structural brain damage, and the majority of children who suffer from brain injuries or neurologic diseases do not develop moderate hyperactive-like behaviors. At the same time, mild, diffuse neurologic abnormalities may be associated with a variety of emotional, learning, and behavioral difficulties. Interestingly, in a recent report, Shaffer et al. (1985) found that neurologic "soft signs" were more associated with anxiety disorders than hyperactivity in adolescence. The point to be made here is that the evidence does not support the validity of a specific MBD syndrome characterized by hyperactive-like behavior problems. Perhaps it would be best to disregard this conceptualization and diagnostic label, both in research and clinical practice, as this conceptualization only perpetuates an inaccurate understanding of the disorder.

Beginning in the 1960s, children with this constellation of behaviors who exhibited learning problems primarily were gradually referred to as having a specific learning disability (Kirk & Bateman, 1962). At the same time, children who exhibited primarily behavioral and conduct disturbances were referred to as hyperactive (Laufer & Denhoff, 1957). The term "Hyperkinetic" was eventually adopted in the formal diagnostic nomenclature, DSM-II (APA, 1968). The DSM-II "criteria" for "Hyperkinetic Reaction of Childhood" consisted of a brief description of the disorder, emphasizing behavioral overactivity, restlessness, distractibility, and short attention span. This disorder was thought to occur primarily in young children and to diminish in adolescence. No attempt was made to provide specific behavioral referents for each area of difficulty nor to account for the wide differences typically evident in each area across age. Other than the recognition that hyperactive-like behaviors may result from organic brain damage (in which case such behavior *should not* be diagnosed as hyperactive), the DSM-II did not identify other issues to be considered in the differential diagnostic process.

Considerable research concerned with hyperactivity was completed between the publication of DSM-II in 1968 and its revision, DSM-III, (APA, 1980). For example, several lines of research concluded that the primary deficits of hyperactive children were their inability to sustain attention and inhibit impulsive responding in structured tasks (e.g., Busby & Broughton, 1983; Douglas, 1972, 1980, 1983; Douglas & Peters, 1979; Gordon, 1979). Largely as a result of this empirical base and corresponding theoretical advances, the presentation of the disorder was substantially altered in DSM-III. Core features of the disorder continued to be inattention, impulsivity, and hyperactivity. However, difficulties with attention were seen as primary, with motor restlessness secondary. The disorder was renamed Attention Deficit Disorder (ADD) to emphasize the primary difficulties with attention. The inattention component was characterized by a short attention span and a deficit in the ability to sustain attention to relevant stimuli, particularly in structured situations such as a classroom. The impulsivity component was characterized by deficits in self-control, rule-governed behavior, and the ability to delay responding in order to consider the various response alternatives or the consequences of one's behavior. The hyperactivity component was characterized by excessive motor restlessness, overactivity, etc. And, consistent with the greater importance given to difficulties with attention and the lesser importance given to hyperactivity, the criteria allowed for a diagnosis of ADD with or without hyperactivity. The diagnostic criteria and clinical description for ADD with hyperactivity (ADD/H) contained in DSM-III are provided in Table 1.1. The criteria for ADD without hyperactivity (ADD) are the same as those for ADD/H, except that the individual never showed signs of hyperactivity (criterion C).

Several additional changes were made in the DSM-III criteria that reflected developments in the literature. First, it was acknowledged that attention span, impulse control, and motor activity normally vary across the age span. Accordingly, a child's behavior was to be considered or evaluated with reference to his or her mental and chronological age. Behaviors must be *developmentally inappropriate* before they may be regarded as meeting the criteria. Second, minimal time parameters (age of onset, duration of signs) were specified. The requirement of an onset before the age of 7 reflected the belief that ADD was a pervasive disorder, often evident early in life, and almost always evident before the child starts formal schooling. This criterion helps to differentiate a behavioral pattern that first emerges later in life, for example at the age of 9 or 10, that might reflect some other difficulty, such as an acute adjustment reaction from an unidentified trauma (e.g., physical or sexual abuse). Similarly, the requirement of a minimum duration helps to differentiate the disorder from other difficulties.

Despite these relative improvements, there has been criticism of the DSM-III criteria for ADD (Barkley, 1981, 1982; Edelbrock, Costello, & Kessler, 1984; Maurer & Stewart, 1980). Perhaps the most controversial issue was the subcategorization of ADD (with and without hyperactivity). Several investigators have examined the validity and clinical utility of this distinction (Edelbrock et al., 1984; King & Young, 1982; Lahey, Shaughency, Frame & Strauss, 1985; Lahey, Shaughency, Strauss, & Frame, 1984; Maurer & Stewart, 1980; Sergeant & Scholten, 1985a, 1985b). This literature was recently reviewed by Carlson (1986). Carlson concluded that some behavioral similarities have been found between ADD/H and ADD children. However, ADD/H and ADD children differ in several important ways, and the research suggests that ADD children may have more in common with those with other diagnoses, such as anxiety disorder. Most importantly, it cannot be assumed

TABLE 1.1
DSM-III Diagnostic Criteria for Attention Deficit Disorder with Hyperactivity

The child displays, for his or her mental and chronological age, signs of developmentally inappropriate attention, impulsivity, and hyperactivity. The signs must be reported by adults in the child's environment, such as parents and teachers. Because the symptoms are typically variable, they may not be observed directly by the clinician. When the reports of teachers and parents conflict, primary consideration should be given to the teacher reports because of greater familiarity with age-appropriate norms. Symptoms typically worsen in situations that require self-application, as in the classroom. Signs of the disorder may be absent when the child is in a new or a one-to-one situation.

The number of symptoms specified is for children between the ages of 8 and 10, the peak age for referral. In younger children, more severe forms of the symptoms and a greater number of symptoms are usually present. The opposite is true of older children.

A. *Inattention*. At least three of the following:
   1. Often fails to finish things he or she starts
   2. Often doesn't seem to listen
   3. Easily distracted
   4. Has difficulty concentrating on schoolwork or other tasks requiring sustained attention
   5. Has difficulty sticking to a play activity

B. *Impulsivity*. At least three of the following:
   1. Often acts before thinking
   2. Shifts excessively from one activity to another
   3. Has difficulty organizing work (this not being due to cognitive impairment)
   4. Needs a lot of supervision
   5. Frequently calls out in class
   6. Has difficulty awaiting turn in games or group situations

C. *Hyperactivity*. At least two of the following:
   1. Runs about or climbs on things excessively
   2. Has difficulty sitting still or fidgets excessively
   3. Has difficulty staying seated
   4. Moves about excessively during sleep
   5. Is always "on the go" or acts as if "driven by a motor"

D. *Onset before the age of seven*

E. *Duration of at least six months*

F. *Not due to Schizophrenia, Affective Disorder, or Severe or Profound Mental Retardation*

Note. From *Diagnostic and Statistical Manual of Mental Disorders* (3rd ed.) by the American Psychiatric Association, 1980, Washington, DC: Copyright 1980 by the American Psychiatric Association. Reprinted by permission.

that ADD/H and ADD children have similar clinical needs or will respond in a similar manner to the same treatments. Overall, the distinction between ADD/H and ADD does not contribute to a clearer understanding of the disorder and may foster further confusion.

Additional criticisms of the DSM-III formulation of ADD have included the failure to address adequately the cross-situational nature of the various problems, the failure to situate the criteria in reference to a pattern of "normal" behavior, the arbitrary use of the age cutoff for onset (i.e., 7 years) and the duration of signs (i.e., 6 months). In view of these criticisms, Barkley (1982, 1988a) has offered more stringent criteria for the diagnosis of ADD. His criteria are consistent with the general model utilized in DSM-III, but offer more precise guidelines, and also require evidence of cross-situational pervasiveness and deviation from age norms on a standardized parent or teacher rating scale of hyperactive behavior. Briefly, Barkley's (1982, 1988a) guidelines are as follows:

1. Parental and/or teacher complaints of inattention, impulsivity, over activity, and poor rule-governed behavior.
2. A score or scores two standard deviations from the mean for same-age, same-sex normal children on factors labeled as "Inattentive" or "Hyperactive" in well-standardized child behavior rating scales completed by parents or teachers.
3. Onset of these problems by 6 years of age.
4. Duration of these problems for at least 12 months.
5. An IQ greater than 85, or if between 70 and 85, comparison with children of the same mental age in using criterion No. 2 above.
6. The exclusion of significant language delay, sensory handicaps (e.g., deafness, blindness), or severe psychopathology (e.g., autism, childhood schizophrenia, etc.).

Recently, the DSM-III criteria were again revised (APA, 1987). The DSM-III-R criteria are presented in Table 1.2. The more current conceptualization has done away with the subtyping of ADD into hyperactive and nonhyperactive categories. Consistent with this reformulation, the name of the disorder has also been changed to Attention-deficit Hyperactivity Disorder (ADHD). The DSM-III-R formulation and criteria also differ from its predecessors in several ways. First, there is a single list of symptoms generated primarily from items of empirically derived rating scales, rather than three groups of symptoms based upon a consensus. Second, the number of symptoms required for a diagnosis was established in a national field trial. The symptoms are presented in descending order of discriminating power based upon data from the field

TABLE 1.2
DSM-III-R Diagnostic Criteria for Attention-Deficit Hyperactivity Disorder

Note: Consider the criterion met only if the behavior is considerably more frequent than most people of the same mental age.

A. A disturbance of at least six months during which at least eight of the following are present:

1. Often fidgets with hands or feet or squirms in seat (in adolescents, may be limited to subjective feelings of restlessness)
2. Has difficulty remaining seated when required to do so
3. Is easily distracted by extraneous stimuli
4. Has difficulty awaiting turn in games or groups situations
5. Often blurts out answers to questions before they have been completed
6. Has difficulty following through on instructions from others (not due to oppositional behavior or failure of comprehension), e.g., fails to finish chores
7. Has difficulty sustaining attention in tasks or play activities
8. Often shifts from one uncompleted activity to another
9. Has difficulty playing quietly
10. Often talks excessively
11. Often interrupts or intrudes on others, e.g., butts into other children's games
12. Often does not seem to listen to what is being said to him or her
13. Often loses things necessary for tasks or activities at school or at home (e.g., toys, pencils, books, assignments)
14. Often engages in physically dangerous activities without considering possible consequences (not for the purpose of thrill-seeking), e.g., runs into street without looking

Note: The above items are listed in descending order of discriminating power based on data from a national field trial of the DSM-III-R criteria for Disruptive Behavior Disorders.

B. Onset before the age of seven

C. Does not meet the criteria for a Pervasive Developmental Disorder

Criteria for Severity of Attention-Deficit Hyperactivity Disorder:

Mild: Few, if any signs in excess of those required to make the diagnosis **and** only minimal or no impairment in school or social functioning.

Moderate: Signs or functional impairment intermediate between mild and severe.

Severe: Many signs in excess of those required to make the diagnosis **and** significant and pervasive impairment in functioning at home and school and with peers.

Note: From *Diagnostic and Statistical Manual of Mental Disorders* (3rd ed., rev.), by the American Psychiatric Association, 1987, Washington, DC: Author. Copyright 1987 by the American Psychiatric Association. Reprinted by permission.

trial (Barkley, Spitzer, & Costello, 1990; Spitzer, Davies, & Barkley, 1990). Finally, a new severity dimension is included based upon pervasiveness (mild, moderate, or severe).

Clinical Description

There has been debate about how to define the disorder. Issues of dispute include the precise inclusionary and exclusionary criteria for ADHD, whether subtyping (with or without hyperactivity) leads to clarity, and the degree of and significance of overlap with similar disorders (such as Conduct and Oppositional Defiant Disorders). However, researchers and clinicians have generally agreed upon the primary difficulties experienced by ADHD children. One of the primary features is a significant deficit in age-appropriate levels of attention. These children may have initial difficulty in orienting to and sustaining their attention to relevant stimuli. In the home setting, these difficulties may manifest themselves in the child's apparent failure to listen when being addressed by others, the failure to finish things he or she has started, such as completing assigned chores or meeting other responsibilities, or an inability to play without supervision or attention from others for more than a brief period. It is not uncommon to hear a parent complain that often the child is given a series of small tasks to complete and "forgets" the second and third task before the first is finished. In the school setting, these difficulties may be manifested in the child's failure to complete in-class and homework assignments, and failure to attend to the teacher during class lectures or instructions. They may also experience a greater than normal tendency to be distracted by and respond to extraneous stimuli, such as sights and sounds eminating from within the classroom, outside the window, or in the hallway.

A second primary feature is poor impulse control, or a significant deficit in the age-appropriate capacity to inhibit response. Various studies have demonstrated that these children respond to stimuli more quickly, and make significantly more errors in responding, than nonhyperative children. Thus, the ADHD child frequently reacts impulsively before considering alternatives or weighing the consequences of his/her behavior. This may be evident in the child experiencing more difficulty than other children of the same age awaiting his/her turn in games or group interactions. For example, the child may frequently disrupt the group by responding out of turn or calling out in the classroom situation. Similarly, the child may have a tendency to shift excessively from one activity to another as a result of failure to inhibit responses to competing stimuli. This can contribute to considerable difficulties organizing oneself in areas such as school deskwork, homework, and social interactions. The child may also have a greater number of accidents or injuries and be in need of more supervision than other children of the same age. Finally, due to their failure to inhibit responding, these children may be more likely than their peers to respond in a verbally and/or physically aggressive manner when they are hurt, frustrated, or angry. Given such difficulties in waiting for their turn in games or group situations, these children may experience the social demands of group situations as unusually frustrating. This, combined with their failure to inhibit aggressive responding when frustrated, may lead to aggressive behaviors in social situations and difficulties maintaining age-appropriate peer relationships.

A third primary feature is excessive motor restlessness or hyperactivity. As noted above, largely because of research developments in the late 1960s and 1970s, hyperactive-like behaviors have been somewhat deemphasized in favor of the primary difficulties of inattention and impulsivity. Briefly, this body of research has demonstrated that ADHD children are not uniformly overactive in all situations, and are not necessarily more active than other children in many situations. Rather, they tend to display increased levels of motor activity and restlessness in situations that require sustained attention and impulse control, e.g., the classroom or similar controlled group activity. However, in relatively unstructured situations, such as free play on the school playground, ADHD children may not always exhibit significantly greater motor activity than their peers. Similarly, evidence suggests these children may display activity levels which are similar to other children in novel or unfamiliar settings, but their activity level may then increase as they become habituated to the setting. In natural settings, this motor activity may be evident in greater than normal tendencies to run about or climb on things, fidget and move about excessively, talk excessively, and have difficulty sitting still when required to do so (in school or in one's chair at mealtime).

A fourth feature characteristic of ADHD children, a deficit in rule-governed behavior, has recently been proposed by Barkley (1981, 1985a, 1985b, 1988a). As described by Skinner (1969), rules are stimuli constructed by the social community or the individual which specify relations (contingencies) among antecedents, behavior, and consequences. Thus, rule-governed behavior refers to the ability of language (instructions, directives, descriptions) and/or other symbolic systems to serve as discriminative stimuli for behavior. Individuals who have normal rule-governed behavior are able to learn verbally mediated (or other symbolic) discriminative stimuli and to modify their behavioral responses in accordance with these discriminative cues. Barkley (1988a) observed that ADHD children have difficulty adhering to rules generated for them by the social community (primarily parents and teachers). This deficit may result from a failure to comprehend the directives due to inattention, or an initial effort at compliance but a failure to follow through due to inattention, distractibility and impulsivity. Barkley (1988a) noted that many research studies reported in the literature using laboratory tasks of attention and impulsivity require the ADHD child to comply with the rules given by the experimenter. Thus, the reported deficits in attention and impulse control may in fact by confounded with deficits in rule-governed behavior. In other words, widely reported deficits in attention span and impulse control may in fact be the results of deficits in an unmeasured construct, rule-governed behavior.

Several additional or secondary behavioral problems are frequently present in ADHD children, although none of these are invariably present. First, these children frequently exhibit low frustration tolerance, general noncompliance, temper outbursts, aggressive behaviors, and conduct problems. These difficulties may be pervasive and severe enough to warrant an additional diagnosis of an Oppositional Defiant or Conduct Disorder. As noted above, there is a substantial overlap between ADHD and Conduct Disorders. For example, Stewart et al. (1981) found that about 65% of the children with ADHD had a coexisting Conduct Disorder, and about 75% of the children with a Conduct Disorder had a coexisting ADHD. Similarly, Safer and Allen (1976) reported that as many as 75% of these children also have Conduct Disorder problems. Additional problem areas may include: below-average cognitive ability, academic underachievement, with perhaps a learning disability, low self-esteem, mild depression, mood lability, low frustration tolerance, vision and language problems, accidental injuries, allergies, chronic health problems, and deficits in social skills with corresponding difficulties developing and maintaining age-appropriate peer relationships. Finally, sleep disturbances, functional enuresis, and functional encopresis are occasionally also present.

Prevalence/Incidence

Estimates of the disorder in the general population have varied widely. It is not uncommon to see estimates ranging from 1% to 20% of the school-age population. This variability is attributable to several factors relating to how the disorder is defined and measured. First, as noted above, there has been debate over what does and does not constitute ADHD. Clearly, the prevalence and incidence will vary with the definition. Second, most agree that the core features (i.e., inattention, impulsivity, and overactivity) are generally normally distributed in the population, and that there are no discrete boundaries between "hyperactive" and "nonhyperactive" children. Obviously, then, where one decides to draw the line (1, 1.5, or 2 standard deviations from the mean on various rating scales) for clinical significance will have a clear impact on the prevalence and incidence estimates that result (Trites, Dugas, Lynch, & Ferguson, 1979). Finally, most of the available diagnostic rating scales and measures do not yield "pure" data concerning hyperactivity. For example, the

Conners Parent and Teacher Rating Scales' Hyperactivity Index, one of the most widely used in addressing hyperactivity, has recently been criticized because it may not be adequately sensitive to the disorder, per se, but may rather tend to identify a mixture of behaviors characteristic of ADHD and Conduct Disorders.

Generally accepted prevalence figures are from 3 to 5% of the school-age population (Barkley, 1981, 1988b; Kerasotes & Walker, 1983; Rapport, 1987; Szatmari, Boyle, & Offord, 1984; Trites et al., 1979). In the recently published DSM-III-R (APA, 1987), the prevalence of ADHD was estimated to be 3%. Comparable rates have also been obtained in the United Kingdom (Gould, Shaffer, Rutter, & Sturge, 1984) and West Germany (Remschmidt, 1984) when similar diagnostic criteria have been used. In most prevalence studies of hyperactivity, two variables, socioeconomic status (SES) and gender, have been identified as significant covariates. First, investigators have reported an inverse relationship between SES and the incidence and severity of hyperactivity. Various hypotheses concerning causes for this overrepresentation of hyperactivity in the lower SES groups have been offered, including the "downward drift" hypothesis, heredity, decreased availability of adequate pre-, peri-, and postnatal medical care, poorer general nutrition, greater economic, social, and familial stress, as well as fewer resources available to cope with such stress. None of these factors has been proven to cause a greater incidence of ADHD in lower SES groups, but all may contribute in a given individual situation.

Second, ADHD occurs much more often in boys than in girls. Again, while estimates vary, it is generally accepted that the disorder is from six to nine times more likely to be found in boys than girls (APA, 1987). There has been a belief that ADHD boys and girls differ in several major ways; for example, boys were considered to have more severe problems with physical aggression and over-activity, and girls were considered to have greater difficulties with low self-esteem, mood, and emotional lability. Although the area of gender differences has only recently been examined, preliminary evidence suggests that there are fewer differences than previously believed (Barkley, 1989b; Befera & Barkley, 1985; Breen, 1989; Breen & Altepeter, 1990a; Breen & Barkley, 1988; de-Hass, 1986; deHass & Young, 1984; Horn, Wagner, & Ialongo, 1989).

Etiology

The causes of this disorder are not entirely clear, and several factors have been proposed in the literature. Each of the causative factors discussed below has some empirical support, but none have sufficient support to enable one to conclude that they are either necessary or sufficient for emergence of the disorder. As noted above, brain damage was the first identified causative factor

(Strauss & Lehtinen, 1947), and initially it was assumed to be synonymous with ADHD. However, recent evidence suggests that only about 5% of these children have evidence of organic dysfunction (e.g., Dubey, 1976; Rutter, 1977), and that most children who suffer brain damage do not develop the disorder (Rutter, Chadwick, & Shaffer, 1983). Some have also suggested that ADHD has a neurochemical basis. The most commonly implicated neurotransmitters are dopamine and norepinepherine (Cantwell, 1975; Shaywitz, Cohen, & Bowers, 1977; Shaywitz, Cohen, & Shaywitz, 1978; Shaywitz, Shaywitz, Cohen, & Young, 1983; Stevenson & Wolraich, 1989; Wender, 1971). However, this line of research has produced conflicting results, and there is no consistent or unequivocal evidence linking ADHD with an increase or reduction in one or more of the neurotransmitters. Finally, some have suggested that symptoms of this disorder are the result of neurological immaturity, although little evidence is available to support this hypothesis.

Recently researchers have begun focusing on other potential causative factors. Evidence has accumulated suggesting a higher incidence of various psychiatric disorders, including ADHD, Conduct Disorder, Antisocial Personality Disorder, Alcoholism, and Depression among biological relatives of these children (Befera & Barkley, 1985; Cantwell, 1975; Morrison & Stewart, 1971, 1973). This literature suggests some hereditary basis for ADHD, although specific mechanisms of transmission have not been identified. Next, some evidence suggests an association between symptoms common to children diagnosed with ADHD and earlier maternal alcohol consumption (Shaywitz, Cohen, & Shaywitz, 1980) and cigarette smoking during pregnancy (Denson, Nanson, & McWatters, 1975; Nichols, 1980). The preliminary evidence is primarily correlational, and it does not allow for causal inferences. One or more other factors may explain the association. For example, since women who are more likely to have such children also have an increased risk of psychiatric disturbance and alcohol abuse, it is possible that the association is due to some other (perhaps hereditary) factor.

Several dietary causes have also been proposed. Most popular has been the hypothesis that hyperactive-like behaviors result from an excess of sugar in a child's diet. A related hypothesis has been that hyperactive-like behaviors result from a toxic or allergic reaction to one of several food additives, such as artificial food colorings. These hypotheses were initially proposed based primarily upon anecdotal data, and gained wide public support after Feingold (1975) published a popular press book suggesting a special sugar- and additive-free diet for children with hyperactivity and other behavioral problems. These hypotheses and Feingold's diet gained wide public support in the late 1970s. Many parents continue to believe that sugar and food additives may adversely effect, perhaps severely, the behavior of their child. Since the sugar/additive hypotheses were first proposed in the mid-1970s, a substantial body of well-controlled research has accrued. In general, the conclusions do not support the initial hypotheses: neither sugar nor food additives appear to affect directly the occurrence or severity of hyperactive behavior in most children (Behar, Rapoport, Adams, Berg, & Cornblath, 1984; Conners, 1980; Furguson, Stoddart, & Simeon, 1986; Gross, 1984; Mattes & Gittelman, 1981; Milich, Wolraich, & Lindgren, 1986; Rosen et al., 1988; Wolraich, Milich, Stumbo, & Schultz, 1985). In particular, several controlled studies that challenged hyperactive children with sugar, using aspartame as a placebo, found no increases in symptoms common to this disorder following the sugar challenges (Gross, 1984; Wolraich et al., 1985). There is evidence that a small percentage of children (about 5%) may be sensitive to additives and that preschool children may be slightly more sensitive than older children (Goldman, Lerman, Contois, & Udall, 1986; Prinz, Roberts, & Hantman, 1980; Weiss, 1984). Even in these studies, however, the effects attributable to additives were relatively small. It has also been suggested that several other toxins can cause ADHD, including various environmental allergens and lead. In each case there is some empirical evidence that the factor in question may be associated with the emergence of ADHD in some children, although sufficient evidence is not available to warrant firm conclusions.

Overall, the available evidence suggests that various genetic/hereditary, neurologic, neurochemical, dietary, and toxic factors may contribute to the disorder in any given child, but that none of these factors appears to be either necessary or sufficient for the emergence of ADHD in most children. At present, the evidence does not allow one to conclude that there is a primary etiology operative in the majority of cases of ADHD. Perhaps the only conclusion that can be reached at the present time is that the disorder apparently has multiple causes, and that the expression of ADHD in the individual child appears to be the final common pathway of one or several of these processes.

Developmental Course

While there are wide individual differences, many children follow a common developmental course. As early as infancy many children with ADHD exhibit a constellation of behavioral and temperamental characteristics, including difficulties with eating, sleep, activity level, and intolerance for stimulation and physical affection. Many display irregularity in sleeping and eating habits and, despite their caretakers' best efforts, do not adjust easily to regular sleeping and eating cycles. They may be very light sleepers who awaken easily at night and then remain awake for several hours. They may be difficult to put down during the day for naps. They may be fussy, irregular eaters who develop milk or other food allergies. They may be more susceptible than other children to chronic infections, such as upper respiratory or ear infections. They may be colicky, fussy, irritable, and may be difficult to calm or soothe. Many of these children are difficult to hold due to their excessive restlessness and overactivity, and some apparently prefer not to be held or cuddled.

During the toddler phase (about 18 months to 3 years) these children exhibit a variety of difficult behaviors. The developmentally normal tendency to explore the environment and begin to exert some independence is compounded by a very short attention span, impulsivity, and a high degree of restlessness and overactivity. Thus, at this stage ADHD children often appear as if their motors are always racing in high gear, as they constantly move from one set of stimuli to another. While most children at this stage are at risk for accidental injuries, the child with ADHD is at higher risk, and extra caution is often needed to ensure the child's safety. At this stage ADHD children are often perceived by their parents or other caretakers as excessively noncompliant and oppositional. Rebellious motives are often attributed to the child. Behaviorally, they are often more noncompliant than other children, owing largely to difficulties with impulsivity and overactivity. At the same time, the child at this age is cognitively incapable of the negative, rebellious motives which are often attributed to him or her, and the tendency in a parent to make these types of attributions can be a warning that the parent lacks appropriate knowledge about child development, is experiencing a high level of stress associated with parenting, and may be at some risk of abusing the child. Finally, earlier sleeping and eating difficulties often continue during this stage.

During the preschool phase (ages 3–6) children with ADHD tend to be increasingly noncompliant and aggressive, begin to display more intolerance for frustrating situations, and experience increasing difficulties with peer relationships. During this stage these children are more likely to become openly defiant of adults, and some escalation of general conduct problems, particularly in public, may occur. Parents often complain that they have tried everything to manage the child's behavior and that nothing seems to work. They may have difficulty finding babysitters or adequate daycare, as others refuse to watch the child. If the parents have used physical forms of discipline such as spanking, often a gradually escalating level of reciprocal aggression in the parent–child relationship occurs during this stage. Such an interaction pattern may terminate in one or more incidents of child abuse (Burgess & Richardson, 1984; Patterson, 1982). Some parents first seek professional assistance to help manage the child's behavior during this phase.

During the elementary school years (ages 6–11) behavior problems generally continue across most settings, including the home, the school, and the neighborhood. Parents find themselves confronted with school personnel who complain about the child's behaviors, and often feel that these problems are the result of their incompetence. This, in turn, contributes to increased parental stress and perhaps the emergence of depression in the parent. Many parents first seek professional assistance to help manage the child's behavior during this phase. Very commonly, identification of deficits in general intelligence and academic problems emerge within the first several years of school. Although estimates vary, some data suggest that as many as 75% of children with ADHD have an associated learning disability (Safer & Allen, 1976). Although the school may identify the child as having special needs, the initial focus is often on the behavior, and as a result the child may be placed in a program for children with behavior disorders. Not uncommonly, the learning disability is not appropriately diagnosed and addressed in educational programming for several years, if at all. Although the types of learning difficulties vary, language and reading disabilities are common in these children. While some make good progress through school, most display below-average progress. During the school years, peer and social problems generally continue. Due to the variety of their aggressiveness and other behavior problems, these children are often rejected by peers. While children with ADHD may have some initial success in making friends, there is considerable difficulty maintaining age-appropriate friendships over time. Finally, minor delinquent behaviors, such as cheating, repetitive lying, and minor stealing may begin during this stage. Often these behaviors are quite impulsive, and if caught the child may deny responsibility and blame others. In addition, these children often fail to learn to inhibit these behaviors through their experience. As noted above, Stewart et al. (1981) found that about 65% of these children had a coexisting Conduct Disorder. Often it is during this stage that more serious conduct problems begin to emerge.

During the middle school years (ages 11–13) the degree of motor restlessness may begin to diminish slightly, so that the external hyperactive-like behaviors may be less apparent. Deficits in general cognitive and academic skills continue, making the degree of school failure more pronounced. Similarly, peer relationships generally continue to be poor. It is common, then, for these children to experience increasing problems with low self-esteem and depression during this stage. An increase in the frequency and severity of conduct problems often occurs during these years as well. There may be an increase in aggressive acting-out behavior, particularly in the form of brief explosive episodes in reaction to mounting stress and frustration. A pattern of delinquent behaviors may begin to emerge, including chronic lying, stealing, and truancy. Parents continue to find themselves confronted with school personnel, and perhaps also juvenile authorities, for various behavior problems and status offenses. Again, the parents may feel rather helpless and believe that the identified behavior problems are their fault. This may maintain and perhaps increase parental frustration and potential for depression.

There is a long-standing belief that problems associated with hyperactivity diminish greatly during adolescence (ages 13–18), and subsequently are minimal to nonexistent in adulthood. Recent research suggests that for most children with ADHD this is not the case. A thorough review of adolescent and adult outcomes was recently provided by Klein and Mannuzza (1989). Much of what follows is a summary of the major trends reported in this review, and the reader is referred to it for more detailed information. Through adolescence, the degree of motor overactivity does diminish to some degree, so that the external hyperactive-like behaviors may be less apparent. However, primary difficulties with attention span, impulsivity, and many of the associated or secondary problems continue. Academic difficulties continue to plague these adolescents throughout this stage, and many drop out or are expelled from school before graduating from high school. Similarly, peer relationships generally continue to be poor. Problems with low self-esteem, low self-confidence, and depression often continue. There may also be continued aggressive behavior in the form of brief explosive episodes in reaction to stress and frustration. There is often an increase in rebelliousness and growing opposition to authority. If delinquent or antisocial behaviors are going to emerge in an individual child, they are most likely to do so during this period. Difficulties might include chronic lying, truancy, theft, assault, alcohol abuse, and promiscuity. For example, in one study where actual arrest records were examined, approximately one-third of the individuals (depending upon social class) had been arrested at least once for moderately serious offenses, such as robbery and assault (Satterfield, Hoppe, & Schell, 1982). Parents may continue to find themselves confronted with juvenile authorities for various problems and status offenses. Often during this stage the parents' frustration continues to mount, and parents may begin to disengage or distance themselves from the adolescent out of their own frustration. These factors, again, may maintain and perhaps increase the risk of parental depression.

A majority (about 60 to 65%) of children with ADHD apparently continue to exhibit difficulties well into adulthood (Henker & Whalen, 1989; Klein & Mannuzza, 1989; Weiss & Hechtman, 1986; Weiss, Hechtman, Milroy, & Perlman, 1985). Common problems include inattention, distractibility, poor impulse control (with impulsive life styles and impulsive personality traits), and some motor restlessness. A substantial minority (about one-third) go on to exhibit antisocial personality features, particularly those who exhibit aggressive behaviors in childhood. Although adequate follow-up data on alcohol and substance abuse are scarce, available evidence suggests a trend toward higher rates of abuse than in the general population. Several lines of research examining the predisposition and development of alcoholism have suggested that ADHD may be one of several predisposing factors. This literature was recently reviewed by Parsons (1987), who concluded that a substantial minority of primary alcoholics acknowledged a childhood history of hyperactivity. Chronic job-related difficulties and inferior occupational adjustment in adulthood are common. These may include inadequate work performance, poor relationships with supervisors, frequent job changes, underemployment, etc. Individuals who display the best occupational adjustment generally select work settings that permit adequate performance in spite of continued inattention, impulsivity, and restlessness (Weiss, Hechtmas, & Perlman, 1978). Although some details remain unclear due to a lack of relevant studies, the available evidence clearly documents that, contrary to previous beliefs, problems associated with this disorder continue well into adulthood for the majority of individuals.

Family Characteristics and Interaction

While considerable research has been reported which examines many behavioral, cognitive, and emotional aspects of children with ADHD, much less has focused upon the families of ADHD children, including their typical interactions. Patterns of parent–child interactions, and the effects of ADHD on various aspects of the family's adjustment, have only recently begun to be studied. Research has demonstrated that biological relatives of ADHD children show a higher incidence of several psychiatric disorders, including ADHD, Conduct Disorder, Antisocial Personality Disorder, Alcoholism, Hysteria, and Depression (Befera & Barkley, 1985; Cantwell, 1975; Morrison & Stewart, 1971,1973). Perhaps the most widely reported and frequently occurring difficulty has been depression in various family members, particularly the mother. There have been several reports of greater marital discord among parents of these children than in the general population. Clinically, it is often apparent that stressors and disagreements associated with parenting, particularly those associated with managing the ADHD child, contribute to greater marital conflict and dissatisfaction. Children with ADHD exhibit significantly more frequent, intense, and pervasive behavioral problems than other children, and this creates many behavior management problems and greater levels of stress associated with parenting (Barkley, 1985b; Barkley, Karlsson, & Pollard, 1985a; Breen & Barkley, 1988). Previous research has demonstrated that parents of these children have difficulty managing the behavior of their children and that generally mothers have more difficulty than fathers. Together these factors may contribute to the increased incidence of maternal depression and increased marital discord. Interactions between the child and his/her parents, as well as in the entire family, can be characterized as being more negative, aggressive, and coercive than within other families. Some evidence suggests that this increased level of negative and coercive interaction may be associated with the severity of behavior problems per se. For example, Cunningham and Barkley (1978) reported that use of stimulant medication reduced hyperactive behavior and increased compliance in children with ADHD, as well as a reduced level of commands given by the mother. These results also suggest a tentative causal relationship, in that the negative and coercive interactions may be, at least in part, caused or exacerbated by the child's behavior problems. Burgess and Richardson (1984) have recently provided an analysis suggesting that such negative and aversive interaction patterns may gradually escalate into incidents of physical abuse. There is evidence that some parents of these children exhibit knowledge and skill deficits in areas necessary for effective parenting, including appropriate knowledge of normal child growth and development, appropriate communication skills, appropriate and effective behavioral management skills, etc. Finally, some research has demonstrated that children of "insular" mothers (i.e., those who were chronically isolated from adequate social supports) have more serious behavior problems than children of "noninsular" mothers. Thus, it has been hypothesized that mothers of these children are more often "insular" than are mothers of non-ADHD children.

CONDUCT AND OPPOSITIONAL DEFIANT DISORDERS

Historical Overview

As previously noted, there is symptom overlap between Conduct and Oppositional Defiant Disorders. This has led several investigators to argue that there is insufficient evidence to substantiate different diagnostic categories (McMahon & Forehand, 1988; Wells & Forehand, 1985; Werry, Methven, Fitzpatrick, & Dixon, 1983). To avoid redundancy in our current presentation, these two disorders will be discussed together, and referred to as "Conduct Disorders." Early references to this set of behavioral signs often referred to "aggressive behavior problems" and "juvenile delinquency." Aggressive behavior problems included excessive physical aggression in the forms of hitting, shoving, kicking, biting, etc., without necessarily violating major societal norms or laws. Juvenile delinquency, on the other hand, included an ongoing behavioral pattern that involved a failure to adhere to major societal norms or laws. This often involved committing a criminal act, or displaying other behaviors that constituted a serious violation of societal norms, such as truancy or curfew violations (Johnson & Fennell, 1983). Herbert (1978) described juvenile delinquents as follows:

> (Those with) delinquent disorders demonstrate a fundamental inability or unwillingness to adhere to the rules and codes of conduct prescribed by society at its various levels. Such failures may be related to the temporary lapse of poorly established learned controls, to the failure to learn these controls in the first

place, or to the fact that the behavioral standards a child has absorbed do not coincide with the norms of that section of society which enacts and enforces the rules. (p. 11)

Early evidence indicated that aggressive child behavior was reasonably stable over time (Beach & Laird, 1968; Eron, Lefkowitz, Walder, & Huesmann, 1974; Olweus, 1979; Robins, 1978) and that early aggressiveness was often associated with future delinquency (Eron, et al., 1974; Robins, 1966).

Quay (1964) developed an empirically based classification scheme for identifying dimensions of delinquent behaviors. He utilized factor-analytic techniques to identify four independent groups of delinquent behaviors: Socialized-Subcultural delinquency, Unsocialized-Psychopathic delinquency, Disturbed Neurotic delinquency, and Inadequate-Immature delinquency. Socialized-Subcultural delinquents were more extroverted, displayed a strong allegiance to a delinquent peer group, were generally well accepted by the delinquent peer group, and engaged in a variety of group-oriented delinquent behaviors. Achenbach (1974) described this type of delinquent as a relatively normal individual living in a sociocultural setting that facilitated the learning of delinquent (as opposed to nondelinquent) norms and values. Unsocialized-Psychopathic delinquents were solitary rather than group oriented, were less accepted by peers, and exhibited irritability, defiance of authority, quarrelsomeness, and verbal and physical aggression. Achenbach (1974) described this type of delinquent as a relatively abnormal individual who did not have good social relationships, even with other delinquent peers, and who sought out trouble and difficulties. Disturbed Neurotic delinquents were not group oriented and were described as shy, timid, unhappy, inhibited, withdrawn, and prone to anxiety and worry. Achenbach (1974) described this group as a heterogeneous class of individuals who have personality or other problems that lead to delinquency but who differ from other types of delinquents in terms of their high levels of anxiety. Finally, the Inadequate-Immature delinquents were passive, not usually accepted by peers, easily frustrated, and with many social skills deficits.

The classification scheme developed by Quay (1964) was partially incorporated into the formal psychiatric diagnostic nomenclature, DSM-II (APA, 1968). The DSM-II included two diagnostic categories, "Group Delinquent Reaction of Childhood," and "Unsocialized Aggressive Reaction of Childhood." Criteria for the "Group Delinquent Reaction of Childhood" consisted of a brief description of the disorder, emphasizing identification with the values, behavior, and skills of a delinquent peer group or gang. This diagnostic category was largely synonomous with Quay's (1964) Socialized-Subcultural delinquency. Criteria for the "Unsocialized Aggressive Reaction of Childhood" consisted of a brief description of the disorder, emphasizing hostile disobedience, quarrelsomeness, verbal and physical aggressiveness, solitary stealing, lying, and hostile teasing of others. This diagnostic category was largely synonomous with Quay's (1964) Unsocialized-Psychopathic delinquency. Quay's (1964) Disturbed Neurotic delinquency and Inadequate-Immature delinquency were not incorporated into the DSM-II.

The presentation of the disorders was broadened and somewhat altered in the subsequent DSM-III (APA, 1980). In all, five separate categories were postulated: four were identified as different dimensions of Conduct Disorders, and the fifth was a new diagnostic category, Oppositional Disorder. The Conduct Disorders were conceptualized along two dimensions, Aggressive–Nonaggressive and Undersocialized–Socialized, so that four separate diagnostic categories were possible (i.e., Aggressive Undersocialized, Aggressive Socialized, Nonaggressive Undersocialized, and Nonaggressive Socialized). The criteria for each dimension of the DSM-III Conduct Disorders are presented in Table 1.3, and the criteria for the DSM-III Oppositional Disorder are presented in Table 1.4.

The core features of Conduct Disorders, as presented in DSM-III, continued to be a repetitive and persistent pattern of behavior in which the basic rights of others and/or major age-appropriate societal norms or rules were violated. The Nonaggressive dimension involved behaviors such as persistent truancy, running away, lying, stealing, and substance abuse. These behaviors typically did not involve a violent confrontation with another person and have been referred to as "covert antisocial behaviors" (Loeber & Schmaling, 1985; Patterson, 1982). The Aggressive dimension involved behaviors such as vandalism, rape, breaking and entering, firesetting, mugging, assault, theft, robbery, or extortion. These behaviors involved a violation of the rights of others, and often included a violent confrontation with another person. These have been referred to as "overt antisocial behaviors" (Loeber & Schmaling, 1985; Patterson, 1982). As is evident in Table 1.3, the Socialized–Undersocialized dimension was concerned with whether an individual displayed evidence of forming an attachment or social bond with others (Socialized) or failed to display such evidence of attachments (Undersocialized).

Several changes were made in the DSM-III criteria that reflected developments in the literature. First, it was acknowledged that the expression of many child behaviors, such aggressiveness, truancy, lying, stealing, etc., vary across the age span. During certain developmental periods these behaviors may occur infrequently in the lives of normal children. Thus, in order to be considered deviant, a child's behavior was to be considered or evaluated in reference to his or her mental and chronological age, and had to be *developmentally inappropriate* before it could be regarded as meeting the criteria. Second, some minimal time parameters (duration of signs) were specified. This requirement reflected the understanding that Conduct Disorders constituted a relatively

TABLE 1.3
DSM-III Diagnostic Criteria for Conduct Disorder

I. *Aggressive–Nonaggressive Dimension*

A. **Aggressive**. A repetitive and persistent pattern of aggressive conduct in which the basic rights of others are violated, as manifested by either of the following:

1. physical violence against persons or property (not to defend someone else or oneself), e.g., vandalism, rape, breaking and entering, firesetting, mugging, assault
2. thefts outside the home involving confrontation with the victim (e.g., extortion, purse-snatching, gas station robbery)

B. **Nonaggressive**. A repetitive and persistent pattern of nonaggressive conduct in which either the basic rights of others or major age-appropriate societal norms or rules are violated, as manifested by any of the following:

1. chronic violations of a variety of important rules (that are reasonable and age-appropriate for the child) at home or at school (e.g., persistent truancy, substance abuse)
2. repeated running away from home overnight
3. persistent serious lying in and out of the home
4. stealing not involving confrontation with the victim

II. *Undersocialized-Socialized Dimension*

A. **Undersocialized**. Failure to establish a normal degree of affection, empathy, or bond with others as evidenced by *no more than one* of the following indications of social attachment:

1. has one or more peer-group friendships that have lasted over six months
2. extends himself or herself for others even when no immediate advantage is likely
3. apparently feels guilt or remorse when such a reaction is appropriate (not just when caught or in difficulty)
4. avoids blaming or informing on companions
5. shares concern for the welfare of friends or companions

B. **Socialized**. Evidence of social attachment to others as indicated by at least **two of** the following:

1. has one or more peer-group friendships that have lasted over six months
2. extends himself or herself for others even when no immediate advantage is likely
3. apparently feels guilt or remorse when such a reaction is appropriate (not just when caught or in difficulty)
4. avoids blaming or informing on companions
5. shows concern for the welfare of friends or companions

III. *Duration of Pattern of Aggressive/Nonaggressive Conduct of at Least Six Months*

IV. *If 18 or Older, Does not Meet the Criteria for an Antisocial Personality Disorder*

Note. From *Diagnostic and Statistical Manual of Mental Disorders* (3rd ed.), by the American Psychiatric Association, 1980, Washington, DC: Author. Copyright 1980 by the American Psychiatric Association. Adapted by permission.

TABLE 1.4
DSM-III Diagnostic Criteria for Oppositional Disorder

A. Onset after 3 years of age and before age 18

B. A pattern, for at least six months, of disobedient, negativistic, and provocative opposition to authority figures, as manifested by at least two of the following symptoms:

1. violations of minor rules
2. temper tantrums
3. argumentativeness
4. provocative behavior
5. stubbornness

C. No violation of the basic rights of others or of major age-appropriate societal norms or rules (as in Conduct Disorder); and the disturbance is not due to another mental disorder, such as Schizophrenia or a Pervasive Developmental Disorder

D. If 18 or older, does not meet the criteria for Passive-Aggressive Personality Disorder

Note. From *Diagnostic and Statistical Manual of Mental Disorders* (3rd ed.), by the American Psychiatric Association, 1980, Washington, DC: Author. Copyright 1980 by the American Psychiatric Association. Adapted by permission.

pervasive behavioral pattern. This criterion helps to differentiate a behavioral pattern that might reflect some other difficulty, such as an acute adjustment reaction from an unidentified trauma (e.g., physical or sexual abuse).

In addition, as noted above, the diagnostic category of Oppositional Disorder was first introduced in DSM-III (see Table 1.4). The criteria for this disorder consisted of a persistent pattern (at least 6 months) of disobedient, negativistic, and provocative opposition to primary and secondary authority figures, including repeated violations of minor rules, temper tantrums, argumentativeness, and stubbornness. The diagnosis could not be made in the presence of a violation of the basic rights of others or major age-appropriate societal norms or rules (as in Conduct Disorder). As proposed, Oppositional Disorder described a relatively mild form of Conduct Disorder devoid of more serious behavior problems or violations of rules or the rights of others.

There have been concerns and criticisms raised about the DSM-III criteria for Conduct Disorders and Oppositional Disorder, as well as other DSM-III child diagnostic categories (Bemporad & Schwab, 1986; Hinshaw, 1987; Kazdin, 1985; McMahon & Forehand, 1988; Quay, 1986; Wells & Forehand, 1985). Perhaps the most widely noted criticism is that the categories have questionable reliability and validity. Much of the available evidence does not support the validity of the DSM-III subcategorization of Conduct Disorder, or the formation of the separate diagnostic category, Oppositional Disorder.

Recently, the DSM-III criteria were again revised (DSM-III-R; APA,

TABLE 1.5
DSM-III-R Diagnostic Criteria for Conduct Disorder

A. A disturbance of conduct of at least six months during which at least three of the following are present:

1. has stolen without confrontation of a victim on more than one occasion (including forgery)
2. has run away from home overnight at least twice while living in parental or parental surrogate home (or once without returning)
3. often lies (other than to avoid physical or sexual abuse)
4. has deliberately engaged in fire-setting
5. is often truant from school (for older person, absent from work)
6. has broken into someone else's house, building, or car
7. has deliberately destroyed others' property (other than by fire-setting)
8. has been physically cruel to animals
9. has forced someone into sexual activity with him or her
10. has used a weapon in more than one fight
11. often initiates physical fights
12. has stolen with confrontation of a victim, (e.g., mugging, purse-snatching, extortion, armed robbery)
13. has been physically cruel to people

Note: The above items are listed in descending order of discriminating power based on data from a national field trial of the DSM-III-R criteria for Disruptive Behavior Disorders.

B. If 18 or older, does not meet the criteria for an Antisocial Personality Disorder

Criteria for severity of Conduct Disorder:

Mild: Few, if any conduct problems in excess of those required to make the diagnosis **and** conduct problems cause only minor harm to others.

Moderate: Number of conduct problems and effect on others intermediate between "mild" and "severe."

Severe: Many conduct problems in excess of those required to make the diagnosis **or** conduct problems cause considerable harm to others, e.g., serious physical injury to victims, extensive vandalism or theft, prolonged absence from home.

Note. From *Diagnostic and Statistical Manual of Mental Disorders* (3rd ed.-rev.), by the American Psychiatric Association, 1987, Washington, DC: Author. Copyright 1987 by the American Psychiatric Association. Reprinted by permission.

1987). The current (DSM-III-R) criteria for Conduct Disorder are presented in Table 1.5. Consistent with the previous formulation, the essential feature is a persistent pattern of behavior in which the basic rights of others and/or major age-appropriate norms or rules are violated. The DSM-III-R formulation has done away with the four subtypes based upon the bipolar dimensions of Aggressiveness–Nonaggressiveness and Socialized–Undersocialized used in

DSM-III. Currently, three subtypes of Conduct Disorder are proposed: Group Type, Solitary Aggressive Type, and Undifferentiated Type. In the Group Type, conduct problems occur primarily in the context of peer group activities. This subtype corresponds roughly with the DSM-III Socialized Nonaggressive subtype, and also with the DSM-II Group Delinquent Reaction. In contrast to the DSM-III subtype, however, physical aggression may be present in the DSM-III-R Group Type. In the Solitary Aggressive Type, conduct problems are largely of a physically aggressive nature, and may be directed at either adults or peers. The behaviors occur primarily at the initiative of the child and not in the context of peer group activities. This subtype corresponds roughly with the DSM-III Undersocialized Aggressive subtype, and also with the DSM-II Unsocialized Aggressive Reaction. Finally, the Undifferentiated Type is identified as a residual group and constitutes a mixture of various behavior problems that constitute a Conduct Disorder, but which cannot be classified precisely as either the Solitary Aggressive or Group Types. Thus, the DSM-III-R criteria for Conduct Disorder differ from their predecessors in several ways. First, there is a change in the subcategorizations. Second, there is a single list of signs, rather than separate groups based upon the bipolar dimensions. Finally, the number of signs required for a diagnosis was established in a national field trial, and are presented in descending order of discriminating power based upon the data from the field trial.

Despite previous criticism that the DSM-III category of Oppositional Disorder lacked empirical support (e.g., Quay, 1986), the DSM-III-R retained this category. While a few minor changes have been made in the revised criteria for this disorder, including the inclusion of several additional behavioral criteria, no substantive changes were made in either the conceptual formulation or the primary features of the disorder. The essential features of the disorder continue to include a pattern of negativistic, hostile, and defiant behavior without the more serious violations of major societal rules and/or the basic rights of others that are seen in Conduct Disorders. The DSM-III-R diagnostic criteria for Oppositional Defiant Disorder are presented in Table 1.6.

Clinical Description

Currently there is ongoing debate concerning the definition of Conduct and Oppositional Defiant Disorders. Issues in dispute include the precise inclusionary and exclusionary criteria, whether subtyping (and which subtypes) contributes clarity or ambiguity, and degree of and significance of overlap with similar disorders, such as ADHD (Hinshaw, 1987; Szatmari, Boyle, & Offord, 1989; Quay, 1986). At the same time, however, researchers and clinicians have generally agreed upon the primary difficulties of the conduct-disordered or oppositionally defiant child/adolescent. (Again, in view of the degree of over-

TABLE 1.6
DSM-III-R Diagnostic Criteria for Oppositional Defiant Disorder

Note: Consider a criterion met only if the behavior is considerably more frequent than that of most people of the same mental age.

A. A disturbance of at least six months during which at least five of the following are present:

1. often loses temper
2. often argues with adults
3. often actively defies or refuses adult requests or rules, e.g., refuses to do chores at home
4. often deliberately does things that annoy other people, e.g., grabs other children's hats
5. often blames others for his or her own mistakes
6. is often touchy or easily annoyed by others
7. is often angry or resentful
8. is often spiteful or vindictive
9. often swears or uses obscene language

Note: The above items are listed in descending order of discriminating power based on data from a national field trial of the DSM-III-R criteria for Disruptive Behavior Disorders.

B. Does not meet the criteria for Conduct Disorder, and does not occur exclusively during a course of a psychotic disorder, Dysthymia, or a Major Depressive, Hypomanic, or Manic Episode.

Criteria for severity of Oppositional Defiant Disorder:

Mild: Few, if any, symptoms in excess of those required to make the diagnosis **and** only minimal or no impairment in school or social functioning.

Moderate: Symptoms or functional impairment intermediate between "mild" and "severe."

Severe: Many symptoms in excess of those required to make the diagnosis **and** significant and pervasive impairment at home and school and with other adults and peers.

Note. From *Diagnostic and Statistical Manual of Mental Disorders* (3rd ed.-rev.), by the American Psychiatric Association, 1987, Washington, DC: Author. Copyright 1987 by the American Psychiatric Association. Reprinted by permission.

lap, and to avoid unecessary repetition, the two disorders will be considered together and referred to as "Conduct Disorders.") Quay (1979, 1986) identified behaviors commonly used to define Conduct Disorders. Behaviors included fighting, hitting, temper tantrums, destructiveness, noncompliance, disobedience, defiance, uncooperativeness, disruptiveness, restlessness, boisterousness, irritability, attention seeking, lying, and stealing. The primary feature that distinguishes Conduct from Oppositional Defiant Disorder is a chronic behavioral pattern in which the basic rights of others and/or major age-appropriate societal norms and rules are repetitively violated (APA, 1980, 1987). The behavioral pattern may consist of various "overt" and "covert" antisocial behaviors (Loeber, 1988; Loeber & Schmaling, 1985; Patterson, 1982). Overt antisocial behaviors involve a violation of the rights of others and may include a violent confrontation with another person. Overt antisocial behaviors include theft, robbery, vandalism, breaking and entering, firesetting, physical cruelty to animals or people, use of weapons when fighting, mugging, assault, rape, or extortion. Physical aggression of one type or another is very often present. Children with this disorder often initiate aggression, may be deliberately and willfully cruel to animals or people, and may deliberately destroy other peoples' property. Covert antisocial behaviors usually do not involve a direct violation of the rights of others and do not include a direct confrontation with another person. Covert antisocial behaviors include frequent truancy, running away, lying, stealing, forgery, and substance abuse.

In the home setting these difficulties may manifest themselves in the child's frequent refusal to comply with various rules or behavioral limits or to meet age-appropriate responsibilities such as completing chores. When parents press the child in an attempt to facilitate behavioral compliance, these children typically do not acquiesce, but escalate their oppositional behavior pattern and may become verbally and physically aggressive with parents. Particularly with early and mid-adolescents, repetitive running away from the home is not uncommon. They may also frequently steal cigarettes, money, credit cards, clothes, or other items from parents or siblings. It is not uncommon to hear a parent complain that the child is very noncompliant, uncooperative, defiant, argumentative, unmanageable, as well as verbally and physically aggressive with the parent, siblings, and peers.

Within the school setting, these difficulties may manifest themselves in the child's refusal to attend or cooperate during class, frequent talking out in class, talking back to teachers, as well as defiance of many classroom and general school rules. As in the home setting, if teachers or others press the child in an attempt to facilitate behavioral compliance, these children often do not acquiesce, but escalate their oppositional behavior pattern, and may become verbally and physically aggressive with teachers or peers. Particularly with adolescents, frequent truancy from school is common. Academic achievement may be negatively affected as well. Often low levels of academic achievement are evident in the primary grades and continue throughout the child's academic career. Grade retention one or more times is very common. Deficits in various academic skills have also been associated with Conduct Disorders; reading disabilities and other language skill deficits are particularly common.

Several additional or secondary difficulties have been reported in the literature as being frequently present in children with Conduct Disorders, although none of these are invariably present. First, these children are often inattentive, impulsive, and overactive. These difficulties may be pervasive and severe enough to warrant an additional diagnosis of ADHD. As noted above, there is a substantial overlap between Conduct Disorders and ADHD (Stewart et al., 1981). Second, these children often exhibit deficits in social skills with corresponding difficulties developing and maintaining age-appropriate peer relationships. Various studies have demonstrated that in comparison with peers, those with Conduct Disorders are often more aggressive, less empathic, more deficient in social problem solving skills, and tend to misperceive their environment, often incorrectly attributing hostile intentions to others. Third, in comparison to peers, conduct-disordered children are more likely to abuse tobacco, alcohol, and/or some other mood-altering chemicals. Fourth, they are often sexually precocious, and sexual behavior may begin unusually early relative to their peer group. Often, they engage in many superficial sexual encounters. Additional difficulties may include: accidental injuries, low self-esteem, mild to moderate depression, mood lability, and low frustration tolerance.

Prevalence/Incidence

Estimates of Conduct and Oppositional Defiant Disorders in the general population are difficult to estimate. Reported estimates range from 5% to 25% of the school-age population. This variability is attributable to several factors relating to how the disorder is defined and measured. First, there has been ongoing debate over what does and does not constitute Conduct Disorder and what are appropriate subtypes. Obviously, the prevalence and incidence will vary with the definition. Second, there is no discrete boundary between conduct-disordered and non-conduct-disordered children. Many of the behavioral features of Conduct Disorders are less frequently present in the general population. For example, in one study in which adolescents themselves reported on their behaviors, the occurrence of oppositional, delinquent behaviors was quite high. More than 60% admitted to engaging in more than one type of antisocial behavior, more than 50% admitted to theft, more than 45% admitted to property destruction, and more than 35% admitted to assault (Feldman, Caplinger, & Wodarski, 1983; Williams & Gold, 1972). Where one decides to draw the line in terms of frequency and severity of behaviors will have a clear impact on the prevalence and incidence estimates which result. Finally, as noted above, there is considerable overlap between Conduct Disorder, Attention-deficit Hyperactivity Disorder, and Oppositional Defiant Disorder. Many of the available diagnostic rating scales and measures do not yield "pure" data concerning Conduct Disorder, but seem to tap a variety of behaviors characteristic of ADHD. Thus, available prevalence/incidence data may be somewhat confounded by other disorders.

Generally accepted prevalence figures are from 4% to 10% of the children under the age of 18 (Kazdin, 1987; McMahon & Forehand, 1988; Szatmari, Boyle, & Offord, 1989). In the recently published DSM-III-R (APA, 1987), prevalence of Conduct Disorders was estimated to be 9% of males and 2% of females under age 18. No prevalence information is provided for the Oppositional Defiant Disorder. Conduct Disorders occur much more often in boys than girls. Again, while estimates vary, it is generally accepted that the disorder is from 4 to 12 times more likely to be found in boys than girls (APA, 1987; McMahon & Forehand, 1988). It is widely recognized that children with Conduct Disorder-type behavior problems represent the largest group of children referred to mental health professionals. It has been estimated that these children account for 35–50% of all clinic referrals (Gilbert, 1957; Herbert, 1978; Robins, 1981; Wolff, 1961).

Etiology

Several causes of Conduct Disorder have been proposed in the literature. A few biological factors have been implicated. Evidence has accumulated suggesting a higher incidence of various psychiatric disorders among biological relatives of children with Conduct Disorders, including ADHD, Conduct Disorder, Depression, Alcoholism, Antisocial Personality, and criminal behavior (Griest & Wells, 1983; Huesmann, Eron, Lefkowitz, & Walder, 1984; Kazdin, 1987; Robins, 1981). In addition, several studies indicate a higher concordance among identical than fraternal twins and a higher incidence of antisocial behavior in the biological versus adopted fathers (Cadoret, 1978; Cloninger, Reich, & Guze, 1978; Jary & Stewart, 1985). These data suggest some genetic predisposition for Conduct Disorders, although specific mechanisms of transmission have not been identified. Other evidence is available linking aggressive conduct-disordered behavior to neurologic abnormalities, including psychomotor seizures, a history of head injuries, etc. However, while these factors may contribute to the development of Conduct Disorder in a small minority of cases, there is no evidence implicating these factors in a substantial proportion of conduct-disordered children (see Wells & Forehand, 1985).

There is considerable evidence for individual differences in "temperament." It has been proposed that there are "temperamentally difficult" children, who exhibit difficult, negative, nonadaptive behaviors starting in early infancy. Children who were temperamentally difficult in infancy tend to exhibit higher levels of aggressive behavior later in childhood (Kolvin, Nicol, Garside, Day, & Tweedle, 1982; Olweus, 1980; Webster-Stratton & Eyberg, 1982); however, the relationship between temperament and subsequent aggressive behavior is not clear. Other variables, such as maternal depression and maternal acceptance of child aggression may contribute as much or more explanatory variance to aggressive behavior than temperament (McMahon & Forehand, 1988). In addition, family variables and patterns of interaction contribute to the emergence of Conduct Disorders in many children. In particular, deficiencies in fundamental parenting skills have been implicated in development of behavior problems and Conduct Disorders. Such deficiencies have included inadequate monitoring of child behavior, insufficient involvement in the child's life, inadequate provision for appropriate positive reinforcement, interaction patterns characterized by negative reinforcement and coercive behaviors, insufficient problem-solving skills, and an overreliance on harsh, aversive methods of physical discipline for behavioral management. Patterson (1982) provided a comprehensive analysis of the family interaction patterns that may contribute to the development of Conduct Disorders in children. He noted the manner in which negative reinforcement contributes to the escalation of reciprocal coercive interaction patterns in the family. Ultimately, negative reinforcement patterns increase the probability of the occurrence of aversive and aggressive behaviors on the part of the child and the parents (Burgess & Richardson, 1984; McMahon & Forehand, 1988; Patterson, 1982, 1986; Patterson & Blank, 1986; Patterson & Dishion, 1985; Patterson & Stouthamer-Loeber, 1984).

Overall, there seem to be several factors that contribute to the emergence of Conduct Disorders in some children. Various hereditary, biologic, temperamental, and family interaction patterns have been implicated as possible causes in some individual cases. At the present time, the evidence suggests that various chronic maladaptive family interaction patterns, particularly deficiencies in fundamental parenting skills, contribute a substantial proportion of the explanatory variance in the majority of cases.

Developmental Course

While not all children who develop Conduct Disorders follow a common developmental course, there are some trends which can be found. As early as infancy, many future conduct-disordered children exhibit a constellation of behavioral and temperamental characteristics, including difficulties adapting to changes, irregularities in sleeping and eating patterns, a high activity level, and a low tolerance of stimulation and physical affection. They may be colicky, fussy, and irritable, and difficult to calm or soothe. Many of these children are difficult to hold due to restlessness and overactivity, and do not show a preference for being held or cuddled. Often the child has one or more features which the parents experience as aversive, such as frequent or high-pitched crying. Patterson's (1982) model suggests that in infancy the parental use of negative reinforcement begins to strengthen the frequency and intensity of aversive child behaviors, thereby teaching the child to behave in an aversive manner.

During the toddler phase (about 18 months to 3 years), these children exhibit a variety of difficult behaviors. The developmentally normal tendency to explore the environment and begin to exert some independence may interact with poor parental monitoring and supervision. As a result, the child may exceed normal limits of exploration before the parent intervenes, and give the parents cause for disciplinary interventions. The parent may then intervene in a negative, punishing, aversive manner which, depending upon the child's response, could easily escalate into a very stressful parent–child conflict. The child may also exhibit short attention span, impulsivity, or restlessness and overactivity and be more difficult to manage than other children of the same age. At this stage these children are often perceived by their parents or other caretakers as noncompliant, negative, and oppositional, with rebellious motives often being attributed to the child. They may be more noncompliant than other children, especially when interacting with the parents, owing in part to difficulties with impulsivity and overactivity and to the history of negative reinforcements in response to their aversive behaviors. Thus, interactions between the child and parent may involve frequent temper tantrums and oppositional behaviors. The coercive behavior interactions the child learns in the home may begin to generalize to daycare and/or neighborhood peer relationships. The child may also begin to exhibit aggressive peer behaviors.

In the preschool phase (ages 3 to 6) these children tend to become increasingly noncompliant and begin to exhibit more difficulties with frustration tolerance, greater displays of aggression, and increasing difficulties with peer relationships. During this stage they are more likely to become openly defiant of adults, and some escalation in general conduct problems, particularly in public, may occur. Parents often resort to harsher physical discipline to control the child's behavior. This may temporarily inhibit the child's negative behavior, (negatively) reinforcing the parent and increasing the probability that harsh physical discipline will continue to be used in the future. Thus, if the parents use physical forms of discipline, such as spanking, a graudally escalating level of reciprocal aggression will often occur in the parent–child relationship. This may give rise to one or more incidents of child abuse (e.g., Burgess & Richardson, 1984). In addition, this may provide ongoing modeling of aggressive behavior for the child, increasing the probability of future aggressive behavior on the part of the child.

During elementary school (ages 6 to 11), behavior problems may continue across the home, school, and neighborhood settings. Parents often find themselves confronted with school personnel who complain about their son or daughter's behaviors. Not uncommonly, the parents are left to feel as though the behavior problems are the result of their inadequacy as parents. This, in turn, may contribute to increased parental stress, increased discipline (often physical) of the child, and the emergence of depressive features in the parent. Very commonly, academic problems emerge within this period. Both behavior disorders and learning disabilities are common. In addition, difficulties with impulsivity and motor restlessness may be identified by the school personnel. Very commonly, the child initially comes to the attention of school personnel as a result of a variety of disruptive and aggressive behavioral difficulties, and the initial reasons for further evaluation are the behavioral problems. The child is often placed in a program for children with behavioral disorders. There may also be associated learning disabilities or ADHD, and, because of the focus on the behavioral problems, these associated difficulties may unfortunately not be identified or addressed in educational programming for several years, if at all. Reading and language disabilities are among the most common in conduct-disordered children, although other learning problems may be present as well. The conduct-disordered child generally continues to display peer and social problems as well. While many conduct-disordered children can be socially engaging and have initial success making friends, they have considerable difficulty maintaining these friendships over time. Typically their aggressiveness and various disruptive behavioral problems create frequent conflicts, and sometimes physical fights, with peers. As a result, many conduct-disordered children are eventually rejected by most non-conduct-disordered peers. They may gradually become more constricted in their social involvement and associate predominantly with other children who have similar problems. Finally, minor delinquent behaviors may begin during this stage, such as cheating, lying, and minor stealing. These behaviors are typically impulsive and may be motivated by strong needs for immediate gratification or oppositional and aggressive acting out. If caught, the child will typically deny responsibility or blame others.

During the junior high school years (ages 11 to 13) as academic difficulties continue to mount, the child often loses interest in school. A pattern of repetitive truancy from school may emerge. Similarly, peer social relationships generally continue to be poor. If ongoing peer relationships are maintained, they are often in the context of other conduct-disordered children. Peer pressure may facilitate the emergence of delinquent group behaviors. There may be an increase in chronic lying, stealing, shoplifting, truancy, running away, alcohol and/or drug abuse, and sexual experiences. There may also be increased aggressive acting-out, particularly in the form of brief explosive episodes in reaction to mounting stress and frustration. Parents continue to find themselves confronted with school personnel, and perhaps also juvenile authorities, for various behavior problems and status offenses. Not uncommonly, these children also experience increasing problems with low self-esteem and depression during this stage.

During adolescence (ages 13 to 18), various behavior and conduct problems generally escalate. Prior to adolescence the child has typically established him/herself in a noncompliant, oppositional, rebellious behavior pattern with a variety of associated problems. This behavior pattern is often exacerbated by the normal developmental movement to separate and individuate during adolescence, which is often enacted in terms of rebelling against authority. Truancy from school may continue to be a problem, and many children drop out or are expelled before graduating from high school. Similarly, general peer relationships continue to be poor. There may be an increased loyalty to the delinquent peer group and greater isolation from other peers. There may be many behaviors that violate major societal rules or norms, including stealing, shoplifting, truancy, running away, alcohol and/or drug abuse, sexual promiscuity, etc. There may also be violent interpersonal behaviors, such as frequent fighting, assault, rape, etc. Problems with low self-esteem, low self-confidence, depression, and expectations of ongoing failure continue during this stage, although these individuals rarely seek mental health treatment for these difficulties. Parents may continue to find themselves confronted with juvenile authorities for status offenses. Often during this stage the parents' frustration continues to mount, and parents may begin to disengage or distance themselves from the child out of frustration. This, again, may maintain and perhaps increase parental depression.

Many conduct-disordered children continue to exhibit difficulties well into adulthood. Among the more common difficulties are antisocial personality disorders and criminal behavior, alcohol and/or drug abuse, and poor marital and occupational adjustment (Kazdin, 1985). Notably, those who exhibit more aggressive behavior problems in childhood, and in more than one setting, are more likely to develop antisocial personality features in adulthood (Loeber, 1982, 1988). Although adequate follow-up data on alcohol and substance abuse are scarce, available evidence suggests a trend toward higher rates of abuse than in the general population. Chronic job-related difficulties and inferior occupational adjustment in adulthood are common, including lower work performance, poor relationships with supervisors, frequent job changes, underemployment, etc.

Family Characteristics and Interaction

Research is now available examining the family characteristics and typical interaction patterns of conduct-disordered children. The major trends of this literature will be summarized here. First, as noted above, research has demonstrated that biological relatives of conduct-disordered children show a higher incidence of several psychiatric disorders, including ADHD, Conduct Disorder, Depression, Alcoholism, Antisocial Personality, and criminal behavior (Griest & Wells, 1983; Huesmann et al., 1984; Kazdin, 1987; Robins, 1981). Perhaps the most widely reported and frequently occurring difficulties have been depression in various female family members, particularly the mother, and antisocial behaviors in various male family members, particularly the father. Second, there have been reports of greater marital dissatisfaction and discord among parents of conduct-disordered children than normals (Griest & Wells, 1983; Kazdin, 1987; McMahon & Forehand, 1988). The pattern also exists in families of children with ADHD, as noted above. Clinically, it is often apparent that stressors and disagreements associated with parenting, particularly those associated with behavior management, may contribute to greater marital conflict and dissatisfaction. In addition, frequently occurring maternal depression and paternal antisocial behaviors would likely contribute to marital discord. Third, conduct-disordered children exhibit significantly more uncooperative, oppositional, disruptive, noncompliant, and defiant behaviors than non-conduct-disordered children. This chronic negative behavioral pattern creates many behavioral management problems and greater levels of stress associated with parenting (Kazdin, 1987; McMahon & Forehand, 1988). Parents of conduct-disordered children have difficulty managing the behavior of their children and often experience considerable distress as a result. Together these factors may contribute to an increased incidence of maternal depression, marital dissatisfaction, and parent-child conflicts and tensions. Fourth, interactions between the conduct-disordered children and their parents, and often among the entire family, are more negative, aggressive, and coercive than those of non-conduct-disordered families. Patterson and his colleagues have examined the interaction patterns in families of conduct-disordered children (Patterson, 1982, 1986; Patterson & Blank, 1986; Patterson & Dishion, 1985; Patterson & Stouthamer-Loeber, 1984). They have reported that such families are characterized by higher levels of aversive interactions, inept parental discipline, more frequent use of extreme forms of physical punishment, and parents who were more distant and less aware of the child's behaviors outside the home. Often there is an underemphasis on the structuring of the child's environment and on attempts to shape the child's behavior in a proactive manner and an overemphasis on aversive, punitive, and more extreme forms of physical punishment in response to child misbehaviors.

Differential Diagnostic Considerations

Before one can plan and implement appropriate treatment interventions, it is necessary to arrive at the appropriate diagnostic formulation. Several other childhood disorders may present with behavioral symptomatology similar to ADHD, Conduct Disorder, or Oppositional Defiant Disorder. Thus, in order to plan appropriate treatment, some consideration must be given to ruling these other disorders in or out. Space does not permit a thorough discussion of each possible childhood disorder that should be ruled out. Instead, in Table 1.7 we provide a brief description of the disorders that should be given differential diagnostic consideration and ruled out. The reader is referred to DSM-III-R and several comprehensive reviews (Herson & Van Hasselt, 1987; Mash & Barkley, 1989; Mash & Terdal, 1988; Ollendick & Hersen, 1989; Quay & Werry, 1986; Walker & Roberts, 1983) for a detailed discussion of these disorders. In many cases, the child may meet the criteria for two or more disorders (e.g., Conduct Disorder and Attention-deficit Hyperactivity Disorder, or Attention Deficit Disorder and a Specific Developmental Disorder). Obviously, in such cases, both diagnoses should be given and treatment planned accordingly.

SUMMARY

This chapter provided a brief overview of Disruptive Behavior Disorders, including ADHD, Conduct Disorder, and Oppositional Defiant Disorder. The discussion included a historical review of these disorders, including the relevant diagnostic guidelines. The diversity and flexibility with which re-searchers and clinicians have applied the DSM guidelines has been alarming. Perhaps of greatest concern here has been the variability with which the guidelines have been interpreted by mental health professionals, and the num-ber of mental health professionals who do not even consult the DSM prior to arriving at a diagnosis. In reviewing this literature, our impression has been that there is a need for a more standardized, systematic, and integrated method of assessing children who present with disruptive, externalizing behavior prob-lems, both in research and clinical settings.

We also reviewed the typical clinical presentation, prevalence, developmen-tal course, and etiologies of these disorders. We also noted the impact that children with Disruptive Behavior Disorders have upon their environments and explicated the importance of understanding these interactions from diag-nostic and treatment perspectives. The reader no doubt noted many similarities across the discussions of the developmental course and etiologies of these disorders and the impact that children with Disruptive Behavior Disorders can have upon their families and larger environments. For example, at certain points the developmental course for ADHD and Conduct Disorder may be very similar. The apparent redundancy through these sections in the current text underscores the considerable overlap among these disorders. Important differences between the disorders were at times evident as well.

It has been our impression that we need to move toward a more consistent,

TABLE 1.7
Differential Diagnostic Considerations for Disruptive Behavior Disorders

1. *Other Disruptive Behavior Disorders*

As noted previously, there is substantial overlap between the Disruptive Behavior Disorders; several estimates suggest that as many as 75% of ADHD children have coexisting Conduct Disorders, and vice versa. Thus, when the tentative diagnosis involves one of the Disruptive Behavior Disorders, the other disorders might also be considered in arriving at a comprehensive diagnostic formulation.

2. *Mood Disorders*

a. Manic or Hypomanic Episode: A period in which the predominant mood is elevated, expansive, or irritable; may include excessive activity and motor restlessness, distractibility, and impulsivity.

b. Major Depressive Episode: A period in which the predominant mood is depressed or irritable; may include psychomotor agitation, difficulties with concentration, attention, distractibility, and indecisiveness.

3. *Anxiety Disorders*

a. Overanxious Disorder: Excessive or unrealistic anxiety or worry; may include nervous, jittery, tense and restless behavior, distractibility, and difficulties with concentration, attention, and indecisiveness.

b. Separation Anxiety Disorder: Excessive anxiety, perhaps to the point of panic, concerning separation from those to whom the child is attached; may include demanding, controlling behaviors, such as temper tantrums, distractibility, and difficulties with concentration and attention.

4. *Adjustment Disorders*

A maladaptive reaction to an identifiable psychosocial stressor, or stressors, that occurs within 3 months after onset of the stressor and that has persisted for no longer than 6 months. Features may include depressed or anxious mood, difficulties with concentration and attention, disturbances in conduct, and/or academic inhibition.

5. *Behavior Problems Secondary to Mental Retardation*

Associated behavior problems are often present, and behavioral symptoms may include low frustration tolerance, poor impulse control, aggressiveness, and/or self-injurious behaviors.

6. *Pervasive Developmental Disorders*

Qualitative impairment in the development of reciprocal social interation, the development of verbal and nonverbal communication skills, and in imaginative activity. Signs characteristic of ADHD are frequently present, but, in such cases, a diagnosis of ADHD is preempted.

7. *Specific Developmental Disorders (e.g., in reading, arithmetic, expressive language, receptive language, etc.)*

Associated features may include deficits in memory, attention, and disruptive behavior problems.

(Continued)

TABLE 1.7 (*Continued*)

8. *Tourette's Disorder*

Involuntary, sudden, rapid, recurrent, nonrhythmic, stereotyped motor movements and vocalizations; associated features may include ADHD and obsessive–compulsive disorders.

9. *Supplementary Conditions*

a. Childhood or Adolescent Antisocial Behavior.

b. Parent–child Problems (e.g., child abuse).

---

systematic, and integrated means of assessing these children in both research and clinical settings. Clinical assessment of Disruptive Behavior Disorders must incorporate multiple sources of information, focus primarily upon the child's typical behaviors across multiple settings (as opposed to focusing on minimal or unrelated theoretical constructs), and be directly tied to subsequent treatment interventions. This type of approach will help to ensure that we identify as homogeneous a cluster of children as possible, and develop focused, individualized treatment interventions that relate directly to the behavioral deficiencies or excesses exhibited by the individual child. Our primary goals in this chapter have been to call attention to the historical course mental health personnel have taken in identifying children with a Disruptive Behavior Disorder, highlight the complexities involved in evaluating these children, and heighten awareness as to the problems inherent in their diagnosis. The need for a systematic, comprehensive, yet practical assessment protocol with a treatment focus is clear. In Chapter 2, we begin to address this need.

2

EVALUATING
DISRUPTIVE BEHAVIOR DISORDERS:
The Interview Process

As noted in the previous chapter, recent surveys of practicing clinicians indicate that a variety of methods are currently used to assess and diagnose children presenting with undercontrolled, externalizing disruptive behavior problems. There is little uniformity regarding the manner with which these diagnostic assessments are conducted. As a result, many children have been underdiagnosed, overdiagnosed, and/or misdiagnosed. While a few of the commonly used assessment methods have direct implications for subsequent treatment, many others are at best tangentially related or unrelated. There is a need for greater uniformity and standardization in the manner with which assessments are conducted. In addition, results of such an assessment should have direct relevance for treatment issues and provide a sufficiently objective baseline against which to assess effects of subsequent intervention. In this text we will present a clinical assessment protocol for use in the evaluation of children presenting with disruptive behavior problems. The protocol has evolved through our research and clinical practice and also reflects the wealth of literature regarding Disruptive Behavior Disorders. We have found it comprehensive, yet sufficiently flexible to accomodate the wide variety of children and families who present with concerns regarding their children's behavior problems. It is our intention that this model will provide the necessary framework to conduct a comprehensive treatment-focused assessment.

It is now recognized that there is considerable cross-situational variation in children's behavior (Barkley, 1988a). Factors such as the relative degree of structure, novelty, or unfamiliarity of the environment, contingencies operative within the environment, presence of caregivers, nature of the task, and prior learning history in similar situations can all contribute to the manner in which the child behaves. Thus, children may behave differently within the home, clinic, and classroom settings. Consequently, in evaluating the intricate and complex behaviors often associated with children exhibiting disruptive behavior, an assessment must derive relevant information from multiple sources and across multiple settings. Such a comprehensive, multi-informant approach also serves a cross-validation function, at times preventing misdiagnoses. For example, a child who is treated in a harsh, overly punitive manner by a parent may exhibit behavior problems in the home but behave relatively normally in the school setting. If information is obtained only from a parent, the child may be diagnosed inappropriately and provided inappropriate treatments.

The major components of our assessment protocol consist of parent, child, and teacher interviews, parent- and teacher-completed child behavior questionnaires, parent and child self-report questionnaires, objective measures of attention span and impulse control, measures of cognitive and academic ability, and direct classroom/clinic behavioral observations. Obviously, not all components would be used in every situation, but where possible we believe it quite appropriate to consider each step of the protocol.

In this chapter we will provide a detailed review and discussion of the clinical interview process with the parent, child, and teacher. Where appropriate, we will provide a research-based rationale for the primary issues to be examined during the interview. In Chapter 3, we will review the more commonly used parent- and teacher-completed child behavior questionnaires, several youth self-report and parent–family questionnaires, psychometric and laboratory measures, and methods of direct observation that have utility in assessing disruptive behavior.

PARENT–CHILD INTERVIEW

The clinical interview with parents is a necessary component in conducting a thorough assessment of child behavior. This process allows the clinician to obtain appropriate background, family, school, and social information regarding the child's functioning. Much has been written regarding general clinical interviews and, more recently, about various semistructured interviews, as to their reliability, validity, and overall utility (Mash & Terdal, 1988; Othmer & Othmer, 1989). The more commonly cited interview formats include The Diagnostic Interview Schedule for Children (Costello et al., 1982), the Diagnostic Interview for Children and Adolescents (Herjanic, Brown, & Wheatt, 1975), The Child Assessment Schedule (Hodges et al., 1982b), and the Schedule for Affective Disorders and Schizophrenia for School-Aged Children (Chambers et al., 1985; Puig-Antich & Chambers, 1978). Typically, such interviews glean information from both parent and child in an effort to increase reliability of the information gathering process. These formats vary relative to the degree of information appropriate for the diagnosis of a Disruptive Behavior Disorder. Our intent here is not to review the efficacy of each format, as this has been provided elsewhere (Edelbrock & Costello, 1988; Hodges, 1987; Morrison, 1988; & Orvaschel, 1988), but rather to acknowledge their existence, their potential, and to suggest that some (particularly students and novice clinicians) may find such orientations useful in certain situations. However, until further research clearly indicates their utility for children with Disruptive Behavior Disorders, we suggest that they be viewed with caution and, if consulted, used in conjunction with other data gathering-strategies.

A thorough evaluation of children with Disruptive Behavior Disorders requires multiple assessment methods, one of which is the clinical interview. As Barkley (1981) articulated, a well-conducted parent interview is necessary for a number of reasons: (1) It provides the clinician with an opportunity to establish rapport with the family, which becomes important later when proposing and implementing treatment strategies; (2) Parents are an important source of information regarding the child's development, level of functioning, and type of parent–child interactions; (3) It assists the parents in viewing their child from a behavioral–interactional perspective, which may facilitate their cooperation if subsequent treatment includes parent training in behavior management; and (4) It provides information necessary in generating meaningful diagnoses and planning subsequent treatment. In keeping with the need for obtaining detailed information focusing upon developmental, behavioral, and interactional variables, we have developed an interview format specific to assessing such issues in children with disruptive behavior. This format is comprised of seven primary categories, each of which represents a general area warranting specific inquiry from developmental, behavioral, and interactional perspectives. A detailed description will be presented in the following section.

The interview process can be greatly enhanced if the clinician has already obtained and reviewed information pertaining to the child's development, behavior, and presenting problems. In addition to pertinent medical and school records and child behavior questionnaires (subsequently discussed), we have found that it is quite helpful to have parents complete a questionnaire highlighting certain information. This may include demographic data, history of motor, language, and physical development, as well as other behavior-related issues. In so doing, pertinent background and current information can be reviewed in a manner that may: (1) assist in directing the focus of the interview, (2) result in a more efficient and cost-effective approach to data gathering, and (3) allow the clinician to spend more time on critical issues for a particular child/family, rather than upon generalities.

Developmental Questionnaire

The general questionnaire (presented in Appendix A) was developed to assist the clinician in obtaining information during the interview. We suggest that this form be sent to parents so they have sufficient time to complete and return the questionnaire prior to their initial appointment. When schedules conflict with this arrangement, parents may bring the completed questionnaire with them to the first appointment, and clinicians may then take a few minutes before the interview to scan this information. The questionnaire was designed to be nonthreatening to parents. Items are generally straightforward and for the most part focus on the child's behavior. Categories are arranged to be consistent with the interview outline. An additional component was the inclusion of two brief checklists. The first checklist is comprised of 18 items that focus on medical, physical, and language issues, although some may have emotional overtones. The second checklist consists of 34 items that allow for more specificity relative to social–emotional, academic, and disruptive behaviors. Neither checklist is meant to be a complete list of potential problem behaviors or concerns that may be uncovered during the evaluation. Rather, both are intended to allow the clinician an opportunity to begin formulating a tentative focus for the upcoming interview. Information obtained by the Developmental Questionnaire can be integrated throughout key sections of the interview in a manner conducive to generating information needed to arrive at appropriate diagnoses and treatment recommendations.

CLINICAL INTERVIEW

Parent Interview

This section will discuss the interview process by category and provide an outline of pertinent issues within each category with a brief explanation as to why these issues are necessary to explore within the context of the interview. Table 2.1 illustrates the basic components of a clinical interview and a brief but succinct outline of critical issues that need to be discussed with parents. We

TABLE 2.1
Clinical Interview Outline: Parent

Name:	Grade:	CA:
Informant(s):	Child's physician:	Date:

Rationale for Referral/Desired Outcome

Source of referral
Brief description of current concerns
Parental expectation of evaluation outcome
Overview to parent(s) of evaluation process

Developmental and Medical History

Pre-, peri-, and postnatal development
Mother's mental and physical health through postnatal period
General physical health of child
General health of family members
Developmental milestones
Eating, diet, and sleeping patterns; evidence of tics
Medical issues contributing to presenting profile
Medications prescribed for child
Contacts with physician

Social Interactions. Approach interactions relative to age clusters, e.g., 0–2, 3–5 (preschool), 6–11 (elementary), 12–14 (junior high school), 15–18 (high school)

Peer interaction (social skills, positive and negative behaviors, ability to maintain friends, social initiative interfering social behaviors)
Parent–child interaction (positive and negative behaviors)
Coercive behavior patterns
Review of Developmental Questionnaire checklist of problem behaviors: severity, pervasiveness, frequency
Manner in which directives are given and behavior expectations expressed
Attempted behavior management strategies
Review sequence of parent–child interaction figure and Home Situations Questionnaire
Review other child behavior questionnaires

General Emotional Development

Emotional maturity
General temperament
Easily angered, ease of frustration
Significant fears or preoccupations
Mood consistent with behavior or expectations; mood swings
Sense of happiness and well-being
Thought processes
Somatic complaints

School History

Academic and/or language delays
Problem school behaviors (classroom, playground, lunchroom)

Parent-perceived teacher–child relations
Review school records and psychoeducational test results
School-based interventions
Review teacher-completed behavior questionnaire and, where possible, initiate
direct contact with the teacher

Family Dynamics and Parent Psychiatric Status

Stressors within family unrelated to the child in question
Intact versus dysfunctional family dynamics
Parental and sibling history of psychiatric disorders
Psychiatric evaluation and treatment of family/individuals
Review marital adjustment

Child Interview

Child's perception of referral
Problem areas, ownership of problems
Peer interaction, problem areas, positive interactions
Parent interaction, problem areas, positive interactions
Degree of academic success
If the child could, what would he change about parents, peers, school, and self?
Willingness to bring about positive change

Individuals and Agencies to Receive Copy of Report

---

have found this form helpful in conducting interviews as it allows for a structured and sequential approach to gathering information. Students and novice clinicians may also find it particularly helpful. We realize there will be instances that require the clinician to explore some issues in more detail. The outline is intended to serve as a structural reminder of issues to be discussed as part of a comprehensive interview and not a rigid format that the interviewer must follow in every situation. Informants, depending upon their mood and/or need, can at times present information in a rather impulsive, disorganized, inconsistent manner and, unless clinicians are effective at redirecting the focus, important information could easily be overlooked or not presented in sufficient detail. In similar fashion, some informants may have difficulty providing behavior specific information, require a great deal of subtle prodding and encouragement, or have difficulty with verbal expression, all of which can easily detract from a smooth clinical interview. In any case, clinicians may find it helpful to follow this format until he/she has conducted enough interviews to feel comfortable in obtaining this information without such structure.

CLINICAL INTERVIEW BY CATEGORY AND RATIONALE FOR INCLUSION

Rationale for Referral/Desired Outcome

We have frequently found that in situations where a father (biological or otherwise) is present within the home and a child's behavior is (one of) the presenting problem(s), the assessment process is greatly enhanced and subsequent treatment is generally more effective when the father is an active participant. Obviously, the father's involvement allows for a more thorough examination of family dynamics (e.g., inconsistencies between parents regarding child management issues, marital discord, etc.) which could easily maintain child behavior problems. Thus, we strongly recommend involving the father as much as possible in every phase of the assessment and treatment process.

Typically, the interview is the first meeting between the parents, child(ren), and the clinician. Family members in attendance may often be somewhat nervous and uncertain as to the procedure and outcome. This initial contact generally sets the tone for subsequent interactions. We typically start by bringing all family members into the office. This is done mostly to ease any anxiety or apprehension the child may experience, which may be heightened by leaving the child and walking away with his/her parents. After a few minutes of casual conversation, the child can be escorted back to the waiting room and told how long the parent interview will last.

Upon returning, it is important to gain a brief understanding from parents as to their rationale for the referral and what they or others hope to gain from the evaluation. Even though parents have already responded to these basic questions by means of the Developmental Questionnaire, it is a good policy to reiterate rationale and expectations, as this can identify inappropriate expectations and facilitate a smooth transition into the interview. At times, parents may begin the interview by expressing frustration about their child's behavior and/or previous attempts to find assistance for their child. If so, they may need to "vent" and should be provided a brief moment to express their frustration, during which the interviewer should offer support and understanding. The clinician should then reassure parents that all of their concerns will be addressed subsequently and refocus them to the task at hand. Finally, parents should be provided with a brief explanation outlining the assessment process. Parents often come to the first interview with an expectation that they will receive answers, specific advice, and appropriate treatment all in the first session, which of course is not always possible. Thus, a brief outline of the assessment process could be helpful and should include such items as expected time parameters, and the need to collect information from a variety of sources. In addition, issues surrounding limits of confidentiality should be discussed.

This is important because it is not uncommon to learn of information during the initial interview which might require the clinician to break confidentiality (e.g., a recent incident of child abuse). Parents can quickly become alienated and fail to return for further evaluation or treatment if confidentiality is broken and they were not forewarned of this possibility. Finally, clinicians should address financial considerations, including the approximate cost of the evaluation, reduced or sliding fees, etc. Often it may not be possible to provide an exact cost for a comprehensive evaluation at the outset. However, we feel strongly that parents should not experience a "financial surprise" due to the clinician's or clinic's failure to address these factors. Parents should be given a realistic range and/or an approximate figure for the evaluation and possible treatment. At this time it may also be helpful to discuss insurance coverage and any obligation parents will encounter should insurance not provide complete coverage. Once these issues have been addressed, the formal interview should begin.

Developmental and Medical History

The next portion of the interview is designed to gain an appreciation of any physical or medical factors that may contribute to the presenting behavior profile. The clinician should inquire as to whether there were any pre-, peri-, or postnatal complications, maternal drug use (prescription or otherwise), and/or atypical stressors during the pregnancy or infancy. Noted irregularities or complications should be further discussed to determine possible implications for current behavior. Relationships between congenital anomalies and/or biological risks and subsequent disturbances in behavior have long been suggested (Kopp & Kaler, 1989; Whalen, 1983). Additionally, children with a Disruptive Behavior Disorder tend to experience more health and physical problems (e.g., motor incoordination, motor tics, enuresis, encopresis, allergies, eating/sleeping problems) than non-DBD children (Barkley, 1988a, b; Hartsough & Lambert, 1985; Herbert, 1978, 1982; Nichols, 1980; Whalen, 1983). When such anomalies exist there frequently are secondary social–emotional features that may play a role in the overall behavior of the child. For these reasons, we believe it important to obtain information regarding the child's general health pattern. Deviations from normal health and development should be explored relative to their impact on child behavior at the time of illness and any adverse or residual effects.

The general health of all family members should be discussed. Significant illnesses or physical complications in another family member, particularly a parent, may be a factor in the degree of a child's attention-seeking behaviors, family dynamics, as well as the capacity of the parents to tolerate and manage difficult child behavior. The clinician should be careful not to lose direction at this point in the interview, as it may be easy to focus on another family member's "problem" rather than on the child in question. Nevertheless, to gain a sense of the general well-being of the child relative to the context of the family can prove very helpful in subsequent diagnostic and treatment considerations.

Developmental milestones (e.g., walking, talking, toilet training, and for older children pubertal development) should be addressed during this phase of the interview. In so doing, the clinician may wish to inquire as to whether there were specific stressors associated with reaching these milestones, note any atypical parental expectations, consequences for developmental immaturity, and continued physical or motor delays. The clinician should also solicit detailed information concerning the child's activity level, peer interactions, compliance with parental instructions/expectations, etc. This phase of the interview can yield information that will be very important in subsequent differential diagnostic procedures. For example, since criteria for ADHD include onset before age seven, evidence as to the presence or absence of difficulties before this age may be very helpful in differentiating this disorder from a moderate to severe adjustment reaction with associated disturbances in behavior.

The child's general temperament should also be discussed from a developmental perspective. Evidence suggests an association between temperament and subsequent behavior problems (Herbert, 1982). Indeed, some children seem inherently difficult to manage, which is often compounded by their sensitive and temperamental nature. It is also important to gain a perspective concerning the degree of "match" between a child's temperament and that of his/her parents. If parents, for example, are easily excited, riled, or impulsive and the child presents in similar fashion, the degree of conflict (almost from day one) is most certainly going to be heightened. It has been our experience that treatment is generally more effective if the degree of match between child/parent temperament is considered and that treatment is individualized to accommodate these considerations.

Eating and diet habits need to be addressed and are important for a number of reasons. First, many parents believe sugar and food additives may adversely effect, perhaps severely, the behavior of their child. Little evidence suggests that either diet or sugar directly effects the occurrence or severity of hyperactive behavior in most children (Behar et al., 1984; Furguson et al., 1986; Gross, 1984; Mattes & Gittelman, 1981; Milich et al., 1986; Rosen et al., 1988; Wolraich et al., 1985). However, there is evidence to suggest that a small percentage of children may be sensitive to additives, and that preschool-age children may be slightly more sensitive than older children (Goldman et al., 1986; Prinz et al., 1980; Weiss, 1984). Clinicians should be aware of this research in order clarify for parents (tactfully), the relationship between diet and hyperactive and disruptive behaviors. Regardless of the sugar–additive issue, a generally poor diet does little to foster mental alertness and appropriate behavior. While diet and eating behavior are important considerations with young children due to potential behavior management issues, during late childhood and adolescence diet and eating behavior should be examined for evidence of other adjustment difficulties. Given the temporal development of anorexic and depressive symptoms with (frequent) onset during the middle-school and high-school years, (Foreyt & McGavin, 1988; Kazdin, 1988), it may be necessary to consider general diet and eating (and sleeping) patterns in relation to the child's presenting profile. Should the child be placed on stimulant medication (given that appetite suppression is one potential side effect), it may prove helpful to have established some type of baseline information regarding eating behavior. In this manner, subsequently assessing the impact of this potential side effect would be more meaningful.

Finally, the interviewer should address any past or present medications prescribed for treatment of significant medical or behavioral problems. This should include a brief review of the parent's impressions concerning therapeutic benefits and adverse side effects experienced with the medications. This is also a good opportunity to note approximately how many times and for what reasons the child has been seen by his/her physician. Some children will have had clear documentation, via medical records, of physician contact due to concerns centering around their behavior and/or physical anomaly. Other children will have had very little contact. In situations where little contact has been made, it may prove helpful to suggest a general physical examination be obtained. A medical evaluation is at times necessary to assist in ruling in/out certain physical or metabolic problems. Such an evaluation would also seem appropriate prior to implementing a trial dose of medication.

Social Interactions

This phase of the interview should focus on the child's interaction with peers and parents. This is undoubtedly the broadest yet perhaps most important (from a behavioral standpoint) category. A somewhat structured developmental-sequential approach to obtaining information may prove the most effective. For example, approaching interactions with respect to age clusters, e.g., 0–2, 3–5 (preschool), 6–11 (elementary school), 12–14 (junior high school), 15–18 (high school) may assist the clinician (and parent) in gaining a necessary perspective relative to onset, frequency, and intensity of problem behaviors and social interactions. Information regarding positive interactions should also be discussed. The clinician should acquire enough information to form an impression concerning any situational variability relative to positive versus negative interaction patterns. This may prove helpful later in planning and conducting treatment, both in building on the factors that foster and maintain positive interaction patterns and in targeting negative patterns. Issues requiring attention here include peer interaction, parent–child interaction, behavior management techniques parents have employed (including their perception of the relative benefits) in attempting to manage their child's behavior, and review of parent-completed child behavior questionnaires.

Peer Interaction

Children with Disruptive Behavior Disorders tend to have poor self-esteem, experience peer rejection, be socially immature, have a repertoire of ineffective social skills, misperceive social cues, and display aggressive, intrusive, and self-centered behaviors (Barkley, 1988a; Gouze, 1987; Lochman & Lampron, 1986; McMahon & Forehand, 1988). These aversive behaviors are typically pervasive in nature, appearing across many situations, and tend to increase in frequency and intensity as the child grows up. Additional issues deserving exploration include peer identification groups, whether the child can make and maintain friendships, and whether any significant community involvement has occurred. Parents of children with Disruptive Behavior Disorders often report that their child is in frequent conflict with neighborhood children (and their parents) due to noncompliant, aggressive, and immature behavior. Community and court involvement may be additional areas of concern when focusing upon adolescent behavior. Where peer and social conflict have been common, the clinician may see a youngster (and perhaps parents) with a self-defeatist or "I don't care, it's hopeless" attitude, or a set of well-ingrained coercive behaviors, all of which will be important factors in understanding the gestalt of this child's behavior pattern and in providing a complete treatment program.

Parent–Child Interaction

Just as children with Disruptive Behavior Disorders can have significant peer interaction problems, so too can parent–child interactions be extremely stressed. Research has indicated that these children pose significant interaction problems to parents by virtue of their negative, oppositional, and defiant behavior as well as their inability to self-monitor and sustain compliant behavior in a manner consistent with age-level expectations. Conversely, parents tend to be more commanding and directive, display more critical behaviors toward their child, be less rewarding and responsive to their child's behavior, and generally have more negative perceptions about their child's behavior than parents of children without these disorders (Barkley, 1981, 1983, 1985a, b, 1988a–d; Barkley et al., 1985a; Mash & Johnston, 1982; McMahon & Forehand, 1988; Rogers, Forehand, & Griest, 1981). Indeed, stress levels generated by mutually coercive behavior in these families can be quite high and the clinician needs to assist parents in sorting through the many bidirectional variables that can adversely affect parent–child interaction (Breen & Barkley, 1988; Brody & Forehand, 1986; Dumas, 1986; Panaccione & Wahler, 1986). At this point it may be advantageous to review with parents the behaviorally oriented checklist found on the Developmental Questionnaire. This would allow specific inquiry as to behaviors central to one or more of the DSM-III-R Disruptive Behavior Disorders. Items identified as problematic should be further discussed in terms of frequency, severity, and relevant antecedent and consequent events. The last issue pertinent to this discussion is the manner in which parental directives are issued to the child and the typical initial responses of the child. Without going into excessive detail, the clinician should explore whether the manner in which requests/directives are given (e.g., unreasonable expectation, impulsively given, too many distractions) contributes to noncompliance and associated stress within the parent–child relationship. It is important to note whether the child, in response to a typical directive, makes (1) an attempt to comply but falls short due to a lack of self-monitoring or parental supervision; (2) makes little attempt to comply or presents with a whiney oppositional manner but eventually completes the directive; or (3) unequivocally defies the directive. Through discussing these issues with parents, the clinician can gain information that facilitates a more complete understanding of the dynamics involved in parent–child interactions. This can be very helpful in formulating diagnostic impressions and targeting appropriate behaviors for subsequent intervention.

Prior/Current Behavior Management

From a behavior management perspective, perhaps most frustrating to parents is the child's relative inability to sustain rule-governed behavior. It is this deficit that contributes to many behavior problems and requires parents to monitor (in some fashion) the child's behavior constantly. The interview should review all methods of behavior management which parent(s) have previously attempted, making careful note of specific strategies, under what conditions (i.e., behaviors) were they effective or ineffective, and approximate length of time any given strategy has been effective. Parents may, for example, indicate that chair time-out has little effect as the child "is right back doing it again," which may then be followed by more aversive parent–child interactions. On the other hand, parents may feel that "grounding" the child for short intervals has been effective or that "absolutely nothing works." The importance of discussing the antecedents and consequences with respect to what has been effective and ineffective with this child should not be overlooked. Differences in parental expectations regarding child behavior, parental ability or willingness to follow up on noncompliant behavior, and the consistency with which expectations and consequences have been adhered to are additional considerations that need to be explored.

It is not unusual to find that parents have attempted various management techniques but have applied these incorrectly or have given insufficient consideration to subtle factors that might adversely impact upon outcome. For example, at the suggestion of a teacher, school counselor, pediatrician, or some other concerned party, parents often devise and attempt to implement positive reinforcement programs, such as a token system with added secondary reinforcers. However, despite their good intentions, when left to their own resources, parents often design ineffective programs or implement them in an inappropriate manner. Adequate attention is often not given to identifying appropriate rewards that are reinforcing to the particular child, with the result that the "reward menu" contains nonreinforcing consequences. Or, the implementation of the program may be done in such a way that positive rewards are confounded with negative, aversive interactions (e.g., parents continuing to hassle or yell at the child if the positive behavior is not emitted), with the end result being noncompliant behaviors continue to be reinforced more than desired behaviors overtly targeted by the program. In such situations, the program is marginally effective if not ineffective, and parents terminate the program in frustration, concluding that such programs will not work with their child. Similarly, parents are often told they can extinguish relatively minor disruptive behavior, such as temper tantrums, by "ignoring" the behavior. Unfortunately, they may not be sufficiently informed that previously reinforced behaviors such as tantrums frequently display a brief increase in frequency and/or intensity when reinforcement is withdrawn (often referred to as the "postextinction burst"). Parents may also not be informed that it could take several weeks to see an appreciable decline in negative behavior. The usual result is that parents attempt to "ignore" the behavior but stop their efforts prematurely in frustration, again with the belief that this approach is ineffective. In addition, given the severity of behavior problems displayed by some children with Disruptive Behavior Disorders, "ignoring" behaviors can be a rather naive attitude to take if not at times dangerous. Many additional examples could be given of situations where parents, despite their best intentions, have applied behavior management techniques inefficiently or incorrectly. Very often, these previous unsuccessful experiences contribute to feelings of demoralization and low confidence in parents and are a cause of subsequent resistance to attempting behavioral management techniques. In order to maximize parental cooperation with subsequent treatment interventions, it will be helpful to identify any such sources of parental demoralization and/or resistance and begin to address these in such a way that parental hope for improvement is increased.

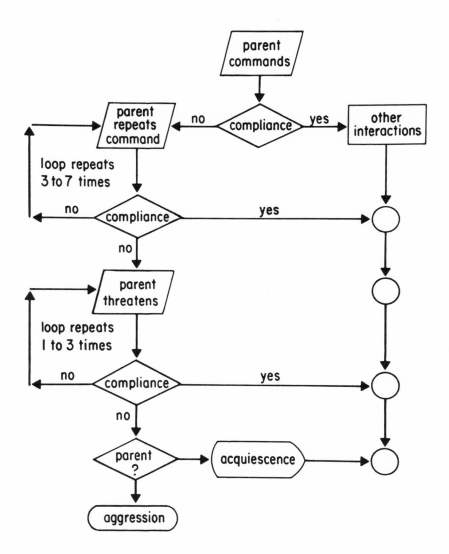

FIGURE 2.1. Diagram of noncompliant interaction. From *Hyperactive Children: A Handbook for Diagnosis and Treatment* (p. 100) by R. A. Barkley, 1981. New York: Guilford Press. Copyright by the Guilford Press. Reprinted by permission.

In facilitating the discussion of parent–child interaction from a behavior management perspective, Figure 2.1 (Barkley, 1981, 1987) may prove useful. This chart illustrates possible sequences of parent–child interactions subsequent to parental directives. Once this chart has been explained, we suggest applying that insight to problem situations parents have identified thus far in the interview and/or by means of the Home Situations Questionnaire (HSQ) (to be discussed below). Review of this questionnaire may also be helpful in noting how pervasive and varied the behavior most difficult to manage seems to be. Children with a Disruptive Behavior Disorder may not display problem behavior across all settings, consistently, to the same degree, or with all caregivers (Barkley, 1988a). Reviewing the HSQ profile often facilitates discussion of parenting roles, disciplinary procedures, expectations for child behavior, and parent–child dynamics.

Review of Child Behavior Questionnaires

At this point in the interview it may be helpful to review contents of those questionnaires (minus the HSQ) which parents have completed. We do not suggest an item-by-item or even factor-by-factor analysis. However, there may be certain behaviors indicated by means of the questionnaire that have not been disclosed thus far or need further clarification. It is often helpful to explore differences between oral reports from parents and trends illustrated through questionnaires. In addition, we have at times found it helpful to ask both parents to complete questionnaires independently. Any discrepancies would then need to be explored, as they might be indicative of significant inconsistencies in parental expectations and ability to manage their child's behavior. It may also be appropriate to explain to parents why they were asked to complete the questionnaire and how this information will be used in the overall assessment of their child.

General Emotional Development

As noted previously, the general development of children having a Disruptive Behavior Disorder is less positive than had once been believed, particularly as the degree of child aggression and family psychopathology increases. Many of these children continue to display problem behaviors inconsistent with age level expectations well into adulthood. In many instances their overall social and emotional adjustment remains poor, and may be characterized by low self-esteem, underachievement, depression, attempted suicide, chemical abuse, and antisocial behavior (Barkley, 1988a; Breen & Barkley, 1983, 1984; Hunt, 1988; Kaplan, 1988; McMahon & Forehand, 1988; Wallander & Hubert,

1985; Weiss & Hechtman, 1986). Given that these associated features typically evolve over a period of time and are a function of many intricate interactions, it is necessary (particularly with older children) for the clinician to gain an understanding of the child's emotional stability. Considerations here might include the child's temperament, general sense of well-being (i.e., happiness, self-contentment, anger, sadness), emotional lability, unusual thought processes, fears or preoccupations, somatic complaints, and degrees of depression and/or anxiety. There may be instances, for example, where parents complain of the child's inability to maintain a conversation. This difficulty could be a function of poor language skills, poor verbal impulse control, and/or elements of a thought disorder. In particular, many children/adolescents with pervasive developmental disorders or peculiar, idiosyncratic thought processes (which are often precursors to adult schizophrenic spectrum disorders) can present with behavioral symptoms similar to children/adolescents with a Disruptive Behavior Disorder. Similarly, while the presenting behavioral symptomatology may appear to be that of a Disruptive Behavior Disorder, it may be a function of an affective disorder, an anxiety disorder, or an acute reaction to significant psychosocial stress. Obtaining historical information can prove very helpful in understanding the onset and course of the child's difficulties. This information will assist in reaching accurate diagnostic conclusions, (i.e., differential diagnoses) and facilitate the development of appropriate treatment.

School History

Discussion within this category should focus on the child's social and academic behavior. While not all children with a Disruptive Behavior Disorder present with significant educational needs, most do (August & Garfinkel, 1990; Barkley, 1988a; Safer, 1984; Sturge, 1982; Tramontana, Hooper, Curley, & Nardolillo, 1990). Problems with behavior in unstructured (and at times structured) situations, poor academic productivity, aggression, disruptive behavior in the classroom, and poor social skills are commonly experienced by these children. Even if academic and social behaviors are not severe enough to warrant exceptional education, many children remain somewhat impaired within the educational setting. The clinician should inquire as to the number of schools the child has attended. Clearly, the more schools the child has attended, and the more adjustments he/she has had to make, the more likely it will be that he/she will experience social and academic adjustment difficulties. The primary elements that children with Disruptive Behavior Disorders need within the academic setting are structure and consistency, both of which would be difficult to maintain when moving from school to school. Parents should then be asked about the child's pattern of school attendance.

It is recommended that a review of the child's social and academic development also follow a sequential process. While there are many instances in which obvious difficulty begins with the onset of formal education (kindergarten), some children with these disorders advance through the first few years in school, or more rarely, through elementary school, before behaviors significantly interfere with expected performance. Such children may still require more than the ordinary number of parent–teacher conferences, some academic and social modifications (e.g., changing the desk, minor behavior management programs), and visits with the school guidance counselor, but behavioral difficulties may not require within-school or outside-the-school referral. However, problem behaviors may intensify and a more comprehensive program of assessment and intervention would then need to be considered. Clinicians should carefully review with parents the types of academic and behavior problems the child has experienced, at what point they became pronounced, what attempts the school has made to intervene, what impact if any the interventions have had, and how positive or negative the parent–child–teacher interaction has been. Parents may comment that they feel that their child has not been given a fair chance or may even have been "set up" for failure, given administrative directives, teacher expectations, and/or the type of classroom structure. Conversely, parents may comment that teachers have been extremely helpful and have made every reasonable attempt to assist their child in being successful. All of these factors must be considered when determining why the child is exhibiting disruptive behaviors and functioning below expected academic and social levels. Should reading, math, language, or general cognitive delays be suspected, discussion should then focus on whether parents would like these domains assessed as part of the current evaluation or whether the school will be conducting a multidisciplinary team evaluation. Some parents will feel quite comfortable with the school completing this assessment, particularly if they have had a generally positive experience thus far. Where there has been mounting tension and poor home–school communication, parents may wish to have the academic–cognitive evaluation pursued concurrently and then take that information back to the school.

If possible, it is recommended that parents obtain and bring with them copies of prior psychoeducational evaluations and Multidisciplinary Team/Individual Educational Plan reports, and that these be reviewed with parents on a somewhat cursory basis. (Alternatively, copies of such reports can be obtained between the first and second appointment, and reviewed briefly during the second appointment.) Discrepant test scores, implications of results, and/or questions parents may have about the test results should be reviewed and discussed. In addition, teacher-completed questionnaires should be reviewed briefly with parents. This provides an opportunity to gain parental insights that may prove consistent or inconsistent with teacher perceptions. Inconsistent perceptions would then need further exploration and clarification. However, clinicians should be sensitive to certain teacher comments that they may not wish to have shared with parents. Obviously, some discretion as to the manner of presentation may be needed at this point.

Family Dynamics and Parent Psychiatric Status

The clinician need not go into a detailed analysis of the family background and psychiatric status of each family member. However, in order to gain a complete understanding of the context in which the child's behavior problems have emerged, it is helpful to review family history and additional within-family stressors. In particular, it is necessary to identify significant contributory factors, such as current parental psychiatric disturbance or history of child abuse, that might be present. Research has suggested that there may be a genetic predisposition increasing the risk of Disruptive Behavior Disorders in children. Parents, siblings, and extended relatives of these children appear to have a higher rate of conduct, learning, and attentional problems than would otherwise be expected. In addition, these parents tend to experience more psychopathology, marital distress, depressive symptomatology (mothers), and extrafamilial distress than do parents of children without Disruptive Behavior Disorders (Befera & Barkley, 1985; Breen & Barkley, 1988; Griest & Wells, 1983; Mash & Johnston, 1983a; O'Leary & Emery, 1984; Wahler, 1980). For example, child behavior problems often emerge in families having recently experienced a parental divorce, reduced earnings or unemployment, a new baby, excessive chemical abuse, child abuse, or psychopathology, and the family may need to deal with the stressors of these situations before interventions focused on child behavior problems will be effective (Jensen, Bloedau, Degroot, Ussery, & Davis, 1990; Reid & Crisafulli, 1990). Thus, the degree to which stressors exist within the family may reflect how responsive and successful parents will be in implementing treatment strategies centering on the child's disruptive behavior. It is therefore quite important that clinicians give proper attention to issues of family dynamics, particularly as they pertain to the behaviors of the child in question. Previous but pertinent psychiatric or mental health interventions in the family should also be discussed. These might include marital or family therapy, individual child and/or adult therapy, or pharmacotherapy, any of which should be explored as to type, length, and outcome of treatment. A cursory review of parental impressions (positive or negative) of such treatments may prove helpful in planning subsequent treatments with the family. This would also be an ideal time to discuss impressions and results of any general family–marital adjustment scale which the clinician may have asked parents to complete. Results should be interpreted and discussed primarily in light of the presenting child behavior profile.

Child Interview

The child being referred for evaluation should also participate in the interview process for a number of reasons. First, children typically realize their behavior is central to the visit. They may not have a clear idea of all the dynamics involved, but most understand that things have not been "calm, cool, and collected" in the home and school settings. The child interview provides an opportunity to clarify the situation for them and to address and dispel any fears or apprehensions they may have. (Will they be given a shot? Is the present appointment a punishment for something that they have done?) The clinician can then solicit their cooperation in the assessment and subsequent treatment processes. Second, it is in everyone's best interest if the child feels a part of this process. After all, the child does have a vested interest in at least a portion of the presenting problem. Third, since parents are likely to seek professional assistance due to the belief that their child "has a problem," they often expect that the clinician will spend sufficient individual time with the "problem child." In fact, it has been our anecdotal impression that some parents more readily accept evaluative feedback and are more willing to comply with subsequent treatment interventions if the "expert" has spent sufficient time individually "evaluating" their child. Fourth, this initial contact allows the child an opportunity to express and discuss his perceptions and feelings about the type and degree of problem behavior and any associated difficulties. For example, the child may be concerned about the frequency and intensity of marital disagreements or the substance use of a parent or sibling. Thus, it is possible that through the child interview the clinician will learn of important family dynamics and stressors parents did not discuss. Finally, this interaction allows the clinician an opportunity to observe the child's general behavior, use of language, thought processes, affect, and general demeanor.

The clinician should keep in mind that depending upon the age, maturity, cognitive development, and degree of defensiveness, information gained from the child may not be representative. As a result, such information must be judiciously interpreted, particularly when the child is below the age of 12 (Barkley, 1988a; Bierman, 1983; McMahon & Forehand, 1988; Sleator & Ullmann, 1981). Children of all ages may present in an apprehensive, negative, insolent, friendly, or cooperative manner, depending upon (in part) their needs and the rationale their parents have provided them for the visit. Clinicians must be sensitive to these factors and make every effort to assist the child to feel comfortable with the interview process. In situations where the child or adolescent presents in an exceedingly distrustful, manipulative, or angry manner, the initial interaction may need to center around easing such hostility. Hopefully, a second interview may then be arranged in order to focus upon other issues.

Where age, maturity, and cooperation permit, the clinician should attempt to gain insight into the child's perception of his/her behavior when interacting with peers, siblings, parents, and teachers. A review of how the child feels about himself/herself, as well as the positive and negative characteristics of each interaction may be helpful. It is also important to ask children what things they would most like to change, if they could, regarding their family, peer, and school interactions, and under what conditions they would be willing to work toward positive change. Admittedly, such information will not always be attained during the initial (or second) interview, but attempts should nevertheless be made. With older children administering a general problem checklist (e.g., Personal Problems Checklist for Adolescents) may be helpful in identifying concerns they may otherwise feel uncomfortable in discussing initially (Schinka, 1985). In so doing, information may be obtained that could facilitate current discussion or be used during subsequent interaction.

Agencies to Receive Report

Clinicians should inquire as to which, if any, agencies or individuals should be sent a copy of the evaluation. There may be instances where the parents and/or child are involved with multiple agencies, all of which have vested interests in this family and which therefore might benefit from a report of the results. It would not be uncommon for the attending physician, school system, one or more social service agencies, judicial system, and/or other private mental health facilities to benefit from the results of the evaluation. On the other hand, parents may state very clearly that certain agencies or individuals are not to receive such information or only portions of results (e.g., oral report to the school). In situations where parent and state child-custody issues are of concern, the clinician must understand to whom and under what conditions information will be released. Parents should also be informed about conditions (e.g., court subpoena) in which the information may be released against their wishes. Parents should then be requested to sign release of information forms so that no confusion can result in the future when reports are completed and ready to be forwarded to appropriate individuals.

Teacher Interview

We believe teachers have all too often been left out of the interview process when evaluating children with a suspected Disruptive Behavior Disorder. This is unfortunate, as we have generally found teachers very willing participants who can provide extremely useful information. If school mental health professionals are conducting the evaluation, an interview with the classroom teacher should not prove difficult, although even within these settings schedule conflicts may make the process inconvenient. For those medical or mental health professionals functioning outside the school setting, a personal interview would probably be difficult to arrange, and in this case a phone conference would be a reasonable alternative. In either situation, certain basic information should be obtained. Whereas the clinical interview with parents may take up to an hour, one cannot expect a classroom teacher to be available for this amount of time. Time spent interviewing the teacher should be streamlined to gather basic information efficiently, and typically the process should not require more than 10–15 minutes. In certain situations it may be necessary to arrange additional time.

Table 2.2 provides an outline of the minimal amount of information that should be discussed with the classroom teacher. We offer this outline as a guide to facilitate the data-gathering process. There may be instances that require a different focus than currently presented, or one may need to detail certain interactions more than others. If the practitioner follows this general guide, a solid foundation of school-based information may be gained in a manner consistent with the parent interview. Ideally, prior to interviewing the child's teacher, a broad-band-behavior questionnaire, such as the Child Behavior Checklist (CBCL) Teacher Report Form, Comprehensive Teacher Rating Scale (ACTeRS), and the School Situations Questionnaire should have been completed by the teacher and reviewed. In this manner, the interview process may focus more productively on specific problem behaviors, the frequency with which they occur, as well as pertinent antecedent and consequent events. Previously attempted academic-oriented interventions and their impact should also be discussed. Just as the behavior of children with Disruptive Behavior Disorders in parent–child interactions may be in part a function of motivation, situational demands, primary authority figure, method of directive delivery, and degree of distractions, so too are behaviors within the school setting mitigated by these variables. That is, the same child may display varied productivity, achievement, and behavior or be quite consistent in degree and manner of presenting problems across situations, teachers, and peer interactions. These are particularly important considerations to be pursued when the child has more than one classroom teacher (e.g., middle and high school students). For these reasons, it is critical to gain teacher insights regarding the child's academic and social behavior.

TABLE 2.2
Clinical Interview Outline: Teacher

Name:	Grade:	CA:
Informant(s):	Teacher:	Date:

Rationale for Referral and Overview of Behavior Problem

Source of referral and relevant explanation to teacher
Specific questions or needs of the teacher that could be addressed through the evaluation
Primary academic and behavior concerns

Medical Background/Implications

How regular is school attendance and/or tardiness?
Does the child appear to be in good general health?
Is the teacher aware of any prescribed medications the child may be taking? If yes, is the teacher aware if the medications are taken regularly as prescribed, or are there compliance problems? Are there any noted side effects?
Are there any tics or twitches present?

Cognitive Issues

Approximate level of academic skills versus report card grades. Are there productivity issues? If so, do they appear a function of motivation, responsibility, organization, inability, etc.? Is motor restlessness an issue at this point?
Does the child receptive/expressive language and memory appear within the norm for his/her age?
Does the child appear to be working at a level commensurate with perceived ability? If not, why not?
Capacity for sustained attention and on-task or goal-directed behavior?

Social Interactions

Peer interaction, e.g., ability to initiate and maintain friends, behaviors that would interfere with or facilitate peer interaction and acceptance.
Teacher-child interaction, e.g., compliance with teacher directives, positive and negative behavior with school-based adult authority figures. Child's response to consequences applied by authority figures
General factors such as aggression/anger, impulsiveness, and destructive behavior which need to be addressed

General Emotional

Self-esteem or sense of well-being
Affect, i.e., generally happy, sad, apathetic, anxious, mood swings, etc.
Basic thought processes
Temperament, ease of frustration, and related behaviors
Child adversely effected by own behavior or oblivious as to ramifications and consequences

Interventions

Type of academic and behavior management programs used with this child. Reasons for such programs. Length of time used and degree of success

(Continued)

TABLE 2.2 (*Continued*)

Within-school counseling programs in which the child may have participated. Degree of success

Child Strengths and Questions Regarding Behavior Questionnaires

Child's strengths and in what condition these are most typically displayed
Specific questions regarding certain items, clusters, or profiles

SUMMARY

In this chapter, we provided a format by which clinical interviews with parents, teachers, and child may be conducted. Our intent was to provide a suitable research-based rationale for the many categories of our outline, so that the reader can understand not just what questions to ask in an interview but why one needs to ask them. We realize that alternative interview formats are available; perhaps, in their own right, they are equally as thorough and task-specific as those presented here. We do believe, however, that our approach will generate the type of information necessary to facilitate appropriate differential diagnoses and structure treatment in a manner conducive to meeting the variety of needs presented by children with Disruptive Behavior Disorders and their families. We cannot stress enough the need to spend quality time in gathering sufficient information from multiple sources. These children usually present many social, emotional, ad cognitive needs, all of which may affect behavior across home, school, and community settings. If the clinician is gathering information from but one source or has a narrow-minded perspective, he/she runs the risk of not obtaining enough information to generate adequate conclusions, thereby limiting the scope of potential treatment. By following the format presented in this chapter, we believe the clinician will obtain the information necessary to arrive at an appropriate diagnosis so that he can use the assessment data to develop and implement a comprehensive treatment program. The following chapter will review measures designed to augment the data-gathering process: child behavior questionnaires, measures of attention span and impulse control, and direct observation of child behavior.

3

EVALUATING DISRUPTIVE BEHAVIOR DISORDERS:
Child Behavior Questionnaires, Laboratory Measurements, and Observations

In this chapter, we will critically review commonly used parent-and teacher-completed child behavior questionnaires and discuss their clinical utility for assessing children with disruptive behavior problems. We will then review several youth self-report and parent/family questionnaires that we believe have potential relevance in assessing certain issues common to children and adolescents with Disruptive Behavior Disorders as well as their families. Next, we will review several psychometric and laboratory measures, including measures of cognitive functioning, academic achievement, attention span, and impulse control, any of which may also have merit in such an assessment. Finally, we will discuss issues related to direct observation of child behavior and review one prototypic coding system.

PARENT-COMPLETED QUESTIONNAIRES

Child Behavior Checklist

The Child Behavior Checklist and Profile (CBCL; Achenbach & Edelbrock, 1983) are parent-completed checklists designed to tap a broad range of children's behavior problems (e.g., overanxiousness, depression, delinquent behavior, hyperactivity, aggression, etc.) and adaptive competencies (e.g., sports, clubs, friendships, school, etc.). The CBCL consists of 138 items; 118 comprise various behavior problem factors, and 20 various social competencies. Parents are asked to rate each behavior item 0 (not true), 1 (somewhat or sometimes true), or 2 (very true). The CBCL typically requires 20–25 minutes to complete and requires at least a 5th-grade reading level (Achenbach & Edelbrock, 1983). Although the same questions are used for all children, six separate sets of factors with corresponding separate norms and profile sheets have been developed based on gender and age (4–5 years, 6–11 years, and 12–16 years). Factors were derived from a series of factor analyses of the responses of 2,300 clinic-referred children. The various factors assessed (depending on the age and gender of the child) include: Schizoid or Anxious, Depressed, Uncommunicative, Obsessive-Compulsive, Somatic Complaints, Social Withdrawal, Immature, Hyperactive, Aggressive, Delinquent, Sex Problems, and Cruel. All six editions include an Aggressive factor and all but the 4 to 5 year-old boys' profile include a Hyperactive factor. All three editions for boys include a Delinquency factor. The checklist also yields two second-order factors, labeled Externalizing and Internalizing. The externalizing factor includes undercontrolled, socially disruptive conduct and behavior problems. The internalizing factor includes overcontrolled, inhibited, or anxious–withdrawn behaviors. Different factors across the age range initially prove somewhat confusing and cumbersome to score and interpret. It is recommended that before using the CBCL, its manual should be read carefully. Caution must be taken in scoring and plotting the profiles to guard against errors. Through experience one quickly becomes familiar with the scoring and plotting procedures.

Norms are available for use with children aged 4 through 16. Subsequent to deriving the various factors, normative data were collected on a representative sample of 1,300 children from an eastern geographic area covering urban, suburban, and semirural areas. The sample was randomly selected and stratified according to SES, race, and age. The standardization process is detailed in the manual (Achenbach & Edelbrock, 1983).

Evidence is available attesting to the psychometric acceptability of the CBCL. Reliability estimates are reported in the manual (Achenbach & Edelbrock, 1983). Briefly, 1-week intraclass coefficients were .95 for the behavior problem items and .99 for the social competence items. Stability estimates for the various factors in a sample of normal children ranged from .61 to .96, with a median value of .89. Average 1-week stability indices for selected factors were reported as follows: Aggressive, .92; Hyperactive, .96; Delinquent, .92. For clinical samples, 3-month stability estimates ranged from .47 to .86, with a mean value of .74; 6-month stability estimates ranged from .44 to .79, with a mean value of about .65; and 18-month stability estimates ranged from .14 to .87, with a mean value of about .60. Reported interrater (between parents) agreement intraclass coefficients were .99 for the behavior problem items and .98 for the social competence items; coefficients for the various factors ranged from .26 to .81, with a median value of .66. Webster-Stratton (1988) reported no significant mean differences between mother and father reports on various CBCL scales.

In the past few years many studies have reported data supporting the CBCL's concurrent and construct validity. It has been shown to correlate significantly with numerous other rating scales and criterion measures of child psychopathology, including the Conners Parent Rating Scale, Revised Behavior Problem Checklist, Werry–Weiss–Peters Activity Rating Scale, and Teacher Report Form and Youth Self-Rreport (Achenbach & Edelbrock, 1983; Kazdin, & Heidish, 1984; Mash & Johnston, 1983b; Phares, Compas, & Howell, 1989). The CBCL factors have been found to correlate significantly with similar factor/dimension scores derived from semistructured clinical interviews (Costello & Edelbrock, 1985; Hodges et al., 1982). Recently, Cohen, Gotlieb, Kershner, and Wehrspann (1985) investigated differences between CBCL internalizing versus externalizing children. Internalizing children had higher general intelligence, higher reading ability, were less egocentric, used more adaptive means of coping with stress, and were viewed by teachers as having fewer conduct problems.

In addition, evidence exists supporting the ability of the scale to discriminate clinic-referred from nonreferred children (Achenbach & Edelbrock, 1983; Breen & Barkley, 1988; Jones, Latkowski, Kircher, McMahon, 1988), psychiatric clinic-referred from learning-disabled and neurologically-impaired (Kindlon, Solle, & Yando, 1988), hyperactive from normal children (Barkley, 1981; Breen, 1989; Breen & Barkley, 1988; Mash & Johnson, 1983b), depressed from nondepressed children (Seagull & Weinshank, 1984), sexually abused from nonabused (Einbender & Friedrich, 1989; Friedrich, Urquiza, & Beilke, 1986), inpatient from outpatient-referred children (Hodges et al.; Jones et al., 1988), children of distressed from nondistressed mothers (Bond & McMahon, 1984), and children with various chronic illnesses from well children (Eyberg, 1985; Hurtig, Koepke, & Park, 1989; Lavinge, Nolan, & McLone, 1988; Morgan & Jackson, 1986; Walker & Green, 1989; Wallander, Feldman, & Varni, 1989; Wallander et al., 1988). Costello and Edelbrock (1985) have provided support for the CBCL's usefulness as a general screening measure in a primary-care pediatric setting. And finally, several reports have provided evidence that the CBCL is sensitive to effects of parent training in child management and to therapeutic interventions with children referred for antisocial behavior (Kazdin, Bass, Siegel, & Thomas, 1989; Webster-Stratton, 1984a; Webster-Stratton, Hollingsworth, & Kolpacoff, 1989; Webster-Stratton, Kolpacoff, & Hollingsworth, 1988).

The CBCL is a well-developed and standardized omnibus parent-completed measure of child psychopathology for use with school-age children. It contains items that tap broad-band behavior dimensions (internalizing, externalizing), narrower behavioral factors within each broader dimension, and social competence scales. Extensive evidence suggests that it has more-than-acceptable reliability and validity. Although different factors emerged as functions of age and gender (which initially proves somewhat confusing), attention to developmental changes in the dimensions of child psychopathology across age and gender is a strength of this scale. The CBCL is one of the more psychometrically sound and clinically useful behavior rating scales currently available for assessing psychopathology and social competence in children.

Revised Behavior Problem Checklist

The original Behavior Problem Checklist (BPC) (Peterson, 1961; Quay & Peterson, 1975) represents one of the earliest attempts to standardize informant ratings of child behavior and emotional functioning. It has been one of the most widely used rating scales in both research and clinical assessment. The BPC is a 55-item scale designed for use with parents, teachers, and other adults who work closely with children. The scale yields four analytically derived factors that tap broad dimensions of child psychopathology. An extensive literature provides support for its reliability and validity (for reviews, see Barkley, 1988a; Quay, 1977; Quay & Peterson, 1975). Briefly, adequate test–retest and interrater (between parents and between teachers) reliabilities have been reported. The BPC has been found to correlate significantly with various parent- and teacher-completed measures of child behavior problems and psychopathology, to discriminate normal from clinic-referred, aggressive, hyperactive, conduct-disordered, and learning disabled children. Finally, the BPC has proven sensitive to changes resulting from psychotherapy and pharmacotherapy. Despite evidence of its acceptable psychometric properties and its widespread use, some weaknesses were evident with the original BPC. In particular, the item pool was limited in scope, resulting in three analytically derived factor scales with very few items. This in turn limited the reliability of the respective factors (Quay, 1983). Consequently, an attempt was made to augment the original item pool and provide additional item coverage for the factors with limited items, which resulted in the Revised Behavior Problem Checklist (RBPC) (Quay, 1983; Quay & Peterson, 1983, 1984, 1987).

The RBPC consists of 89 items of problem behaviors. Like its predecessor, it was designed for use with parents, teachers, and other adults who work closely with children. Informants are asked to rate each behavior 0 (not a problem), 1 (a mild problem), or 2 (a severe problem). The RBPC typically requires 15–20 minutes to complete. Six factors were derived from a series of factor analyses of the responses of 760 children, including inpatient and out-patient psychiatric, learning-disabled, and developmentally disabled children. The various factors assessed included: Conduct Disorder, Socialized Aggressive, Attention Problems–Immaturity, Anxiety–Withdrawal, Psychotic Behavior, and Motor Excess (Quay, 1983; Quay & Peterson, 1987). The first three factors tap "externalizing" behavior problems, the fourth factor taps "internalizing" problems, and the last two factors tap specific, narrow-band problems. Norms by gender and grade/age are available for use with children ages 5 through 17. Normative data were collected from samples that were diverse in terms of geographic area, racial, and socioeconomic-status representation. The standardization process is reviewed in the manual (Quay & Peterson, 1987).

Evidence is beginning to accumulate attesting to the psychometric acceptability of the RBPC. Alpha coefficients for the six factors across several samples have ranged from .70 to .95 (Quay, 1983; Quay & Peterson, 1987). Two-month stability estimates of teacher ratings for the factors ranged from .49 to .83 (Quay & Peterson, 1987), and 5-month stability estimates across two samples from .01 to .92, with most coefficients in the .50 to .85 range (Hogan, Quay, Vaughn, & Shapiro, 1989). Interrater agreement across the factors has ranged from .52 to .85 for teachers and .55 to .93 for parents (Quay, 1983; Quay & Peterson, 1983, 1987). The checklist has been shown to correlate significantly with the CBCL (Achenbach & Edelbrock, 1983; Kazdin & Heidish, 1984; Mash & Johnston, 1983b), to discriminate normal from clinic-referred children (Aman & Werry, 1984; Quay, 1983; Quay & Peterson, 1987), conduct-disordered children (Lahey, Russo, Walker, & Piacentini, 1989), and attention-deficit-disordered children, with and without hyperactivity (Lahey et al., 1984), and adolescents from high parental conflict homes (Forehand et al., 1987; Forehand et al., 1988; Long, Slater, Forehand, & Fauber, 1988).

The RBPC is a recent revision of a widely used multi-informant measure of child psychopathology for use with school-age children. Evidence is available attesting to the psychometric acceptability of the original BPC. Preliminary evidence suggests that the RBPC is equally acceptable.

Conners Parent Rating Scale (Three Forms)

The Conners Parent Rating Scales are among the most widely used questionnaires for research and clinical assessment of children with ADHD (Barkley, 1981, 1988a, 1988c; Edelbrock, 1988; Edelbrock & Rancurello, 1985). There are three versions of the Conners Parent Rating Scales: the original 91-item version developed by Conners (1970, 1973), the 48-item revision published by Goyette, Conners, and Ulrich (1978), and the 10-item Abbreviated Symptom Questionnaire. Each of these will be reviewed.

Original Conners Parent Rating Scale

The original Conners Parent Rating Scale (CPRS) was developed to provide a brief assessment of deviant behaviors, including hyperactivity, conduct problems, learning problems, aggression, anxiety, and depression. The scale consists of 93 items, most of which describe disruptive and other externalizing-type behaviors characteristic of conduct problems and hyperactivity. Parents are asked to rate the presence and severity of each behavior from 0 (not at all) through 3 (very much). The CPRS typically requires 10–15 minutes to complete.

An investigation of the factor structure of the CPRS has been provided by Conners and Blouin (1980). The CPRS was found to assess the following factors: Conduct Disorder, Fearful–Anxious, Restless–Disorganized, Learning Problem–Immature, Psychosomatic, Obsessional, Antisocial, and Hyperactive–Immature. Normative data (means and standard deviations) for 683 children, aged 6–14 were also provided by Conners and Blouin (1980). Unfortunately, separate norms were not reported by age and gender. An Australian modification of the scale has been developed by Glow and her colleagues (Glow, 1979; Glow, Glow, & Rump, 1982), with normative data on 1,900 children.

Despite its widespread use, only limited evidence exists at this time concerning the reliability of the CPRS. Moderate to high two-month stability estimates for the various factors have been reported, with most estimates ranging in the .70's and .80's (O'Connor, Foch, Sherry, & Plomin, 1980). There is evidence suggesting that an initial practice effect may cause scores on several factors to decline from the first to the second administration, although apparently not on subsequent administrations. As a result, it has been recommended that the scale be administered at least twice before assessing treatment effects, so as to minimize the impact of testing effects (Conners, 1985; Barkley, 1988a). Estimates of internal consistency and interrater (between parents) agreement have not been reported. On the other hand, considerable evidence exists supporting the CPRS's concurrent, construct, and discriminative validity. It has been shown to correlate significantly with numerous other rating scales and criterion measures of child psychopathology, including the Werry–Weiss–Peters Activity Rating Scale (Broad, 1982), The Child Behavior Checklist (Achenbach & Edelbrock, 1983; Mash & Johnston, 1983b), the original Behavior Problem Checklist (Arnold, Barnebey, & Smeltzer, 1981; Campbell & Steinert, 1978), and the Revised Behavior Problem Checklist (Quay & Peterson, 1983). In addition, the CPRS has been shown to discriminate clinic-referred from nonreferred children as well as neurotic from conduct-problem children (Conners, 1970), normal from hyperactive children (Prior, Leonard, & Wood, 1983; Ross & Ross, 1982), and depressed from non-depressed children (Leon, Kendall, & Garber, 1980). Finally, several studies have demonstrated the CPRS's sensitivity to treatment effects of stimulant medication and diet management with hyperactive children (Barkley, 1977; Cantwell & Carlson, 1978; Harley et al., 1981).

Conners Parent Rating Scale—Revised

Conners and his colleagues modified the original Parent Rating Scale (CPRS-R) (Goyette et al., 1978). The revised scale was shortened to 48 items. Some items from the original were omitted and other similar items combined and/or reworded to increase clarity. In particular, many items assessing internalizing behaviors and symptoms (i.e., psychosomatic, obsessional, overanxious, and depressive symptoms) were omitted, so that the CPRS-R would be more specific to externalizing, disruptive behavior problems and symptoms. Thus, the CPRS-R would seem to have its greatest utility in the assessment of Disruptive Behavior Disorders. As with the original version, parents are asked to rate the presence and severity of each behavior from 0 (not at all) through 3 (very much). The CPRS-R typically requires 5–10 minutes to complete. Goyette et al. (1978) also reported factor structures of the CPRS-R, which were identified as: Conduct Problems, Learning Problems, Psychosomatic, Impulsive–Hyperactive, and Anxiety. A separate Hyperactivity Index, not factorially derived, was also developed (see below). Normative data (means and standard deviations by age and gender) for each factor and the Index were based on 578 children, aged 3–17 (Goyette et al., 1978).

Like the original CPRS, the CPRS-R enjoys widespread use despite only limited evidence concerning its reliability. There have been no reports of stability estimates for the various factors. It has been suggested (Barkley, 1988a) that in the absence of evidence concerning temporal stability and possible practice effects, the same precautions used with the CPRS be taken when using the CPRS-R to assess treatment effects (i.e., multiple preadministrations to minimize testing effects). Estimates of interrater (between parents) agreement have been reported, with coefficients ranging from .46 to .56

across the five factors. Although some evidence is available concerning the CPRS-R's validity, it has not been sufficiently examined. Voelker, Carter, Sprague, Gdowski, & Lachar (1989) have recently reported that all CPRS-R factors and the Hyperactivity Index discriminated normal from ADHD children. Barkley (1981) reported that the hyperactivity factor did not correlate significantly with objective measures of activity or attention, but did correlate with measures of child noncompliance. Given the similarity in item content and factor structure between the original and revised CPRS, it has been presumed that the evidence of validity for the externalizing factors of the original CPRS would be consistent with comparable factors on the CPRS-R (see Barkley, 1988a). Several recent studies have demonstrated that the CPRS-R is sensitive to stimulant medication effects (Barkley et al., 1988; Pelham et al., 1988), parent training, and self-control training with hyperactive children (Horn, Ialongo, Popovich, & Peradotto, 1984, 1987; Pollard, Ward, & Barkley, 1983; Pelham et al., 1988).

Abbreviated Symptom Questionnaire

Several abbreviated indices commonly referred to as the "Abbreviated Symptom Questionnaire" (ASQ), the "Hyperkinesis Index," and the "Hyperactivity Index" were originally reported by Conners (1973) and subsequently described in the revision of the CPRS (Goyette et al., 1978). The ASQ consists of the ten items most commonly endorsed by parents of hyperactive children. The ASQ was developed in order to provide a brief, highly sensitive means of assessing treatment effects in hyperactive children (Conners, 1985, 1989). It has been used primarily to select/screen hyperactive children for research and to assess treatment effects in research studies. Little independent investigation into the psychometric properties of the ASQ has been undertaken. Recently, Horn et al. (1989) reported that the CPRS-R Hyperactivity Index discriminated normal children from those with Attention Deficit Hyperactivity Disorder. Normative data by age and gender for 578 children, ages 3–17, are presented by Goyette et al. (1978). Unfortunately, several different abbreviated questionnaires or indices have been utilized by researchers, with different subsets of items from the CPRS and CPRS-R, leading to considerable inconsistency and confusion (Ullmann, Sleator, & Sprague, 1985). Conners (1985) has recommended that only the form discussed by Goyette et al. (1978) be utilized. There has also been some question as to whether the ASQ is sufficiently sensitive to subtle intricacies of ADHD, per se. For example, Ullmann et al. (1985) argued the ASQ is not a pure measure of hyperactivity, noting that it assesses conduct problems as well as hyperactivity. Similarly, Barkley (1988a) concluded the ASQ most likely assesses parent–child interaction conflicts and conduct problems in children, rather than hyperactivity, per se. Consequently, it appears that one is likely to identify a mixed sample of conduct- and attention-deficit-disordered children if the ASQ is utilized. Given the existence of more than one Abbreviated Questionnaire, varied item content, and the availability of different norms, continued use of the ASQ in research, particularly as a criterion to identify/define a sample of hyperactive children, is likely to contribute to further confusion and inconsistency. On the other hand, given its brevity, availability of normative data, and evidence suggesting it is sensitive to general treatment effects, the continued use of the form discussed by Goyette et al. (1978) may prove useful in certain well-defined clinical situations. A similar conclusion has been reached by Edelbrock (1988) and Conners (1989).

The Conners Parent Rating Scales are brief questionnaires with demonstrated utility in discriminating children with Disruptive Behavior Disorders from normal children. However, none of the scales has demonstrated the sensitivity to discriminate between the specific Disruptive Behavior Disorders (e.g., hyperactive children from conduct-disordered children). Where a broadband rating scale such as the CBCL is already being utilized, the Conners Parent Rating Scales seem to contribute little unique information. On the other hand, due to its brevity, ease of completion, and the empirical evidence concerning the scale's general sensitivity to treatment effects with hyperactive children, the CPRS-R may prove useful in monitoring and assessing treatment effects in certain research and clinical protocols. If it is to be used in this manner, several cautions are warranted. First, the CPRS-R is recommended over the CPRS, given its relative brevity. Second, it is suggested that the Goyette et al. (1978) version of the Hyperactivity Index be utilized if such a measure is appropriate. Finally, given prior comments concerning initial practice effects, it is recommended that the scale be administered at least twice before it is used to assess treatment effects.

Eyberg Child Behavior Inventory

The Eyberg Child Behavior Inventory (ECBI) (Eyberg, 1980; Eyberg & Ross, 1978; Robinson, Eyberg, & Ross, 1980) was developed to assess oppositional behavior and conduct problems in children ages 2–16. The scale consists of 36 items, most of which describe the disruptive and externalizing behaviors characteristic of conduct disorders. The few remaining items refer to developmental and attentional difficulties. Parents are asked to indicate (yes or no) whether or not each behavior is a problem, and rate the frequency from 1 (never) through 7 (always) of each behavior. The inventory yields two scales, the Problem Scale (the total number problem behaviors identified) and the Intensity Scale (the sum of the frequency ratings for all items). The ECBI requires approximately 10 minutes to complete.

Insufficient normative data are available at this time. Preliminary data were reported for 512 children ages 2–7 (Robinson et al., 1980). However, even though significant gender differences were reported, with boys scoring higher than girls, data are reported by age only. Thus, caution is indicated for clinical use of these data. Further comparison data derived from a referred sample of adolescents, ages 13–16, were provided by Eyberg and Robinson (1983). Preliminary evidence examining the inventory's psychometric properties has been reported. An internal consistency coefficient of .98, split-half reliability estimates ranging from .90 to .94, three-week stability estimates of .88 for the Problem score and .86 for the Intensity score, and an estimate of interrater (mother–father) agreement of .79 have been reported (Eyberg & Robinson, 1983; Robinson et al., 1980). Webster-Stratton (1987) reported similar mean differences between mother and father reports on the ECBI Total Problem and Intensity scores. Robinson and Anderson (1983) have demonstrated that responses on the ECBI are independent of social desirability. Two reports of factor-analytic investigations have suggested that ECBI is a unidimensional scale measuring conduct and behavior problems in children (Eyberg & Robinson, 1983; Robinson et al., 1980). In several studies the ECBI was able to discriminate conduct-disordered from normal nonreferred and other clinic-referred children (Aragona & Eyberg, 1981; Eyberg & Robinson, 1983; Eyberg & Ross, 1978; Robinson et al., 1980), and to correlate significantly with clinic observations of parent–child interactions (Robinson & Eyberg, 1981). In addition, the ECBI appears sensitive to the treatment effects of parent training (Eyberg & Robinson, 1982; Packard, Robinson, & Grove, 1983; Webster-Stratton, 1982a,b, 1984a,b; Webster-Stratton et al., 1988, 1989).

While preliminary evidence suggests the ECBI shows promise as a rating scale for behavior/conduct problems, several factors suggest caution concerning use of the instrument in assessment situations. Perhaps the greatest cause for concern at this time is the lack of adequate normative data. Also, most of the evidence concerning its psychometric characteristics is derived from a limited number of studies. Additional investigations that replicate and extend the evidence of reliability and validity are needed. Finally, given that the ECBI is apparently a unidimensional measure of behavior and conduct problems, it has limited utility in broad-based screening and comprehensive assessment situations. Perhaps it is most useful as one of several measures to assess the effectiveness of treatment with behavior-disordered children.

Home Situations Questionnaire

The Home Situations Questionnaire (HSQ) (Barkley, 1981) was developed as a means of assessing situational variability and severity of behavior problems in children with Disruptive Behavior Disorders. A detailed account of the questionnaire's development and rationale for clinical use has been provided by Barkley and Edelbrock (1987). (The questionaire appears in Appendix B.) The HSQ consists of 16 situations in which informants (e.g., parents) observe and manage child behaviors. Parents are asked to indicate whether problem behaviors occur in these situations and, if so, to rate the severity from 1 (mild) through 9 (severe). The HSQ yields two summary scores: Number of Problem Situations, and Mean Severity.

The HSQ is novel in its approach to behavior assessment in that it assesses situational variability in behavior rather than specific types of problem behaviors. No other available child behavioral checklist or rating scale specifically considers the situation-specific determinants of behavior. At the same time, the HSQ retains the simplicity and brevity common to many parent rating scales. In this manner, useful information concerning problem behaviors may be obtained with a minimum of professional time and expense.

Altepeter and Breen (1989) have provided normative data and psychometric analyses for the HSQ. Briefly, the HSQ normative sample included 995 children ages 4 through 11. Stability estimates for the HSQ summary scores ranged between .83 and .89 for mothers and .60 and .63 for fathers. Individual item stability coefficients for mothers ranged from .38 to .94 (median value of .76) and for fathers from .10 to .85 (median value of .69). Alpha coefficients ranged between .82 and .88 for the HSQ. Item-to-summary score coefficients typically fell within a moderate range (.40 to .70). Finally, concurrent validity was examined by comparing the HSQ summary scores with selected factors from the CPRS-R. The HSQ Number of Problems and Mean Severity ratings were significantly correlated ($p < .01$) with the Conners Conduct Problems factor (.60/.60), Impulsive–Hyperactive factor (.56/.58), and Hyperactive Index (.49/.46), respectively.

A few additional studies reported data on the psychometric properties of the HSQ. Barkley et al. (1988) reported stability estimates of .66 for the Number of Problems and .62 for Mean Severity ratings. Barkley (1981) reported data suggesting the HSQ discriminated hyperactive from normal children. Breen (1990) reported significant and moderately high correlations between the HSQ summary scores and several of the Child Behavior Checklist P-factors (Aggressive, Hyperactive, Delinquent, Depressed, Social Withdrawal), ranging from .46 to .83 with a median value of .60. Breen and Barkley (1988) presented correlations between HSQ summary scores and subtests from the Parenting Stress Index, ranging from .22 to .78 with a median value of approximately .60. Recently, Breen and Altepeter (1990b) factor-analyzed the HSQ normative data. The four factors emerging were: Non-Family Transactions, Custodial Transactions, Task-Performance Transactions, and Isolate

Play. Means, standard deviations, and significant cutoffs for each factor by gender and age are presented in Appendix B.

The HSQ is a brief and psychometrically acceptable measure of situational variability in children's behavior. Given that it specifically taps situational variability, its inclusion in a standardized assessment protocol augments the more traditional measures of child behavior. Even more important, its inclusion provides a brief and efficient method of identifying specific situations that are disruptive within the home setting and that are potentially the most useful targets for subsequent treatment.

TEACHER-COMPLETED QUESTIONNAIRES

Child Behavior Checklist

The Teacher Report Form of the Child Behavior Checklist (TRF) (Achenbach & Edelbrock, 1986) is a teacher-completed questionnaire intended to obtain teachers' reports of students' behavior problems and adaptive competencies. The TRF consists of 118 items that concern various behavior problems and several items that assess social adjustment. Teachers are asked to rate each behavior 0 (not true), 1 (somewhat or sometimes true), or 2 (very true). The TRF typically requires 20–25 minutes to complete. Similar to the CBCL-P, the same questions are used for all children. Separate sets of factors have been developed based upon gender and age (6–11 years and 12–16 years), with corresponding norms and profile sheets. TRF factors were derived from a series of factor analyses of the responses of 1,700 students referred for behavioral and/or social–emotional problems. The various factors assessed (depending upon the age and gender) include: Anxious, Social Withdrawal, Unpopular, Self-Destructive, Obsessive–Compulsive, Immature, Depressed, Inattentive, Nervous–Overactive, Aggressive, and Delinquent. As with the CBCL-P, the use of different factors initially proves somewhat confusing and cumbersome. It is recommended that one read the TRF manual carefully and use caution when initially scoring and plotting profiles. Attention to developmental changes in the dimensions of child psychopathology, as reflected by the different factors across age ranges, is a positive feature. Norms are available for children ages 6–16. Subsequent to deriving the various factors discussed above, normative data were collected for these same factors on a representative sample of 1,100 children. The standardization process is discussed in detail in the manual. Normative data were collected from teachers in three diverse geographic areas. The sample is well distributed in terms of the children's SES and race.

Because the TRF has only recently been developed, investigations into its psychometric properties are ongoing. Preliminary data available at this time are quite favorable. Reliability estimates are reported in the manual (Achenbach & Edelbrock, 1986). One-week stability estimates for the various factors in a sample of 55 special-education students ranged from .76 to .99, with a median of .90. Two-week stability estimates in a sample of 117 special-education students ranged from .65 to .89, with a median of .84. Two-month stability estimates in a sample of 21 special-education students ranged from .63 to .88, with a median value of .74, and four-month estimates for the same sample ranged from .25 to .82, with a median of .68. Interrater (between teachers and teachers' aides) agreement for the various factors ranged from .30 to .84, with a median of .57. Some evidence in support of its validity is available. Phares et al. (1989) reported significant correlations between the total behavior problems, the internalizing and externalizing scales on the TRF and the CBCL, and between the externalizing scale on the TRF and the Youth Self-Report. Edelbrock, Greenbaum, and Conover (1985) reported coefficients between similar factors on the TRF and the CTRS-R ranging from .62 to .90, and a correlation of .85 between the total problems score of both scales. Similarly, the TRF factors have been found to correlate significantly with similar factor/dimension scores derived from direct observations of school behavior (Reed & Edelbrock, 1983). In addition, evidence exists supporting the ability of the scale to discriminate clinic-referred from nonreferred children (Achenbach & Edelbrock, 1986), attention-deficit-disordered from other clinic-referred children (Edelbrock et al., 1984; Kazdin, Esveldt-Dawson, & Loar, 1983), and emotionally disordered from learning-disabled children (Harris, King, Reifler, & Rosenberg, 1984).

The TRF is a recently developed, well standardized, omnibus measure of child psychopathology for use with school-age children. Similar to the CBCL-P, it contains broad-band behavior problem measures (i.e., internalizing, externalizing), several narrow-band behavior factors within each broad dimension, and social competence scales. Evidence available thus far suggests it has acceptable reliability, although additional independent evidence would be beneficial. While the process of validation is still underway, preliminary evidence supports its validity. It is apparent the TRF has many strengths and may prove to be one of the most psychometrically acceptable and clinically useful teacher-completed behavioral rating scales available.

Revised Behavior Problem Checklist

The Revised Behavior Problem Checklist (RBPC) (Quay, 1983; Quay & Peterson, 1983,1984,1987), a recent revision of the widely used Behavior Problem Checklist, is an 89-item checklist of problem behaviors. As noted above, it was designed for use with parents, teachers, and other adults who work closely with children, such as residential treatment staff. It requires

15–20 minutes to complete and yields six factors: Conduct Disorder, Socialized Aggressive, Attention Problems–Immaturity, Anxiety–Withdrawal, Psychotic Behavior, and Motor Excess (Quay, 1983; Quay & Peterson, 1987). Norms, by gender and grade/age are available for use with children ages 5–17. Evidence is available attesting to the psychometric acceptability of the original BPC, and preliminary evidence suggests that the RBPC is equally acceptable.

Conners Teacher Rating Scales (Four Forms)

The Conners Teacher Rating Scales have been among the most widely used teacher rating scales for both research and assessment of Disruptive Behavior Disorders (Barkley, 1981, 1988a,c; Edelbrock, 1988; Edelbrock & Rancurello, 1985; Trites, Blouin, & Laprade, 1982). There are currently four versions of the Conners Teacher Scales: the original 39-item version developed by Conners (1969, 1973), the 28-item revision (Goyette et al., 1978), several 10-item Abbreviated Symptom Questionnaires adopted from the Goyette 28-item revision, and the recently developed IOWA Conners Teacher Rating Scale (Loney & Milich, 1982). Each of these will be briefly reviewed.

Conners Teacher Rating Scale

The original Conners Teacher Rating Scale (CTRS; Conners, 1969, 1973) was developed to assist in the diagnosis and treatment of hyperactivity. The scale consists of 39 items which describe a variety of overt, disruptive behaviors characteristic of conduct problems and hyperactivity (e.g., fidgeting, restless, inattentive, etc.), as well as some internalizing behaviors characteristic of anxious and depressive disorders (e.g., shy, fearful, submissive, anxious, etc.). Teachers are asked to rate the presence and severity of each symptomatic behavior from 0 (not at all) through 3 (very much). The CTRS typically requires 5–10 minutes to complete.

The original CTRS has been widely researched and considerable evidence attesting to its psychometric acceptability is available. Far too many studies are available for a comprehensive review here. In brief, moderate to high test–retest estimates for the various factors have been reported, with short-term (1 month or less) estimates typically ranging from .70 to .80 (Conners, 1973) and long-term (1 year or more) estimates typically ranging from about .35 to about .60 (Trites, Blouin, Ferguson, & Lynch, 1981). Estimates of interrater (between teacher) agreement have been high for the total scale and moderately high (from about 0.45 to about 0.80) across factors (Trites et al., 1982; Vincent, Williams, Harris, & Duvall, 1977). Evidence also exists supporting the CTRS's concurrent, construct, and discriminative validity. It has been shown to correlate significantly with numerous rating scales and criterion measures of child psychopathology, including the Child Behavior Checklist (Achenbach & Edelbrock, 1983) and Behavior Problem Checklist (Arnold et al., 1981; Campbell & Steinert, 1978). In addition, various studies have reported the CTRS to discriminate hyperactive from normal, learning-disabled, and speech/language-impaired children, (Ackerman, Elardo, & Dykman, 1979; Baker, Cantwell, & Mattison, 1980; Conners, 1969; Copeland & Weissbrod, 1978; Kupietz, Bialer, & Winsberg, 1972; Sandoval, 1977; Taylor & Sandberg, 1984; Werry, Sprague, & Cohen, 1975), depressed from nondepressed children (Leon et al., 1980), and children with high academic and social competence from those with low competence (Cohen, Kershner, & Wehrspann, 1988). Finally, the scale has been shown to be sensitive to treatments used with hyperactive children, including stimulant medication (Barkley, 1977; Cantwell & Carlson, 1978; Conners, 1969, 1970), behavior modification (Abikoff & Gittelman, 1984; O'Leary & Pelham, 1978), diet (Harley et al., 1981), and self-control training (Horn, Chatoor, & Conners, 1983).

Several investigators have examined the CTRS factor structures, with some inconsistencies. For example, Conners (1969) identified five factors in a sample of clinic-referred behavior-disordered children. Werry, Sprague, & Cohen (1975) identified six factors in a sample of normal children, while Trites et al. (1982) identified six factors in a large stratified random sample of normal children. Although there were some similarities in factors across these studies (e.g., in all analyses a hyperactivity factor emerged), important discrepancies and inconsistencies were also present. For example, items on the Conners (1969) Tension–Anxiety factor loaded as four separate factors in Werry et al.'s (1975) analysis. Several translations, modifications, and normative data have been developed, from Australia (Glow, 1979), French-Canada (Trites & Laprade, 1984), West Germany (Sprague, Cohen, & Eichlseder, 1977), Great Britain (Taylor & Sandberg, 1984; Thorley, 1983), New Zealand (Werry & Hawthorne, 1976), and Italy (O'Leary, Vivian, & Nisi, 1985).

It has been recommended (Barkley, 1988a,c; Conners, 1989; Edelbrock, 1988), and we concur, that factors derived from Trites et al. (1982) be utilized, given the large and randomly selected normative sample from which they were derived. The six CTRS factors, as reported by Trites et al. (1982), are Hyperactivity, Conduct Disorder, Emotional Overindulgent, Anxious–Passive, Asocial, and Daydream/Attendance Problems. Normative data (factor means and standard deviations) delineated by gender and age for 9,583 children ages 4–12 are available.

The CTRS is a psychometrically acceptable and widely used questionnaire. It has proved effective in discriminating hyperactive from normal and other clinical samples of children as well as sensitivity to treatment effects with hyperactive children. We suggest normative data reported by Trites et al.

(1982) be utilized for assessment purposes. Finally, as noted above with the CPRS, there has been some concern about practice effects with the CTRS (Ullmann et al., 1985). Accordingly, we suggest the scale be administered at least twice before using it to assess treatment effects.

Conners Teacher Rating Scale—Revised

Conners and colleagues modified the original Teacher Rating Scale (CTRS-R) (Goyette et al., 1978). The revised scale was shortened to 28 items, with some items from the original scale being either omitted, shortened, or reworded. As in the original version, teachers are asked to rate the presence and severity of each behavior from 0 (not at all) through 3 (very much). The CTRS typically requires 5 minutes or less to complete. Goyette et al. (1978) reported the following factors: Conduct Problems, Hyperactivity, and Inattention–Passivity. Normative data (factor means and standard deviations) presented according to age and gender were provided for 383 children, ages 3–17 (Goyette et al., 1978).

Like the original CTRS, the revised form has been widely used in research and clinical practice. Evidence as to its psychometric characteristics is available. High test–retest estimates over a 1-week period have been reported by Edelbrock and Reed (1984), with coefficients ranging from .94 to .98 for all factors. Estimates of interrater (between teacher) agreement have not been reported. The CPRS-R's concurrent, construct, discriminant, and predictive validity have not been thoroughly investigated. Given the similarity in item content and factor structure with the original CTRS, it has been presumed that the CTRS-R would be equally valid (Barkley, 1988a). At the same time, however, some evidence addressing the CTRS-R validity is available. Edelbrock et al. (1985) reported coefficients between the CTRS-R factors and similar factors on the Teacher Report Form of the Child Behavior Checklist ranging from .62 to .90, and a correlation of .85 between the total problems score on both scales. Several recent studies have reported data indicating that the CTRS-R can discriminate hyperactive from normal, clinic-referred nonhyperactive, or learning-disabled children (Breen & Barkley, 1988; Horn et al., 1989). In addition, there is evidence that the CTRS-R is sensitive to the treatment effects of stimulant medications and behavior therapy (Barkley et al., 1988; Pelham et al., 1988).

Abbreviated Symptom Questionnaire

Several abbreviated indices commonly referred to as the "Abbreviated Symptom Questionnaire" (ASQ), the "Hyperkinesis Index," and the "Hyperactivity Index" were originally reported by Conners (1973) and subsequently described in the revision of the CPRS (Goyette et al., 1978). The ASQ consists of the ten items most commonly endorsed by teachers of hyperactive children. As with the previously described parent ASQ, the teacher ASQ was developed to provide a brief, sensitive means of assessing treatment effects in hyperactive children (Conners, 1985, 1989). It has been used primarily to select/screen hyperactive children for research and to assess treatment effects in research studies. Normative data are presented by Goyette et al. (1978). Several independent investigators have reported test–retest reliability coefficients in the .90's (Edelbrock & Reed, 1984; Zentall & Barack, 1979). Parent–teacher agreement of .49 was reported by Goyette et al. (1978). Finally, it has been demonstrated that the scale is sensitive to the treatment effects of stimulant medications (Douglas, Barr, Amin, O'Neill, & Britton, 1988; Sprague & Sleator, 1977) and self-control training (Kendall & Wilcox, 1980; Kendall & Zupan, 1981).

Unfortunately, as with the parent version, several different abbreviated questionnaires or indices have been utilized by researchers and this has led to a degree of inconsistency (Ullmann et al., 1985). There has also been some question as to whether the teacher ASQ is sufficiently sensitive to hyperactivity, per se. For example, Ullmann et al. (1985) have suggested the ASQ is not a pure measure of hyperactivity, noting that it assesses conduct problems as well as hyperactivity. It would appear one is likely to identify a mixed sample of children with aggressive conduct problems and coexisting attentional deficits if the ASQ is utilized to identify children for research and/or clinical purposes.

IOWA Conners Teacher Rating Scale

A shortened modification of the original CTRS is the recently developed IOWA Conners Teacher Rating Scale (Loney & Milich, 1981). The IOWA Conners was developed to discriminate among pure hyperactive, pure aggressive, and mixed hyperactive-aggressive children. It consists of 10 items, five taken from the Inattentive–Overactive factor, and five from the Aggressive factor of the original CTRS. The items were chosen for their factor "purity" and discriminative power. That is, they had high loadings on the original respective factors and did not load on other factors. Thus, the IOWA Conners provides a 5-item hyperactivity scale and a 5-item aggression scale. Normative data for the IOWA Conners are not available at this time; similarly, there is little information concerning the scale's psychometric properties. Currently the scale is used primarily as a means of identifying subjects for research purposes. The scale has potential clinical utility, particularly as a brief and rapid means of gathering supplementary data to aid in differential diagnosis and subsequent treatment planning. However, evidence concerning its psychometric properties, particularly its construct and discriminative validity, are needed before it can be recommended for clinical use.

The four versions of the Conners Teacher Rating Scales are brief, reliable behavior rating scales that have demonstrated utility in discriminating children with Disruptive Behavior Disorders from those without. However, none of the scales have demonstrated the ability to discriminate between the specific disruptive behavior disorders (e.g., hyperactive children from conduct-disordered children). Thus, in diagnostic situations where a broad-band teacher rating scale such as the TRF is already being utilized, the Conners Teacher Scales seem to contribute little or no unique information. On the other hand, due to its brevity, ease of completion, and the evidence of the scale's sensitivity to treatment effects, continued use of the CTRS may prove useful in monitoring and assessing such effects. If it is to be used in this manner, several cautions are warranted. First, Trites' normative data are recommended, given the larger sample and the superiority of sampling procedures. Second, care should be taken to ensure that when using the ASQ, one realizes the item overlap and potential for misdiagnosis. Third, given the previous comments concerning practice effects, the scale must be administered at least twice before assessing treatment effects. Finally, while the IOWA Conners offers considerable promise as a brief measure capable of discriminating hyperactive from aggressive behavior, its use in assessment situations cannot be recommended at this time due to the limited evidence concerning its normative characteristics.

ADD-H Comprehensive Teacher Rating Scale (ACTeRS)

The ADD-H Comprehensive Teacher Rating Scale (ACTeRS) (Ullmann, Sleator, & Sprague, 1984a, 1988) was designed as a brief teacher rating scale to assist in the diagnosis of ADD-H and the subsequent monitoring of treatment effects. The scale consists of 24 behavioral items rated by teachers from 1 (almost never) to 5 (almost always). Items load on four empirically derived factors: Attention, Hyperactivity, Social Skills, and Oppositional. Total raw scores for each factor are obtained by summing the scores for items that load on the factor. The scores are then converted into percentiles. The normative sample ($N = 1,339$; 694 boys, 645 girls) is evenly distributed across students in grades K through 5. Separate norms are provided by gender but not age. Current efforts are underway to collect additional normative data through grade 8. Preliminary evidence examining the scale's reliability is reported in the test manual. Internal consistency (alpha) coefficients for each factor ranged from .93 to .97, stability estimates for each factor from .78 to .82, and interrater agreement for each factor from .51 to .73. Preliminary evidence addressing the scale's validity is also available. The ACTeRS has been shown to discriminate normal nonreferred children from those diagnosed as ADD-H

(Ullmann, Sleator, & Sprague, 1984b) and learning-disabled from ADD-H (Ullmann, 1985; Ullmann et al., 1988). Finally, in several recent studies, the ACTeRS has been shown to be sensitive to the therapeutic effects of methylphenidate (Douglas et al., 1988; Ullman & Sleator, 1985; Ullman & Sleator, 1986).

The ACTeRS offers promise as a brief teacher rating scale to assist in the diagnosis, treatment, and monitoring of children with disruptive behavior disorders. While sufficient evidence exists regarding the ACTeRS's psychometric acceptability to justify its use in assessment situations, additional independent evidence would be beneficial.

The School Situations Questionnaire

The School Situations Questionnaire (SSQ) (Barkley, 1981) is the teacher counterpart to the HSQ. A detailed account of the questionnaire's development and rationale for clinical use has been provided by Barkley and Edelbrock (1987). (The questionnaire appears in Appendix B.) Briefly, it was developed as a means of assessing situational variability and the severity of behavior problems in children with Disruptive Behavior Disorders. It consists of 12 situations in which teachers routinely observe and manage child behaviors. Teachers are asked to indicate whether problem behaviors occur in these situations and, if so, to rate the severity. Like the HSQ, the SSQ yields two summary scores: the Number of Problem Situations and the Mean Severity.

Altepeter and Breen (1989) recently provided normative data and psychometric properties for the SSQ. The SSQ normative sample included 615 children, aged 6–11. Stability estimates for the SSQ Number of Problem Situations ranged from .64 to .77, and for Mean Severity from .77 to .82. Alpha coefficients ranged between .84 and .92 for the SSQ. Item-to-summary score coefficients ranged from .65 to .81. Additional studies have reported data on the psychometric properties of the SSQ. Barkley et al. (1988) reported stability estimates of .78 for the Number of Problems and .63 for Mean Severity rating. Breen (1990) reported significant moderate correlations between the SSQ summary scores and the Conners Teacher Questionnaire in Conduct, Inattentive, and Hyperactivity factors and CBCL's Aggresive, Self-Destructive, Inattentive, and Nervous–Overactive factors (.50 to .63). Breen (1989) reported the SSQ summary scores discriminated hyperactive from normal children. Recently, Breen and Altepeter (1990b) factor-analyzed the SSQ normative data. The three factors identified were: Unsupervised Settings, Task Performance, and Special Events. Factor means, standard deviations, and significant cutoffs by age and gender are presented in Appendix B.

The SSQ is a brief, psychometrically acceptable, well-normed measure regarding the situational variability of children's behavior. Given the nature of the SSQ, its inclusion in a standardized assessment protocol augments the more traditional teacher-completed measures of behavior problems. Even more important, its inclusion provides a brief, efficient method of identifying specific situations that are most disruptive in the classroom and which potentially are the most useful targets for subsequent treatment.

SNAP Checklist

The SNAP checklist is a brief teacher-completed scale developed by Pelham and colleagues (Atkins, Pelham, & Licht, 1985; Johnson, Pelham, & Murphy, 1985; Pelham, Atkins, Murphy, & White, 1981; Pelham, Atkins, Murphy, & Swanson, 1984). It is the translation of DSM-III criteria for Attention Deficit Disorder with Hyperactivity (ADD-H) into a rating scale. Each SNAP item (i.e., DSM-III criterion) is rated by teachers as being present "not at all," "just a little," "pretty much," or "very much." Consistent with the DSM-III, any child who receives a rating of "pretty much" or "very much" on two or more of the hyperactive criteria and three or more of the inattentive and impulsive criteria is classified as having ADD-H. The SNAP also includes a few additional items describing social behaviors and peer relationships that are informative but not directly used in scoring. Recent evidence suggests the SNAP can discriminate normal from ADHD children (Horn et al., 1989) and that higher scores on the SNAP checklist are associated with increased conduct problems (Walker, Lahey, Hynd, & Frame, 1987). This type of approach to identifying "pure" subjects for research purposes has appeal. Recently the SNAP checklist has become more widely used in research to identify children with ADD-H.

The SNAP is a quick and appealing measure used to identify DBD children. However, there is insufficient independent evidence examining the reliability or validity of the diagnostic decisions reached through the use of the SNAP checklist. In particular, further documentation of test–retest and interrater reliability as well as discriminative validity seem indicated. Without further corroboration concerning these issues, there is little reason to recommend it over other available teacher rating scales in clinical assessment situations, and with the recent publication of the DSM-III-R, the SNAP checklist in its present form has become outdated.

The Stony Brook Scale

The Stony Brook Scale (SBS) (O'Leary & Steen, 1982) was developed as a brief, practical method of identifying subcategories of hyperactive children based upon prior work of Loney, Langhorne, and Paternite (1978). Briefly,

Loney et al. (1978) developed a procedure for identifying independent dimensions of hyperactivity and aggression in a group of behavior disordered boys referred for a trial of stimulant medication. O'Leary and Steen (1982) attempted to build on the conceptual framework of Loney et al. by developing a more practical, clinically useful scale. The SBS was based on 12 of the 13 symptom dimensions proposed by Loney et al. (1978). It consists of 68 teacher-completed items covering the 12 dimensions; 33 were selected from the Conners Teacher Rating Scale (CTRS) (Conners, 1973) and 35 from the Peterson-Quay Behavior Problem Checklist (BPC) (Quay & Peterson, 1975). Items were selected for inclusion in the SBS based on the similarity of the item content and Loney's symptom descriptors. In the original report by O'Leary and Steen (1982), four factors emerged (Aggression, Anxiety–Depression, Hyperactivity, and Uncoordination) and three of the same four factors emerged in a replication sample (Aggression, Anxiety–Depression, and Hyperactivity). Interestingly, and consistent with the model developed by Loney et al. (1978), separate factors tapping aggression and hyperactivity emerged in both samples.

There has been little further examination of the psychometric properties of the SBS. Currently the scale is used primarily as a means of identifying and subcategorizing subjects for research purposes. The scale has potential clinical utility, particularly as a means of gathering supplementary data to aid in differential diagnosis (e.g., hyperactive versus conduct disordered versus mixed) and subsequent treatment planning. However, further evidence concerning its psychometric properties is needed before it can be recommended for clinical assessment purposes.

Self-Control Rating Scale

The Self-Control Rating Scale (SCRS) (Kendall & Wilcox, 1979) was developed as a brief teacher rating scale to assess self-control in elementary school age children. The scale is based on a cognitive–behavioral conceptualization of self-control. That is, self-control is assumed to require both cognitive (e.g., deliberation, problem-solving, planning, and evaluation) and behavioral (e.g., execution of chosen behavior, inhibition of other behaviors, etc.) components. The SCRS consists of 33 questions about child behaviors rated by teachers on a scale from 1 (indicating maximum self-control) to 7 (indicating maximum impulsivity). The scale contains 10 items that indicate self-control, 13 descriptive of impulsivity, and 10 that denote both possibilities. The scale requires 5–10 minutes to complete. In the original paper (Kendall & Wilcox, 1979) norms (means and standard deviations) were reported by gender for a sample of 110 (59 boys, 51 girls) randomly selected children attending a middle-class elementary school. The sample ranged in age from 8 through 12 years, distributed across grades 3–6. A modified version of the scale was recently developed, with normative data on 763 children in grades 4–5 (Humphrey, 1982).

Preliminary evidence addressing the psychometric properties is available. Internal consistency (alpha) in the normative sample was 0.98, whereas test–retest reliability over 3–4 weeks, derived from a subsample ($n = 24$) was .84 (Kendall & Wilcox, 1979). Interrater (teacher–parent) agreement has been reported as .66 (Kendall & Braswell, 1982). Again, based on the normative sample, the SCRS correlated significantly with the Kagan Matching Figures Test, the Porteus Mazes, and observation ratings of off-task, inattention, and out-of-seat behaviors. The scale did not correlate with the Peabody Picture Vocabulary Test. Factor analysis of the normative sample produced a one-factor solution labeled cognitive–behavioral self-control. In a subsequent study reported in the same paper, the SCRS differentiated children referred by teachers due to problems with self-control from nonreferred (normal) matched controls (Kendall & Wilcox, 1979). It has also been demonstrated that the SCRS differentiated children referred to mental health clinics from children referred to medical clinics (Robin, Fischel, & Brown, 1984), and that high SCRS scores were associated with disruptive classroom behaviors (Kendall, Zupan, & Braswell, 1981). Evidence is also available indicating that the SCRS is sensitive to the effects of cognitive–behavioral interventions in children with self-control problems (Kendall & Braswell, 1982; Kendall & Wilcox, 1980; Kendall & Zupan, 1981).

The SCRS is a brief teacher rating scale designed to assess self-control deficits in elementary school children. Although not thoroughly researched, the evidence available indicates acceptable reliability. In several independent studies it has proved sensitive to cognitive–behavioral interventions with impulsive children. Perhaps the greatest limitation of this scale is the normative sample, which has a limited age range and is relatively small. Based on the moderate interrater (teacher–parent) agreement, the SCRS can be employed by both teachers and parents (Kendall & Braswell, 1982,1985). However, given the lack of parental normative data, use of the SCRS in this manner should be done with caution.

YOUTH SELF-REPORT QUESTIONNAIRES

Child Behavior Checklist: Youth Self-Report Form

The Youth Self-Report and Profile of the Child Behavior Checklist (YSR) (Achenbach & Edelbrock, 1987) is an individually completed checklist intended as a youth counterpart to the parent- and teacher-completed CBCL.

The YSR was designed to obtain reports from adolescents regarding their interests, experiences, and behaviors, including various behavior problems and adaptive competencies (e.g., social, organizational, employment activities, etc.). The YSR consists of 103 items that assess various behavior problems and 17 items that assess social adjustment. Individuals are asked to indicate whether items reflect their typical behavior, either 0 (not true), 1 (somewhat or sometimes true), or 2 (very true). The YSR is designed for youths who are 11 to 18 years old, and it requires a 5th-grade reading level. Alternatively, it can be administered orally to those with a lower reading level. The YSR typically requires about 20 minutes to complete.

Similar to the parent- and teacher-completed CBCL, the same questions are used for all youths. Separate sets of factors, with corresponding norms and profile sheets, are available based upon gender. YSR factors were derived from a series of factor analyses, based on the responses of 927 youths referred for mental health services because of behavioral and/or social–emotional problems. Factorial dimensions are as follows: Depressed, Unpopular, Somatic Complaints, Thought Disorder, Self-Destructive, Aggressive, and Delinquent (Achenbach & Edelbrock, 1987). Subsequent to deriving the factors outlined above, normative data were collected for the same factors on a representative sample of 686 children. The standardization process is detailed in the manual. Briefly, normative data were collected from youths randomly selected from 34 residential census tracts within the Worcester, Massachusetts metropolitan area. The sample is well distributed in terms of the children's SES and race.

Since it was developed only recently, independent reports on the psychometric properties and clinical utility of the YSR are largely unavailable at this time, although investigations are ongoing and additional information should be available in the near future. Preliminary data available at this time are favorable. Reliability estimates are reported in the manual. Briefly, 1-week stability estimates for the various factors in a sample of 50 nonreferred adolescents ranged from .33 to .94, with a median of .81. Correlations were slighly higher for girls (mean was .84) than for boys (mean was .77). Eight-month stability estimates in a sample of 102 nonreferred 12- to 14-year-olds ranged from .28 to .78, with a median of .51. Again, the correlations were slightly higher for girls (mean was .65) than for boys (mean was .46). The authors report moderate correlations between the YSR factors and comparable factors on the CBCL (averaging .41 for boys and .45 for girls) and moderate correlations between the YSR factors and comparable factors on the TRF (averaging .43 for boys and .45 for girls). Phares et al. (1989) reported significant correlations between the total behavior problems and the internalizing and externalizing scales of the YSR and the CBCL, and between the externalizing scales of the YSR and the TRF. Finally, the manual reports data indicating that the scale discriminated clinic-referred from nonreferred youth.

The YSR is a recently developed, well-standardized, omnibus self-report measure of child/adolescent psychopathology for use with youths aged 11 through 18 years. Similar to the parent- and teacher-completed CBCL, it contains broad-band behavior problem measures (internalizing, externalizing), several narrow-band factors within each broad dimension, and social competence scales. Evidence to date suggests that it is reliable. While independent evidence is currently unavailable concerning its validity, the preliminary information reported in the manual is favorable. Further evidence is needed concerning its reliability, criterion, construct, and discriminative validity, and its clinical utility, as well as studies which determine its sensitivity to various treatment interventions. The YSR offers promise of providing a much needed self-report measure for youth.

Child Depression Inventory

The Child Depression Inventory (CDI) (Kovacs, 1981, 1983, 1985) is reported to be the most thoroughly researched and widely used measure of depression in children (Finch, Saylor, & Edwards, 1985; Kazdin, 1981; Saylor, Finch, Spirito, & Bennet, 1984). The CDI is a 27-item self-report questionnaire designed as a downward extension of the Beck Depression Inventory (BDI) (Beck, Rush, Shaw, & Emery, 1979). The CDI assesses cognitive, behavioral, and physical/vegetative signs and symptoms of depression. For each item the individual is instructed to choose one of three statements that best describes him or her for the past 2 weeks. Items are scored on a three-point scale (0 through 2) of increasing severity and scores for all items are summed to provide a total score. Total scores are interpreted to reflect severity of depression (Kovacs, 1981, 1985). Kovacs (1981) reported that a cutoff of 19 identified the upper 10% of the distribution in a sample of nonclinic children, a finding recently replicated (Doerfler et al. 1988). Several sets of normative data reported in the literature have been highly consistent (Doerfler et al., 1988; Finch et al., 1985; Kovacs, 1983; Smucker, Craighead, Craighead, & Green, 1986). The CDI is intended for children between the ages of 8 and 13, and requires 10–15 minutes to complete.

Research examining the psychometric properties of the CDI has been reviewed by several investigators (Saylor et al., 1984; Slotkin et al., 1988). Briefly, internal consistency estimates have ranged from .80 to .94. Stability estimates have ranged from .50 to .87 for psychiatric patients, and .38 to .84 for other non-psychiatric subjects. There is general consensus supporting the CDI's content validity, particularly for Major Depressive Disorder. Concurrent validity has been investigated by comparing CDI scores with various measures of depression. Correlations have generally ranged from .40 to .90. CDI scores have also been found to correlate significantly with adolescent-completed indices of parent–child conflict (Forehand et al., 1988). The CDI has been shown to discriminate clinical from nonreferred control samples (Carey et al., 1987; Morgan & Jackson, 1986; Romano & Nelson, 1988; Saylor et al., 1984; Walker & Green, 1989; Worchel et al., 1988); depressed from non-depressed psychiatric patients (Carey et al., 1987; Kazdin, Colbus, & Rodgers, 1986; Knight, Hensley, & Waters, 1988; Kovacs, 1985; Lobovits & Handal, 1985; McCauley, Mitchell, Burke, & Moss, 1988; Romano & Nelson, 1988; Saylor et al., 1984); acutely suicidal psychiatric inpatients from other psychiatric inpatients (Spirito et al., 1978); and psychiatric from nonpsychiatric medical patients (Worchel et al., 1988). Considerable evidence for convergent and divergent validity also exists. The CDI has been found to correlate negatively with self-esteem, adaptive social functioning, and overall adjustment. Positive correlations have been found with loneliness, suicidal ideation and behaviors, a variety of physical symptoms (such as headaches and upset stomachs), and stress. Finally, the CDI has been found to have low to moderate correlations with various measures of anxiety.

The factor structure of the CDI has been examined by several investigators (Carey et al., 1987; Hodges, Siegel, Mullins, & Griffin, 1983; Saylor et al., 1984). Each investigation produced different results, with the number of factors ranging from 2 to 8 depending on the type of sample (i.e., nonreferred normal, depressed, conduct disorder) and the factor analytic technique employed. Perhaps the only conclusion that can be reached at this point is that no clear factor structure has been established for the CDI.

The CDI offers a brief, reliable, valid means of screening for cognitive, behavioral, and physical/vegetative signs and symptoms of depression in children aged 8 through 13. Overall, the CDI has proven to be a good discriminator between clinical and nonreferred samples. In addition, there is evidence supporting the CDI's capacity to discriminate depressed from non-depressed psychiatric patients. However, some ambiguity remains over the appropriate interpretion of the instrument. While Kovacs (1981) recommended a cutoff of 19, Lobovits and Handal (1985) found that discriminative power could be increased by using an alternative method of double-weighting the 5 items that tap the major symptom of dysphoria. Given the added discriminative power, the alternative method employed by Lobovits and Handal (1985) seems preferable, although it should be used with some caution until additional evidence is available replicating their results.

Reynolds Adolescent Depression Scale

The Reynolds Adolescent Depression Scale (RADS) (Reynolds, 1987) is a 30-item self-report questionnaire intended for use with adolescents aged 12 through 18. The RADS assesses cognitive, behavioral, affective, and physical/vegetative signs and symptoms of depression. It was designed to cover the depressive symptom domain of DSM-III (APA, 1980), as well as the adult and child versions of the Schedule for Affective Disorders and Schizophrenia (SADS) (Endicott & Spitzer, 1978); K-SADS (Puig-Antich, Orvaschel, Tabrizi, & Chambers, 1980). Each RADS item contains a symptom-related statement, and the individual is instructed to respond on a 4-point scale, indicating whether the symptom has occurred almost never, hardly ever, sometimes, or most of the time. Responses are then summed to provide a total score. Total scores are interpreted to reflect increasing severity of depression. A score of 77 or more indicates a level worthy of further assessment (Reynolds, 1986, 1987). In addition, 6 items are identified as "critical" on the basis of their empirically determined ability to discriminate depressed from nondepressed adolescents (Evert & Reynolds, 1986; Reynolds, 1987). Normative data are available for a sample of 2,460 adolescents, ages 12 through 18, and were derived from one urban/suburban community in the midwest, containing appropriate representation of minorities. The RADS requires about 10 minutes to complete. Factor structure of the RAD's normative sample has been examined and reported in the manual (Reynolds, 1987). Analyses produced a 5-factor solution. Virtually identical factor structure and loadings were found in separate analyses by gender. The following factors were identified: Generalized Demoralization, Despondency and Worry, Externalized Somatic–Vegetative symptoms, Anhedonia, and Self-Worth.

Evidence concerning the psychometric properties of the RADS is available. Briefly, internal consistency (alpha) for the normative sample was .92, with coefficients ranging from .90 to .94 by gender and grade level. Additional internal consistency (alpha) estimates for 15 separate samples reported in the manual ranged from .90 to .96, with a median value of .93. Reported stability estimates were .80 for 6 weeks, .79 for 3 months, and .63 for 1 year (Reynolds, 1987). The overlap of RADS items with DSM-III and SADS criteria supports the RADS's content validity, particularly for symptoms of Major Depressive Disorder. Concurrent validity has been investigated by comparing RADS scores with various measures of depression. Reported correlations between the RADS and the Beck Depression Inventory have ranged from .68 to .76, with a median value of .72 (Reynolds, 1987; Reynolds & Anderson, 1986; Sullivan, 1985); between the RADS and the CDI, 0.73; and between the RADS and the Zung rating scale, .72 (Reynolds, 1987). In addition, Reynolds (1986) reported correlations of .83 and .84 between the RADS and ratings derived from the Hamilton Rating Scale, a semistructured interview. Preliminary evidence for the convergent and divergent validity of the RADS exists. Several studies have reported significant correlations between the RADS and measures of anxiety, loneliness, hopelessness, and suicidal ideation, as well as negative correlations between the RADS and measures of self-esteem (reviewed in Reynolds, 1987). Several studies have demonstrated that the RADS could discriminate depressed from nondepressed adolescents (Evert & Reynolds, 1986; Reynolds, 1986), and acutely suicidal from chronically maladjusted adolescents (Spirito et al., 1987). Finally, the RADS has proven sensitive to treatment with moderately to severely depressed adolescents (Reynolds & Coats, 1986).

The RADS offers a brief means of screening for cognitive, behavioral, and affective signs and symptoms of depression in adolescents aged 12 through 18. Preliminary investigations indicate that it has adequate reliability and validity, although further evidence establishing its discriminative validity and treatment sensitivity would be useful.

PARENT AND FAMILY QUESTIONNAIRES

Beck Depression Inventory

The Beck Depression Inventory (BDI) was first introduced by Beck and his colleagues in 1961 (Beck et al., 1961). It was modified in 1971 and copyrighted in 1978 (Beck et al., 1979). Over the years, the BDI has become one of the most commonly used instruments for assessing the presence and intensity of depression in psychiatrically diagnosed patients and screening for depression in normal populations (Beck, Steer, & Garbin, 1988; Piotrwoski, Kashani, Sherman, Parker, & Reid, 1990; Sherry & Keller, 1985; Steer, Beck, & Garrison, 1986). Several versions are currently available, including the 1971 21-item modified version, a 13-item short form (Beck & Beck, 1972), a Spanish translation (Conde, Estaban, & Useros, 1976), and a German translation (Mayer, 1977). The 1971 21-item modified form is the most commonly used version, and will be the focus of the brief review here. The reader is referred to a recent comprehensive review of the BDI (Beck et al., 1988) for more detailed information.

The BDI consists of 21 items that assess various signs and symptoms of depression, including mood, pessimism, sense of punishment, feelings of guilt, failure, fatigue, loss of appetite, weight, libido, sleep disturbance, crying and irritability, social withdrawal, etc. Each item consists of four statements from which the individual is instructed to choose the one that best describes him or her for the past 7 days. Items are scored on a 4-point scale (0 through 3) of increasing severity, and scores for all items are summed to provide a total score. Cutoffs are interpreted to reflect absence of depression, mild to moderate, moderate to severe, and severe depression (Beck & Beamesderfer, 1974). It has a 6th grade reading level (Berndt, Schwartz, & Kaiser, 1983), and requires 5–10 minutes to complete. Women tend to score about 2 points higher than men, and BDI scores are inversely related to educational level (Oliver & Simmons, 1984, 1985).

Evidence for the reliability and validity of the BDI has been exhaustively reviewed by Beck et al. (1988). Briefly, internal consistency estimates have ranged from .73 to .95, with a mean value of about .83. Stability estimates have ranged from .48 to .86 for psychiatric patients, and .60 to .90 for nonpsychiatric subjects. There is a general consensus supporting the BDI's content validity. In fact, one criticism of the BDI has been that it is relatively easy to fake in either a normal or more pathological direction because of its strong content validity (Beck & Beamesderfer, 1974). Concurrent validity has been investigated by comparing BDI scores with various independent measures of depression. Correlations have ranged from .41 to .96, with most reported coefficients in the .60 to .80 range. A series of studies have demonstrated that the BDI is able to differentiate depressed psychiatric patients from nonpsychiatric individuals. It is generally not able to differentiate among persons with mixed depressive diagnoses (e.g., endogenous, involutional depression versus reactive depression), although some evidence suggests that it does accurately discriminate severity of depression (e.g., major depressive episodes versus dysthymic disorders). Evidence for convergent and divergent validity exist. The BDI has correlated positively with a variety of physical symptoms, such as headaches, upset stomachs, etc., suicidal ideation and behaviors, overall adjustment, loneliness, and stress. Low to moderate correlations have been reported with various measures of anxiety. Several investigators have examined the factor structure of the BDI, with the number of factors that have emerged ranging from 3 to 7. Beck et al. (1988) reviewed these studies and concluded that the inconsistencies were attributable partly to the use of different factor analytic procedures and partly to the characteristics of the samples used (e.g., normal, depressed, or alcoholic). They interpreted the trend across these studies to suggest that the BDI measures a general first-order factor of depression with 3 highly intercorrelated second-order factors reflecting negative attitudes, performance difficulties, and somatic complaints.

The BDI is a brief, psychometrically acceptable, and widely used rating scale of depression in adolescents and adults. It has repeatedly been found to discriminate depressive psychiatric patients from nondepressed individuals and to be sensitive to the severity of depression. In addition, it has proven to be an effective screening device for depression in the normal population. Given the greater incidence of depression in parents, especially mothers, of children with Disruptive Behavior Disorders, use of the BDI to screen for depressive symptomatology in parents may prove helpful.

Parenting Stress Index

The revised (Form 6) Parenting Stress Index (PSI) (Abidin, 1986; Burke & Abidin, 1978; Loyd & Abidin, 1985) was developed by Abidin and colleagues as a means of identifying and measuring stress associated with parenting. In particular, it was designed to assess various characteristics in the child–parent dyad and the parenting subsystem that are most commonly associated with dysfunctional parenting behaviors. In developing the PSI it was assumed that stressors are multidimensional, both as to source and kind, and that the effects of various stressors are cumulative. What emerged, then, were three major source domains: (1) Child Domain, (2) Parent Domain, and (3) Situational/Demographic Life Stress. In the revised (Form 6) PSI, there are 47 items comprising 6 subscales in the Child Domain; 54 items comprising 7 subscales in the Parent Domain; and 19 items in the optional Life Stress Scale. Thus, the PSI (Form 6) contains a total of 120 items. The 6 Child Domains (i.e., Adaptability, Acceptability, Demandingness, Mood, Distractibility/Hyperactivity, Reinforces Parent) tap temperament and behavioral characteristics of children that create stress for parents. The seven Parent Domains (i.e., Depression, Attachment, Restriction of Role, Sense of Competence, Social Isolation, Relationship with Spouse, Parent Health) tap parent characteristics and family context variables that have been identified as impacting upon the parent's ability to function as a competent caregiver (Abidin, 1986). The PSI requires a 5th-grade reading level to complete and can be finished by most parents in 15–20 minutes.

The normative sample contained 534 parents, primarily from central Virginia, of both normal and problem children. The sample was 92% white, 6% black, 2% other, with ages of parents ranging from 18 to 65 (mean of about 30). Alpha coefficients for the normative sample were .95 for the Total Stress Score, .89 for the Child Domain, and .93 for the Parent Domain; alphas ranged from .62 to .70 for the Child Domain subscales and from .55 to .80 for the Parent Domain subscales (Loyd & Abidin, 1985). Nearly identical coefficients were recently reported for the subscales, Domains, and Total Stress Scores in a cross-cultural validation of the PSI (Hauenstein, Scarr, & Abidin, 1986). Three-week to 3-month stability estimates for the Domain and Total Stress Scores have ranged from .63 to .96, with a median value of about .80 (Abidin, 1986; Loyd & Abidin, 1985). Webster-Stratton (1987) reported significant differences between mothers and fathers of conduct-disordered children on most Parent and Child Domain scores, with mothers consistently obtaining higher scores.

Evidence supporting the concurrent, construct, discriminant, and predictive validity of the PSI is reviewed by Abidin (1986). Several studies have demonstrated that one or more PSI Domain scores were effective discriminators between normal and hyperactive children (Breen & Barkley, 1988; Mash & Johnson, 1983a, b) and abusive, nonabusive/neglecting, and nonabusive parents (Holden, Willis, & Foltz, 1989; Johnson, Floyd, & Isleib, 1983; Mash, Johnston, & Kovitz, 1983). Factor analyses of the normative sample (Abidin, 1986) and a cross-cultural validation sample (Hauenstein et al., 1986) have been reported. Each produced 2 general factors similar to the child and parent domains, 6 second-order child domain factors, and 7 second-order parent domain factors, with loading patterns very similar to the domain subscales. These data suggest that each subscale measures a moderately distinct source of stress. Finally, it has been demonstrated that the PSI is sensitive to treatment effects of parent training programs (Webster-Stratton et al., 1988, 1989).

The PSI was developed as a means to identify stress associated with various characteristics in the child–parent dyad and parenting subsystem. It is adequately normed and has acceptable psychometric properties. Relatively brief and easy to complete, it provides useful information about the degree of subjective distress the parent has been experiencing and the potential sources of the stress. The PSI has proved effective in discriminating normal from hyperactive children and abusive from nonabusive parents. In addition, it is sensitive to treatment effects of parent training programs.

Conflict Behavior Questionnaire

The Conflict Behavior Questionnaire (CBQ) (Prinz, 1977; Prinz, Foster, Kent, & O'Leary, 1979) was developed by Prinz and colleagues as a means of estimating the degree of conflict and negative communication experienced within the family system. Comprehensive reviews of the CBQ, including copies of the items and scoring procedures, have recently been published (Foster & Robin, 1988; Robin & Foster, 1989). The CBQ was intended primarily for use with the families of adolescents. Parents and adolescents independently complete parallel versions of the CBQ, rating their interactions over the past several weeks. The parent version contains 75 items. Of these, 53 are concerned with parent perception of the adolescent's behavior and 22 with their perceptions regarding parent–adolescent interaction. The adolescent version contains 73 items, 51 dealing with the adolescent's perception of the parent's behavior and 22 with perceptions of adolescent–parent interaction. All items endorsed in the conflictual direction are scored with 1 point. Points are summed to yield 8 separate indices: Maternal Appraisal of the Adolescent, Maternal Appraisal of the Mother–Teen Dyad, Adolescent Appraisal of the Mother, Adolescent Appraisal of the Mother-Teen Dyad, Paternal Appraisal of the Adolescent, Paternal Appraisal of the Father–Teen Dyad, Adolescent Appraisal of the Father, and Adolescent Appraisal of the Father–Teen Dyad.

Standardized norms are not available at this time, although comparison data are available. Each version requires 10–15 minutes to complete.

Six- to 8-week stability estimates for the various CBQ indices have ranged from .37 to .85 for distressed dyads (Foster, Prinz, & O'Leary, 1983; Robin, 1981). Internal consistency (alpha) coefficients have reported to be .90 or above for mother and teen reports on each of the indices. All 8 indices have discriminated distressed from nondistressed families (Foster & Robin, 1988; Prinz et al., 1979; Robin & Foster, 1984, 1989; Robin & Weiss, 1980). Although standardized norms are not available, Robin and Foster (1984, 1989) recommend these data (i.e., means and standard deviations for distressed and nondistressed families) be used for comparison purposes. Evidence is also available indicating that the CBQ is sensitive to the effects of therapeutic interventions (Foster et al., 1983; Robin, 1981).

Two shortened versions of the CBQ have also been developed. The CBQ-44 is a 44-item modification developed by Prinz et al. (1979). This form was developed by extracting items from the original CBQ that best discriminated distressed from nondistressed families. It requires about 10 minutes to complete. Separate normative or comparison data for the CBQ-44 are not available. Scoring of the CBQ-44 follows the same rules as the long form. Total scores for each index are multiplied by a correction factor to produce totals that are assumed to be equivalent with those of the long form. CBQ-44 indices correlated .98 or above with those from the long form. The CBQ-20 is a 20-item modification developed by Robin & Foster (1989). This was accomplished by extracting an even smaller subset of items from the original CBQ that discriminated distressed from nondistressed families. The CBQ-20 requires about 5 minutes to complete and yields a single summary score for each respondent. The CBQ-20 correlates .96 or higher with indices from the original CBQ.

The CBQ, in its various forms, offers a means of estimating the degree of conflict and negative communication present in families with adolescents. It seems particularly promising in providing a quick method of identifying distressed family systems and perhaps specific areas of distress within the family. Although only limited data are available concerning its reliability and validity, existing data suggest the questionnaire has adequate psychometric properties. The questionnaire does not have acceptable standardized norms, but comparison data are available. This may be of less concern if the questionnaire is utilized to monitor changes in the degree of conflict and negative communication within a family through the course of treatment or where comparisons with previous data are of concern. At the same time, additional evidence for its temporal stability, what effects if any are produced by multiple retestings, and the degree to which the questionnaire is sensitive to treatment effects would be helpful.

Issues Checklist

The Issues Checklist (IC) (Prinz, 1977; Robin & Foster, 1989), a modification of an earlier version (Robin, 1975), is a 44-item checklist that has been developed as a means of estimating both the presence of conflictual issues and the perceived intensity of anger regarding those issues. Reviews of the IC, including copies of the items and scoring procedures, have recently been published (Foster & Robin, 1988; Robin & Foster, 1989). The IC was intended primarily for use with families of adolescents. Parents and adolescents independently complete identical versions of the IC, rating their interactions over the past 4 weeks. The IC contains 44 items, each of which deals with a separate issue that is often an area of conflict between adolescents and parents, such as curfew, smoking, drinking, talking back to parents, etc. For each topic, the informant indicates whether it has been broached over the past 4 weeks, and if so, to rate the intensity of the discussions from 1 (calm) to 5 (angry). The IC yields three scores for each informant: Quantity of Issues (total number of issues endorsed), Mean Anger Intensity (mean of intensity rating for all issues endorsed), and a Weighted Average of Frequency and Anger Intensity. Standardized norms are not available at this time, although comparison data are available. The IC requires about 10 minutes to complete.

One- to 2-week stability estimates for IC indices have ranged from .47 to .80, with a median of about .70 for nondistressed dyads (Enyart, 1984). Six- to 8-week stability estimates for IC indices have ranged from .15 to .90, with a median of about .50 for distressed dyads (Foster et al., 1983; Robin, 1981). All indices discriminate distressed from nondistressed families (Forehand et al., 1987; Foster & Robin, 1988; Prinz et al., 1979; Robin & Foster, 1984, 1989). Although standardized norms are not available, Robin and Foster (1984, 1989) recommend these data (i.e., means and standard deviations for distressed and nondistressed families) be used for comparative purposes. Evidence is also available indicating that the IC is sensitive to the effects of therapeutic interventions (Foster et al., 1983; Robin, 1981).

The IC offers a means of estimating both the presence of conflictual issues and the perceived intensity of those disputes. It seems very promising in providing a quick method of identifying specific areas of conflict in parent–adolescent disputes, and focusing subsequent treatment interventions on high-priority behavioral targets. Although limited data are available concerning reliability and validity, data that do exist suggest that the questionnaire has adequate reliability. Currently, the questionnaire does not have acceptable standardized norms, but comparison data are available. This may be of less concern if the questionnaire is utilized informally, perhaps as an adjunct to the clinical interview or to monitor changes in conflictual issues through the course of treatment.

LABORATORY MEASUREMENTS

In addition to information gleaned from the interview and behavior questionnaires, the clinician may need to gain additional insights through administering objective measures of cognitive ability, academic achievement, attention span, or impulse control. Our purpose here is to provide an overview of the more commonly utilized laboratory measurements used when assessing children with disruptive behavior.

Intelligence and Achievement

Measures of general intelligence may prove helpful if one of the questions to be answered relates to the child's learning ability. Where one suspects language, cognitive, or academic delays as a contributing factor to the overall behavior profile, then administration of an appropriate measure would be in order. Perhaps the most commonly used measures are the Kaufman Assessment Battery for Children (KABC) (Kaufman & Kaufman, 1983) and Wechsler Intelligence Scale for Children-Revised (WISC-R) (Wechsler, 1974).

Aside from the global assessment of verbal and nonverbal reasoning, the WISC-R and KABC each have a cluster of subtests that would appear to be of interest in assessing children with Disruptive Behavior Disorders, i.e., the KABC's Sequential and the WISC-R's Freedom From Distractibility scores. The KABC Sequential scale is comprised of the Hand Movements, Number Recall, and Word Order subtests, all of which in some fashion involve, at minimum, sequencing, memory, and concentration skills. Similarly, the Freedom From Distractibility factor consists of the Arithmetic, Coding, and Digit Span subtests, which would seem to require many of the same types of skills necessary for success on the KABC scale. On the surface, it may be tempting to speculate that children experiencing difficulty with attention and impulse control would perform poorly on these tasks. While some children with Disruptive Behavior Disorders may indeed display deficient skills across these subtests, such tasks have not consistently been shown to discriminate children with Attention Deficits or Conduct Disorders from other children (Breen, 1989; Sattler, 1988). This may be due to a number of factors. First, attention and impulse control are comprised of many intricate processes, many of which may not be assessed by the Sequential or FFD measures. Second, children with Disruptive Behavior Disorders do not display deficits in attention and impulse control across all tasks or situations. Third, the degree of structure or stimulus control surrounding the performance of these tasks may actually be to the child's benefit, and poor performance may well be a function of deficits in other psychological processes and not due strictly to lack of attention or impulse control. Last, far too many "other" skills are necessary for success across these subtests (e.g., language, listening, motor, and visual perception) to support their efficacy as a measure suited for assessing attention and impulse control. In short, where the task is to provide an estimate of general intellectual functioning, the KABC or WISC-R should prove an appropriate measure. However, neither appears sensitive to the intricacies of attention or impulse control and as a result should not be used in the assessment of such processes as in the diagnosis of a Disruptive Behavior Disorder.

Given the high frequency of learning problems observed in children with Disruptive Behavior Disorders (Barkley, 1988a; Hunt, 1988; Kaplan, 1988; McMahon & Forehand, 1988), it is important to assess general academic skills as part of a comprehensive assessment protocol. This would also allow the clinician time to observe and interact with the child in a manner perhaps less threatening than during the interview process. If, however, the clinician is to conduct a thorough academic assessment, including suspected specific developmental disabilities, then a more complete assessment approach must be done. A detailed account of learning disabilities and instruments appropriate for their assessment and diagnosis are presented elsewhere (Sattler, 1988; Taylor, 1988).

In providing a cursory evaluation of basic reading, math, and spelling skills, we suggest use of either the Kaufman Test of Educational Achievement (KTEA) (Kaufman & Kaufman, 1985) or the Peabody Individual Achievement Test-Revised (PIAT-R) (Markwardt, 1989). Each manual presents a detailed account of psychometric characteristics, content rationale, and administrative considerations. The KTEA has recently been studied regarding its relation to more specialized academic measures and found to be quite appropriate as a screening measure of academic skills (Breen & Drecktrah, 1989). Due to its recent publication, such data are not yet available regarding the PIAT-R, though the original version did appear consistent with this intention (Sattler, 1988). Both the KTEA and the PIAT-R assess a common core of academic skills, are appropriate for school age children, and generate similar interpretive metrics. The PIAT-R also provides an estimate as to the child's general information and written expression ability. The two measures differ, however, in administrative format across a number of subtests; this may be an important consideration in determining which measure to employ. For example, the PIAT-R retained its multiple-choice answering format whereas the KTEA is not structured to allow the child a choice of answers. This difference is perhaps most obvious for the spelling and math subtests. If one were conducting a detailed academic assessment (or if time permits) it would make sense to administer both types of measures as each utilizes a different modality or process in generating the answer. This process along with perhaps the administration of other measures assessing academic skills, can certainly be helpful in understanding the mechanisms by which a child processes academic information. Due to scaling procedures and item content, the PIAT-R may be more suited for use with very young children. In general though, both appear to be appropriate in screening for academic ability.

Objective Measures of Attention Span and Impulse Control

Continuous Performance Task

With children for whom attention deficits are suspected, it may prove beneficial to assess attention span and impulse control by means of objective analysis in addition to the more subjective impressions formed through the interviews and rating scales. Administration of these measures may not always be necessary, particularly with older children and for those displaying more defiant than inattentive and impulsive behaviors. By far the most popular and sensitive measure of attention and impulsivity has been the continuous-performance test (CPT). CPT tasks are varied in nature and many clinicians have developed their own versions of this paradigm for research and clinical use. Essential characteristics are the presentation of rapidly occurring letters, numbers, or figures onto a computerlike screen. The participant is required to press a button when a predetermined stimulus or pair of stimuli appear. Interpretation is based upon the number of omissions (number of misses), commissions (incorrect responses), and number correct. Number correct and number of omissions appear to assess sustained attention while commissions may reflect impulse control and sustained attention. CPT tasks have been shown sensitive to attention deficits and stimulant drug effects (Barkley, 1977; Campbell & Werry, 1986; Gordon, 1987; Shapiro & Garfinkel, 1986; van der Meere & Sergeant, 1988). However, others have raised questions regarding the degree to which such tasks discriminate those with attention deficits from normals (Breen, 1989; Draeger, Prior, & Sanson, 1986; Davidson & Prior, 1978), though these concerns seem more related to issues surrounding length of task and degree of controlling/motivational factors (e.g., examiner presence) than necessarily to the CPT task. Thus, the CPT task itself does seem to have clinical utility in assessing children with possible attention and impulse control problems.

Gordon Diagnostic System

The Gordon Diagnostic System (GDS) (Gordon, 1982) is the only commercially available measure of this sort we could identify. The GDS is a microprocessor-based portable unit purporting to assess elements of sustained attention and impulse control. This measure is comprised of Delay, Vigilance, and Distractibility tasks. The Delay Task consists of instructing the child to press a button, wait, and then press the button again. The child is told that if he/she waits long enough between button presses, a light will appear. If the child waits for the appropriate length of time (a minimum of 6 seconds) before depressing the button a light will appear; if the response is premature, no reinforcement or credit is provided. Scores are calculated at 2-minute intervals and for the entire 8-minute duration of this task. The Vigilance Task requires the child to press a button every time a certain number sequence (e.g., 1/9, 3/5, 1, or 0, depending on the child's age) appears on the screen. Digits are randomly presented for 9 minutes at the rate of one per second, although for preschool children they are presented for 6 minutes at the rate of one per two seconds. The Distractibility Task is similar to the Vigilance Task in all features except that random sets of numbers are additionally flashed, at random intervals, on the outer two (of three) columns. The child is instructed to watch for the predetermined number sequence and when it appears in the middle column to press the button. For all tasks, the microprocessor calculates scores without being obvious to the participant.

The GDS was normed on 1,300 boys and girls, ages 4 through 16. As reported by Gordon & Mettelman (1988) test–retest reliability indices for the Delay, Vigilance, and Distractibility Tasks ranged from .60 through .85. One-year stability estimates ranged from .52 through .94 for the Delay and Vigilance Tasks, respectively. In all cases, indices for the Vigilance Task tended to be greater than for the Delay Task.

The GDS has been shown sensitive to stimulant drug effects, attention deficits, and to correlate moderately well with child behavior questionnaires commonly used in research with ADHD children (Aylward, Verhulst, Bell, Kelly, & Dorry, 1988; Barkley, Fischer, Newby, & Breen, 1988; Fischer, Barkley, Edelbrock, & Smallish, 1989; Gordon, 1987; Gordon, DiNiro, Mettelman, & Tallmadge, 1989; Gordon, Mettelman, & DiNiro, 1989; Hall & Marks, 1988; McClure & Gordon, 1984). Correlations with measures of general intelligence have generally been low, accounting for less than 10% of the variance. More recently however, the number Correct and Commission subtests from the GDS Vigilance Task correlated significantly with the KABC Sequential, Simultaneous, Mental Processing Composite, and Achievement scales (.49/−.38, .29/−.24, .44/−.37, .42/−.27), respectively (Gordon, Thomason, & Cooper, 1989). This may suggest performance on the GDS is a function of skills relatively independent of general cognitive ability. The actual contribution of general cognitive ability to performance on the GDS appears to vary considerably and remains in question, though differences here may be a function of the measure of general ability and the sample utilized within each investigation.

The GDS generates a number of scores. The Delay Task yields three scores:

number of responses, number of correct responses, and the percentage of correct responses (known as the efficiency ratio). Performance on the Vigilance Task is assessed relative to errors of omission (failure to press as appropriate), errors of commission (extraneous presses), and the number of correct presses. The Distractibility Task and Vigilance Task yield identical scores. Raw scores may be converted into percentile ranks.

The GDS is a well-normed, constructed, standardized, and objective measure appearing to assess variants of vigilance and impulse control. Clinicians should guard against overgeneralization and dependence on a measure such as the GDS in identifying children with Disruptive Behavior Disorders. While we believe the GDS can certainly stand on its own merit and will probably continue to be used in research and clinical situations, it is but one measure appropriate for use in a comprehensive clinical protocol, evaluating disruptive behavior disorders.

Matching Familiar Figures Test

The Matching Familiar Figures Test (MFFT) (Kagan, Rosman, Day, Albert, & Phillips, 1964) is a frequently employed measure purporting to assess a dimension of reflection-impulsivity. The MFFT is administered by allowing the participant visual inspection of a common and easily recognized picture (e.g., cowboy, giraffe, leaf), subsequent to which the child is shown six very similar pictures. The child is to choose a picture identical to the stimulus design. There are five alternate sets, each comprised of 12 stimulus pictures. Performance is based upon mean time taken to the first response (latency) and total number of errors (pictures identified incorrectly).

Undoubtedly the most popular measure of impulse control used in research with hyperactive children, the MFFT has undergone revisions (Cairns & Cammock, 1978; Kagan et al., 1964; Salkind, 1978) and has been the subject of discussion regarding the theoretical concepts governing its development (Block, Block, & Harrington, 1975; Kagan & Messer, 1975; Milich & Kramer, 1984). Briefly, initial norms and estimates of reliability for the MFFT were fairly poor by current standards. In an attempt to improve the technical characteristics of this scale, Cairns & Cammock (1978) expanded the 12 stimulus pictures to 20 (MFF20) and selected only those items with an appropriate discriminative index. The goal was to improve the reliability and discriminative power of the test. The authors presented four separate studies, each investigating a different aspect of the MFF20. Their data suggested the expanded version was reliable and appropriate for use with children aged 9 through 11, although it should be used judiciously with children under the age of 9 and not used with children under the age of 7. More recently, Messer &

Brodzinsky (1981) offered support for use of the MFF20 with children up to age 14. Salkind (1978) provided a much more extensive data base, norming the MFFT on more than 2,800 children aged 5 through 12.

Research with the MFFT and MFF20 has supported their clinical utility. They have been shown to discriminate children with Disruptive Behavior Disorders from normal children, correlate with clinic observations of activity level and attention, correlate with the GDS's Efficiency Ratio, and be sensitive to stimulant drug effects (Barkley, 1977; Campbell, Douglas, & Morgenstern, 1971; McClure & Gordon, 1984; Milich, Landau, & Loney, 1981). Despite widespread use of this measure, current thinking based upon more sophisticated research methodologies and review of literature suggests the scale may more appropriately be thought of as an index sensitive to general cognitive ability or information processing competence rather than strictly a measure of impulsivity (Fischer, Barkley, Edelbrock, & Smallish, 1989; Milich & Kramer, 1984). This is not to diminsh its rich clinical background but only to suggest that the MFFT/MFF20 may not be quite the "all-encompassing" measure of impulsivity it was once perceived to be and that it may well be assessing many related cognitive processes.

DIRECT OBSERVATION

Several observational coding systems have been developed for use within clinic and school settings. These systems allow for the direct observation of many behaviors that would not otherwise surface during the typical interview or review of child behavior questionnaires. While parents or teachers could report a child as being noncompliant, not listening, and/or as having problems with sustained on-task behavior, to observe such behavior may serve to heighten the clinician's overall sense as to the degree, severity, or pervasiveness of the problem behavior. Coding systems have been found useful in diagnostic and treatment approaches and can be used in the home, clinic, or school environments. Typically, systems identify a series of behaviors or interactions, and each is observed relative to frequency and duration. Sampling of specific behaviors varies depending upon need and type of system employed, although most approaches will use a continuous- or interval-sampling technique. There is little doubt that where time and physical constraints permit, direct observation can provide meaningful information.

Many clinicians have recently advocated the use of direct observations when assessing disruptive behavior disorders. Coding systems have consistently been found to discriminate between children with Disruptive Behavior Disorders and those without and to be sensitive to changes due to behavior/stimulant drug therapy (Barkley, 1989a; McMahon & Wells, 1989). Indeed, their potential value seems to be without question. However, conducting observations outside the academic setting is not always possible. It may prove rather cost-ineffective for clinicians to observe within the home setting. In order for within-clinic observations to occur, one needs an adequate observation room with a one-way mirror and an intercom system. While many of the larger child guidance centers may have this capacity, it is likely many clinicians do not have access to such physical accommodations. Even though an academic setting would appear to be the most consistently available source of direct observation, it may be cost-ineffective to send a clinician to observe within the school. School mental health personnel are frequently quite busy themselves and may not have the time to collect these data. While direct observation of child behavior is desired, such a process is less likely to consistently occur as part of an assessment protocol for children with Disruptive Behavior Disorders than those techniques previously discussed. For this reason, and because there are far too many coding systems available to review within this text, we have chosen to limit our discussion to one easy system that can be used in clinic and school settings and that typifies the majority of such coding systems. Extensive reviews of observation coding systems have recently been provided (Foster, Bell-Dolan, & Burge, 1988; Gross & Wixted, 1988; Reid, Baldwin, Patterson, & Dishion, 1988) and the reader is referred to these sources for detailed information.

For illustrative purposes, we will discuss the Restricted Academic Situation coding system developed by Barkley (1981, 1988a). We believe this system has several advantages. First, it encompasses many of the primary behaviors commonly displayed by children with Disruptive Behavior Disorders. Second, it is a simple and straightforward approach to behavior observation and requires relatively little time to learn. Third, it has been shown sensitive to stimulant drug effects, to discriminate between hyperactive and nonhyperactive children, and to have adequate test–retest and interrater reliability (Barkley et al., 1988; Breen, 1989; Fischer et al., 1989). Last, the coding system can easily be used in conducting classroom observations. This might improve the likelihood that school mental health professionals would be able to find the necessary time to conduct a few observations and forward results to the attending clinician (particularly if the clinic does not have this capacity). Because of its relative simplicity and brevity, the system can also be used to monitor treatment effects. When using this system the same relative set of behaviors can be observed in clinic and school settings. This is an important point since one key consideration in evaluating and then monitoring children with Disruptive Behavior Disorders is to maintain as much consistency within and across assessment strategies as possible. Where the intent is to obtain a measure

indicating degree of deviance from an established norm, an analysis of antecedent and consequated behaviors, or a more comprehensive observation of
negative/positive behavior, the Restricted Academic Situation system may
not be appropriate. However, we do believe the system has merit as one avenue of data gathering when the intent is to obtain a basic observation of
certain behaviors found problematic in children with Disruptive Behavior
Disorders.

The Restricted Academic Situation instructions and protocol for coding
behaviors are presented in Tables 3.1, 3.2, and 3.3. We have slightly modified
the protocol and instructions from Barkley (1988a), to better accommodate
in-school observations. For example, we have added a column for each of the
30 intervals so that simultaneous observation of a control subject is possible.
This type of format is particularly appealing when observing children in the
academic setting, as multiple observations can be conducted across various
settings using either the same child as the control or a different control for each
observation. The only other modification we made was to include the word
"teacher" after the word "mother" throughout the instructions. This simply
allows for an easier transition from clinic (mother–child) to school (teacher–
child) observations. R. A. Barkley (personal communication, 1989) has suggested deleting three of the original items from his observation protocol (talks
to mother, negative behavior, and mother commands). The rationale for
removing them was that they tend to elicit defiant behavior from the child and
are not necessarily sensitive to attention deficits. Accordingly, Table 3.3 presents the Restricted Academic Situation coding system as recently proposed for
in-clinic observation. However, we believe including these three items in an
in-school observation would be advantageous (Table 3.2), particularly if considering the educational diagnosis of emotional disturbance. Thus, by including these items, the clinician may generate a broader understanding of certain
teacher–child interactions that could prove helpful in developing diagnostic
and treatment recommendations.

For simplicity's sake, we have kept the directions for these observations the
same for the clinic and the school setting. However, separate observation
protocols have been provided. In conducting observations in the school settings, one need not adhere to the first two paragraphs of the instructions, as
they pertain to clinic observations. It is however important that the clinician
wait approximately 5 minutes, even if observing within the classroom, as it
does take a short period for children to settle down from the previous activity
and/or habituate to the clinician's presence in the room. The Restricted Academic Situation coding system is a short, adaptable, and concise way to observe
behaviors and interactions that frequently pose difficulty for children with
Disruptive Behavior Disorders.

TABLE 3.1
Restricted Academic Situation: Instructions for Coding Behavior

Instructions for Conducting Observation

Place the child in a playroom having a one-way mirror and intercom facilities, a small table and chair at which the child will work, a larger chair or sofa and magazines for the mother, and a number of toys available for play. Instruct the child to play with the toys as he or she might do at home. Allow 5 minutes for play. This is a habituation period and is not used for recording behavior. (The same habituation period should be provided when conducting a classroom observation.)

At the end of the 5 minutes, enter the room and instruct the child to complete a set of math problems (at least five pages in length). The child is to work at the small table and is not to get up, play with toys, or leave the room. Math problems should be appropriate for the child's developmental level. When conducting observations within the academic setting, care must be taken to ensure that the activity lends itself to a sustained performance level.

After the instructions, the examiner returns to the observation room and begins the audiotape containing the interval-coding cues. This tape merely contains voice prompts indicating the beginning of each 30-second interval (i.e., Begin 1, Begin 2, Begin 3, Begin 30). When the tape sounds the interval number, the coder proceeds to that column and places a check mark in that block corresponding to each behavior category observed during that time interval. Each category is scored only once during a 30-second interval, regardless of how often it may occur. When the tape recorder sounds the next interval number, the coder moves to the next column and begins marking any behaviors that occur in that interval. Use of an audiotape when conducting observations within the academic setting may be cumbersome and, in this instance, the clinician may wish to use a stopwatch.

The following behavior categories may be recorded for either the in-clinic or in-school observation protocol: Off Task, Fidgeting, Vocalization, Talks to Teacher-Peer (school only), Plays with Objects, Out of Seat, Negative Behavior (school only), and Teacher Commands (school only). It is possible to score a child as showing any or all of these behaviors within any 30-second coding interval. There are 30 intervals to be coded, for a total of 15 minutes. The following definitions are used for each behavior category.

Definitions of Behavior Categories

1. *Off Task*: This category is checked if the child interrupts his or her attention to the tasks to engage in some other behavior. Off-task behaviors are looking around the room, playing with the pencil, looking at or playing with clothing, talking to mother/teacher or peer, or any other behavior where the child is not looking at the worksheets. A child can hum or whistle while working, kick his or her legs, or even stop using the pencil, and still remain "on task" as long as he or she maintains eye contact with the task. It is essentially the breaking of eye contact with the worksheets that constitutes off-task behavior.

2. *Fidgeting*: Any repetitive, purposeless motion of the legs, arms, buttocks, or trunk. Remember, it must occur at least twice in succession to be considered repetitive, and it should serve no purpose. Examples: swaying back and forth, kicking legs back and forth, swinging arms at sides, shuffling feet from side to side, or shifting buttocks about in the air.

(Continued)

TABLE 3.1 (*Continued*)

3. *Vocalization*: Any vocal noise or verbalization made by the child, excluding statements made toward the mother/teacher/peer. Statements made out loud but to no one in particular (talking to self) are scored in this category. If the child initiates any verbal interaction with the mother/teacher/peer, or responds to her interactions verbally, it is scored in the next category (Talks to Mother/Teacher/Peer). Examples of vocalizing might be humming, whistling, clicking teeth together, making odd mouth noices, or throat clearing. Sniffling is not a vocalization.

4. *Talks to Teacher/Peer*: Any verbal statement, question, comment, remark, or command directed toward the teacher/peer. Eye contact with the teacher/peer need not be made, so long as it is clear that the statement or question is directed toward that person.

5. *Plays with Objects*: If the child manually touches any other object in the room (except mother/teacher/peer) that is not related to the task (paper, pencil, desk) it is scored in this category. Playing with body parts or clothing or touching the mother is not scored here. Examples: touches other chairs, tables, curtains, cabinets, toys, etc.

6. *Out of Seat*: Any time the child's buttocks break the flat surface of the seat in which he or she is sitting, it is coded in this category.

7. *Negative Behavior*: Any verbal or nonverbal display of anger, refusal, opposition, or discouragement toward the teacher/peer.

8. *Teacher Commands*: Any imperative or interrogative statement directed toward the child that directs the child to perform some behavior or stop an ongoing behavior is scored here.

Scoring Dependent Measures

The score for each behavior category is derived by counting the number of check marks for that category, dividing by 30 (or the actual number of intervals of observation), and multiplying by 100 to yield a percentage correct.

Note. From "Attention Deficit Disorder with Hyperactivity" by R. A. Barkley (1988). In E. Mash and L. Terdal (Eds.), *Behavioral Assessment of Childhood Disorders* (2nd ed., p. 91). New York: Guilford Press. Copyright 1988 by The Guilford Press. Adapted by permission.

TABLE 3.2
Restricted Academic Situation Coding Chart: In-School

Interval	Off Task	Fidget-ing	Vocaliz-ing	Talks to Teacher Peer	Plays w/ Objects	Out of Seat	Negative Behavior	Teacher Com-mands
1a								
1b								
2a								
2b								
3a								
3b								
4a								
4b								
5a								
5b								
6a								
6b								
7a								
7b								
8a								
8b								
9a								
9b								
10a								
10b								

TABLE 3.2 (Continued)

11a								
11b								
12a								
12b								
13a								
13b								
14a								
14b								
15a								
15b								
16a								
16b								
17a								
17b								
18a								
18b								
19a								
19b								
20a								
20b								
21a								
21b								

22a								
22b								
23a								
23b								
24a								
24b								
25a								
25b								
26a								
26b								
27a								
27b								
28a								
28b								
29a								
29b								
30a								
30b								

Off Task (__/30) × 100 = __%   Fidgeting (__/30) × 100 = __%

Vocalizing (__/30) × 100 = __%   Talks to Teacher (__/30) × 100 = __%

Plays w/ Objects (__/30) × 100 = __%   Out of Seat (__/30) × 100 = __%

Child Negative (__/30) × 100 = __%   Teacher Commands (__/30) × 100 = __%

Child's Name_____   Observer's Name_____   Date_____

TABLE 3.3
Restricted Academic Situation Coding Chart: In-Clinic

Interval	Off Task	Fidgeting	Vocalizing	Plays with Objects	Out of Seat
1a					
1b					
2a					
2b					
3a					
3b					
4a					
4b					
5a					
5b					
6a					
6b					
7a					
7b					
8a					
8b					
9a					
9b					
10a					
10b					

11a					
11b					
12a					
12b					
13a					
13b					
14a					
14b					
15a					
15b					
16a					
16b					
17a					
17b					
18a					
18b					
19a					
19b					
20a					
20b					
21a					
21b					
22a					
22b					

TABLE 3.3 (*Continued*)

23a					
23b					
24a					
24b					
25a					
25b					
26a					
26b					
27a					
27b					
28a					
28b					
29a					
29b					
30a					
30b					

Off Task (__/30) × 100 = __%   Fidgeting (__/30) × 100 = __%

Vocalizing (__/30) × 100 = __%   Talks to Teacher (__/30) × 100 = __%

Plays w/ Objects (__/30) × 100 = __%   Out of Seat (__/30) × 100 = __%

Child Negative (__/30) × 100 = __%   Teacher Commands (__/30) × 100 = __%

Child's Name_____ Observer's Name_____ Date_____

SUMMARY

This chapter focused upon data gathering procedures that supplement information obtained during the clinical interview. We presented information regarding several child behavior questionnaires, psychometric measures of attention span and impulse control, as well as an in-school and in-clinic observation format. We highlighted relevant psychometric characteristics and research for each questionnaire so that one may determine which scale seems to fit the general scope of assessment needs best. It was extremely difficult to review only those presented. Indeed, many other well-designed instruments are available for clinical use. We chose these because they tend to be the most commonly referenced measures in research with children identified as having a Disruptive Behavior Disorder. We cannot stress enough that one or two well-developed and broad-band measures of general child psychopathology appear to be a necessary component in any well-structured and comprehensive evaluation. While no single questionnaire should ever be the sole criterion on which to base a diagnosis, it can prove quite helpful in validating certain behaviors or concerns gleaned from parent and teacher interactions, provide information not gained through the interview, and provide a psychometric perspective as to the relative degree of deviant behavior. We also included several narrow-band questionnaires that may prove useful when one questions very specific aspects of psychopathology, e.g., child/adolescent/adult depression, parent stress, or issues that may need to be resolved within the confines of family interaction. We then focusd our review upon measures of attention span, impulse control, and direct observation. There is little doubt these procedures can greatly enhance the data-gathering process and offer new insights into behavior. However, few well-developed and commercially available measures of attention span or impulse control exist. Direct observation of behavior within a clinic setting is not always possible, given physical constraints. In-school observations would appear the most feasible from a time-management and consistency standpoint. Where possible, direct observations of child behavior should be conducted, but one must be careful not to overinterpret the results. That is, just because a child is observed for 15 minutes and not seen as particularly active, impulsive, noncompliant, etc., or for that matter does well on a measure of attention span, should not be construed as suggesting the child does not have a Disruptive Behavior Disorder. Conversely, one could observe these behaviors and account for their occurrence in a manner not consistent with a Disruptive Behavior Disorder. The key to using the methods discussed in this chapter is to use them in conjunction with other measures and then to interpret them in a sensible and judicious manner.

4

TREATMENT OF DISRUPTIVE BEHAVIOR DISORDERS

In the previous two chapters we have reviewed in some detail various methods of gathering data that might assist the clinician in reaching more reliable and valid diagnostic conclusions. Perhaps the primary reason for undertaking a comprehensive clinical assessment of any presenting condition or situation is to clarify the nature of the presenting concerns so that appropriate treatment may be implemented. While there are occasions in clinical practice where the pattern of presenting concerns clearly suggests one type of difficulty or disorder, and not others, these occasions are infrequent. More commonly, one or more persons present in some subjective distress, complete with an array of behavioral, cognitive, emotional and/or physiological symptoms. The situation can seem confusing and perhaps overwhelming, particularly to the student or novice clinician. This is particularly true when the child or adolescent presents with a Disruptive Behavior Disorder. In this instance, the primary informant is typically an adult (parent or teacher) and the child gives little or no report of subjective distress. In addition, in the clinic or office the child may not exhibit the behavior problems or other difficulties about which the parent or other adult expressed concern. In clinical practice, then, the primary focus of assessment is to bring order to a confusing and perhaps inconsistent situation, so as to facilitate appropriate and minimize or avoid inappropriate treatment. If the clinical evaluation is conducted in too brief and cursory a fashion, one runs the risk of gathering insufficient information, reaching incorrect diagnostic impressions, and implementing inappropriate treatments. For example, we have unfortunately observed situations where a relatively normal child exhibited mild to moderate behavior problems in the context of some family-based stressor (e.g., moderate marital discord or the death of a grandparent), was briefly evaluated by a physician at the request of the parent, and subsequently placed on Ritalin. In this instance, the child was placed on a medication which was not warranted and the real problem remained undetected and untreated. Ideally, comprehensive clinical evaluation will lead to appropriate and effective treatment.

Once a thorough assessment has been conducted and appropriate diagnostic impressions formed, the clinician then needs to focus on unique features or characteristics of *this* child and family which might serve as moderator variables that may facilitate or impede treatment. For example, a child diagnosed as having an Attention deficit Hyperactivity Disorder may theoretically derive some benefit from medication, a parent training program, a home–school behavior management program, and/or changes in educational placement and programming. However, not all ADHD children will benefit equally from such interventions and in some cases there may be significant contraindications to one or more of the interventions. For example, as noted below in more detail, there are several different types of medications commonly used with children diagnosed as having Disruptive Behavior Disorders. None are effective with all such children, as each presents with some contraindications and adverse side effects. Thus, after initial diagnostic impressions are formed, the clinician must go one step further and design a treatment program that accommodates the unique needs of the child, parent(s), family, and teacher. Clinical evaluation should lead to appropriate, effective, and individualized treatment. In this chapter we will review the major treatments commonly used with children who exhibit Disruptive Behavior Disorders. Treatment orientations receiving attention will be educational, pharmacological, parent training in behavior management, individual cognitive–behavioral training, and family therapy. We will attempt to provide an overview of the nature and effectiveness of each treatment.

EDUCATION

It is common that a child or adolescent diagnosed as having one or more of the Disruptive Behavior Disorders will need some type of educational or classroom adjustment. Evidence suggests that children diagnosed as having a Disruptive Behavior Disorder frequently present with concomitant learning problems, many times to the point of necessitating some form of exceptional educational (APA, 1987; Barkley, 1988a, 1989a; Douglas & Peters, 1979; Halperin, Gittelman, Klein, & Rudel, 1984; Hinshaw, 1987; Holborow & Berry, 1986; McMahon & Wells, 1989; Rutter et al., 1976; Sandoval & Lambert, 1985; Taylor, 1989). Although many forms of exceptional education exist (e.g., programs for children with mental retardation, speech/language impairments, physically handicapping conditions, etc.), the two programs to which children with Disruptive Behavior Disorders are most often assigned are for those with a learning disability (LD) or an emotional disturbance (ED). It is often thought that these programs have the potential to "help" the student because of their structure and design. Space limitations preclude providing a detailed analysis of the historical development and current lines of thought concerning the relative efficacy of exceptional education. Rather, we will discuss certain issues we believe are important in understanding the role that regular and exceptional education may play in a comprehensive treatment program for disruptive-behavior-disordered children. We will limit discussion to the following issues: (1) differences in the definition of (and resulting confusion between) DSM-III-R's Disruptive Behavior Disorders and Academic Skills Disorders and the federal guidelines (Public Law 94-142) that educational systems are required to follow in implementing exceptional education programs (e.g., LD and ED); (2) the concept of a handicapping condition applied to a least-restrictive learning environment and the regular education initiative (REI); (3) the Children-At-Risk Initiative (CAR); and (4) classroom management of children with Disruptive Behavior Disorders.

Definitions

If all clinicians and exceptional education teachers, regardless of whether they were employed in or outside of the school setting, followed the same set of working guidelines to identify clinical and educational disorders, less confusion would result concerning which children should or could obtain services. This obviously is not the case. There have long been, and will probably always be, differences of opinion concerning which set of guidelines should serve as the focal point in the assessment of educational needs and how best to interpret the intent or "spirit" of such guidelines. Unfortunately, parents and to some extent educators are frequently caught in the middle of "our" debates and inconsistencies. Of particular interest here are the similarities and differences in guidelines that may overlap when working with children identified from a clinical perspective as having one or more of the Disruptive Behavior Disorders, and from an educational perspective as having a learning disability or an emotional disturbance.

Table 4.1 presents DSM-III-R's criteria for the Academic Skills Disorders. Guidelines for emotional disturbance and learning disability as presented through *Public Law 94–142* are as follows:

Specific learning disability means a disorder in one or more of the basic psychological processes involved in understanding or in using language (spoken or written) and may manifest itself in an imperfect ability to listen, think, speak, read, write, spell, or to do mathematical calculations. The term includes such conditions as perceptual handicaps, brain injury, minimal brain dysfunction, dyslexia, and developmental aphasia. The term does not include children who have learning problems that are primarily the result of visual, hearing, or motor handicaps, of mental retardation, of emotional disturbance, or of environmental, cultural, or economic disadvantage.

Seriously emotionally disturbed is defined as a condition exhibiting one or more of the following characteristics over a long period of time, to a marked degree, and adversely affecting educational performance:

1. An inability to learn that cannot be explained by intellectual, sensory, or health factors.
2. An inability to build or maintain satisfactory interpersonal relationships with peers and teachers.
3. Inappropriate types of behavior or feelings under normal circumstances.
4. A general pervasive mood of unhappiness or depression.
5. A tendency to develop physical symptoms or fears associated with personal or school problems.
6. The term includes children who are schizophrenic. The term does not include children who are socially maladjusted, unless it is determined that they are seriously emotionally disturbed. (Code of Federal Regulations, 1984)

Since guidelines for the Disruptive Behavior Disorders have been presented in Chapter 1, they will not be listed here. In reviewing Table 4.1, a number of observations can be made. First, in both the DSM-III-R and federal guidelines, criteria that need to be followed by clinicians are somewhat vague and may facilitate differences in the "functional" manner with which clinicians conduct assessments and reach conclusions. In some cases, it may be that the particular state criteria (LD and ED) that are adapted from the federal guidelines are more specific. However, it has been our experience that state criteria vary from state to state (and even from school district to school district), are subject to varied interpretation, and also lead to differences and inconsistencies in the assessment style and conclusions that are reached. The DSM-III-R guidelines for Disruptive Behavior Disorders and Academic Skills Disorders, as we have suggested, also contain sufficient ambiguity to allow for varied interpretation. Since children diagnosed as having one of the Disruptive Behavior Disorders may be at risk for developing, if not presenting with, exceptional education

TABLE 4.1
DSM-III-R Diagnostic Criteria for the Academic Skills Disorders

DSM-III-R: Developmental Arithmetic Disorder

1. Arithmetic skills, as measured by a standardized, individually administered test, are markedly below the expected level, given the person's schooling and intellectual capacity (as determined by an individually administered IQ test).
2. The disturbance in (1) significantly interferes with academic achievement or activities of daily living requiring arithmetic skills.
3. Not due to a defect in visual or hearing acuity or neurologic disorder.

DSM-III-R: Developmental Expressive Writing Disorder

1. Writing skills, as measured by a standardized, individually administered test, are markedly below the expected level, given the person's schooling and intellectual capacity (as determined by an individually administered IQ test).
2. The disturbance in (1) significantly interferes with academic achievement or activities of daily living requiring the composition of written texts (spelling words and expressing thoughts in gramatically correct sentences and organized paragraphs).
3. Not due to a defect in visual or hearing acuity or a neurologic disorder.

DSM-III-R: Developmental Reading Disorder

1. Reading achievement, as measured by a standardized, individually administered test, is markedly below the expected level, given the person's schooling and intellectual capacity (as determined by an individually administered IQ test).
2. The disturbance in (1) significantly interferes with academic achievement or activities of daily living requiring reading skills.
3. Not due to a defect in visual or hearing acuity or a neurologic disorder.

Note: From *DSM-III-R* by the American Psychiatric Association, 1987, Washington, DC: Author. Copyright 1987 by the American Psychiatric Association. Adapted by permission.

needs, clinicians need to be sensitive to both the clinical and the educational guidelines. While federal guidelines for exceptional education are an important point of interest, criteria proposed by the local Department of Public Instruction must also be followed by educational M-Teams. Therefore, mental health professionals in the position of assessing children suspected of having a Disruptive Behavior Disorder should make an effort to become familiar with state guidelines for exceptional education services and learn to work within those guidelines to become an effective child advocate. In particular, if the rationale for an outside-the-school evaluation is to consider the presence of an exceptional education need (or perhaps to form a second opinion), clinicians should conduct the evaluation in a manner consistent with the local school guidelines and perspectives on cognitive, academic, and social–behavioral assessment. This is not to suggest that one type of service or professional perspective necessarily dictates to another (regardless of the direction) the method and style of the clinical assessment. Clearly, that defeats the purpose of a second opinion. Rather, we suggest an effort be made to ensure that the assessment, interpretation, and treatment be fairly compatible. Such a process would facilitate consistent and clear communication among all parties (mental health professional, school, and parents) as well as helping to identify and meet the child's needs.

The second observation is concerned with the lack of conceptual agreement between guidelines proposed in the DSM-III-R and those contained in the federal standards (and likely state criteria). While we appreciate that uniform agreement involving terminology, concepts, and diagnostic criteria across medical, mental health, and education professions is not possible, the current lack of consistent diagnostic criteria can foster inconsistency in communication. This serves only to confuse and frustrate all parties concerned, particularly parents. For example, it is not uncommon for a clinician, based upon the results of a clinical evaluation (and often not fully cognizant of existing state educational guidelines), to suggest to parents that the child's behavior and/or academic productivity could be more effectively managed through an LD or ED program. However, the child may not meet school guidelines for placement in an LD or ED program, as suggested by an M-Team. Parents may then be quite confused and angry at the school's failure to place the child in an exceptional education program. Clearly greater agreement in concept and terminology between the medical, mental health, and educational professionals would be helpful. While it is likely that many students in an ED program would be given a DSM-III-R diagnosis of Conduct Disorder, Oppositional Defiant Disorder, or Attention-deficit Hyperactivity Disorder, not all children diagnosed as having one of the Disruptive Behavior Disorders need exceptional education. Such children/adolescents may indeed present with behaviors that could be helped through the structure and small teacher–student ratio of an exceptional education program. However, unless behaviors have clearly facilitated or resulted in academic (LD), or social, emotional, or behavioral deficits (ED), and interfered with attaining expected levels of academic performance, exceptional education is not generally an appropriate consideration.

The issue of academic deficits associated with a Disruptive Behavior Disorder and the legitimacy of a program for the learning disabled becomes a more delicate issue as the child matures chronologically. For example, while the guidelines assume significant academic deficits in relation to the child's expected level of performance, none offers methods to determine exactly what constitutes a significant deficit. This is the point where confusion often develops. In adapting federal guidelines, most state guidelines include a specific method of determining "significant" deficits, although methods vary from state to state. In Wisconsin, for example, when identifying a learning disability, evaluation teams are to use as a *guide* the formula, "IQ × years in school × .5"

(Wisconsin Department of Public Instruction, 1983). Thus, a 50% lag be-tween functional and expected levels of achievement must exist before the child is identified as handicapped and entitled to exceptional education services. There are, of course, other considerations and exclusionary factors that enter into the educational definition of a learning disability. Given the relative sim-plicity of such guidelines, a sensitive yet practical issue is the selection of measures assessing academic skills. Not all such measures are developed with similar rigor, share similar methodology, or generate "comparable" metric indices (i.e., grade level estimates); (Breen, 1984; Breen, Lehman, & Carlson, 1984; Breen & Drecktrah, 1989).

If, for example, we were to apply this approach to a youngster with a Disruptive Behavior Disorder in the third grade with an average IQ, he would have to display approximately a 1 1/2-year lag in functional achievement in order to "qualify" for the LD program. An eighth-grade student with average cognitive ability would need to display functional skills approximating a 4-year lag. This same eighth-grade student may present with deficits approximating a two-year lag, certainly enough to facilitate frustration, problems completing homework, and perhaps some degree of avoidant or acting-out behaviors, all of which could easily exacerbate presenting disruptive behaviors. While this lag in achievement may be sufficient to warrant one or more of the DSM-III-R Academic Skills Deficit diagnoses, it does not approach the magnitude re-quired by the state guidelines for exceptional education placement. Unless an M-Team were to view this student's profile as indicative of an emotional disturbance due to concomitant behavior problems, exceptional education would likely not be available as an academic intervention.

Parents often become confused and frustrated at this point because of the "system's" inability to provide services to meet their child's needs. They may be told by a mental health clinician that their child has a Disruptive Behavior Disorder and an Academic Skills Disorder, perhaps implying that Exceptional Education Needs (EEN) and services are required. They may then be told by school personnel that while the child does exhibit academic deficits, these are not of sufficient severity to warrant exceptional education, programs that on the surface would appear to benefit the child (i.e., small group instruction, individualized program, structure, potential for a greater degree of follow-through and consequences for behavior, etc.).

Although such a perspective may appear unsympathetic if not callused rel-ative to the child's needs, the issue of whether a child could benefit from a highly structured program and the issue of adhering to educationally oriented guidelines for exceptional education are, unfortunately, not always synono-mous. The point we would like to make is that within most elementary, middle, or high school programs for the emotionally disturbed or learning disabled, there will likely be a number of students who would clinically be viewed as having one or more of the Disruptive Behavior Disorders and legitimately belong within such parameters. Whether a child is enrolled in an exceptional education program depends upon the severity, pervasiveness, and degree of academic skill deficit rather than a clinical diagnosis and impression of whether such a program would be helpful to the child. Children identifed as having a Disruptive Behavior Disorder or an Academic Skills Disorder do not necessarily need or qualify for exceptional education. It is only when behaviors clearly interfere with the ability to function within regular education parameters, prove resistant to regular education intervention, and cause or lead to significant academic skill deficits, that exceptional education should be considered. This method of scrutinizing the need for EEN services is in keeping with the idea that children should be educated within the least restrictive learning environment.

Least-Restrictive Learning Environment

Another exceptional education issue of concern to all clinicians who work with children diagnosed as having Disruptive Behavior Disorders, whether employed within or outside of a school setting, is that of least restrictive learning environment. One theme central to PL 94–142 is that all handicapped children have a right to a free and appropriate education. Implicit is the notion that educational services are not to be provided at the cost of exclusion of interaction with nonhandicapped students; the rationale is that to segregate handicapped children by educating them separately from other students is to violate their due process and educational rights. On the surface, this may be difficult to implement fully, as the notion that "we have specialized teachers, so let them help the child with special needs" appears to be well ingrained throughout clinical and educational settings. Children with severely handicapping conditions who cannot function in a normal educational setting belong in specialized environments. However, one must be careful to ensure that exceptional education does not become a dumping ground for mildly handicapped children whose educational needs do not mesh exactly with existing methods of instruction. To consider these children appropriate candidates for exceptional education is to violate the spirit of PL 94–142.

Perhaps during the initial developmental stage of special or exceptional education, it was more appropriate to consider EEN programs as a method of "helping" children, with less emphasis on the legal and social ramifications. While mainstreaming was certainly an ultimate goal, perhaps it did not occur to the degree that it should have or to the degree it now does. Exceptional education has not only expanded in the number of students served, but it has also (appropriately) become more sophisticated regarding the children enrolled within such services. The goal of providing services to handicapped children within the regular education setting is important. While some may still view exceptional education as a "catchall" program for children regular education cannot (or chooses not to) handle, the pendulum appears to be swinging in the direction of even more integration within regular education rather than more of a "pull-out" from regular to exceptional education (Lieberman, 1984).

This has recently been discussed in terms of the Regular Education Initiative (REI) (Davis, 1989; Reynolds, Wang, & Walberg, 1987; Will, 1986). Central to the theme of this initiative is that children with exceptional educational needs should have an opportunity to participate in a restructured regular education program rather than a restructured exceptional education program. This is not to suggest an abandonment of the concept of or of the practical efficacy of exceptional education. Rather, where realistically appropriate, regular education may better accommodate children with handicapping conditions than is currently observed. Debate over the practical application of REI will probably continue for some time (Hallahan, et al., 1988; Kauffman, Gerber, & Semmel, 1988). The point of contention is not so much the concept but rather how to successfully implement such a program, which of course is no easy task at any level of educational service.

We raise these issues as applied to children with Disruptive Behavior Disorders because many may be in the process of being considered for or already placed in either an LD or ED program. Mental health professionals in and outside of the school settings who evaluate and treat these children should be sensitive to these issues. Parents will look to professionals for guidance, direction, and treatment of their child. Unless we can collaborate in a consistent manner with each other while effectively discussing such issues and implications with parents, we may be offering them less than a thorough means by which to intervene with their child. Where the child's needs are so pervasive, clearly handicap educational performance, and have proven resistant to all reasonable intervention, exceptional education is a viable alternative and should be pursued on behalf of the child. However, from an educational perspective and within reason, such services should be the last alternative or method of intervention and not the first to be considered.

Children At-Risk Initiative (CAR)

Since exceptional education may not always be an appropriate consideration for children with Disruptive Behavior Disorders, regular education will have to accommodate these students. One means of identifying and then addressing the needs of such students (as well as many others) would be to utilize the At-Risk process recently developed by many state departments of public instruction, commonly known as the Children-At-Risk Initiative (CAR). In essence, this is a process designed to reduce the number of students at risk of failing within the academic and/or social domains by attempting to deal with the issues that seem to impair the student's ability to learn, and therefore to make appropriate progress through school and graduate from high school. The CAR process identifies a series of factors viewed as contributing to school failure and attempts to modify the educational experience to best accommodate the child's needs. Certainly, the majority of children identified as having a Disruptive Behavior Disorder could be viewed as being at-risk for not being academically successful or even completing school.

In many instances, the at-risk process is an appropriate first step in working with families and teachers of children with Disruptive Behavior Disorders. Although each school's adaptation of their state's administrative rules governing the at-risk process will vary, central to each program is the identification of variables that contribute to the student's lack of success within an academic setting. These may include *educational variables* (e.g., achievement below grade or ability level expectations, displaying disruptive behavior in or outside the classroom setting, a number of unexcused absences, failing a certain number of subjects, having an exceptional education need, or being a school dropout) and/or *health/social variables* (e.g., displaying ineffective or poor interpersonal skills, low self-esteem, dysfunctional family, being a victim of physical/sexual/emotional abuse, substance use/abuse, teenage parent, adjudicated delinquent). Usually the school system will have a referral form with these variables listed. Teachers and/or parents complete the referral and a meeting with appropriate school personnel (or other professionals) is arranged. The purpose of this meeting is to discuss the student's unique needs and those issues requiring resolution. The end product should be the development of a Student's Educational Plan (SEP), which consists of methods that will be used to assist the student in being more successful within the academic setting. Factors within the SEP may include alternative programs, support services, curriculum adjustment, methods of monitoring behavior, implementation of a home–school behavior management program, referral for psychological, medical, or EEN assessment, or the implementation of suggestions from a recently conducted outside-the-school evaluation. The At-Risk process is a helpful and ongoing way to meet the needs of these children within the regular (and, where appropriate exceptional) education setting. It is a process that, when implemented carefully, can facilitate communication between professionals and parents as well as accountability for all involved with service delivery to the child in question.

As noted, the SEP may suggest an exceptional educational needs referral be generated for a suspected learning disability or emotional disturbance. Should the child or adolescent display the appropriate need and meet necessary standards for enrollment, an Individual Educational Plan (IEP) is then developed. It is the IEP that governs the method, type, and degree of intervention. Students enrolled within an EEN program are frequently subjected to a fairly structured academic program complete with response cost procedures designed to assist in managing behavior. There is little doubt that such procedures are both necessary and effective when working with DBD children (Atkeson & Forehand, 1979; Barkley, 1989a; Jones & Kazdin, 1981; McMahon & Wells, 1989; Rapport, Murphy, & Bailey, 1982; Safer & Allen, 1976). A more rigorous program could certainly be established within the confines of exceptional education, given the smaller number of students and the availability of a teacher and usually a teacher's aid. In addition, EEN teachers are trained in behavior management principles. It is not our purpose to review the variety of methods used to manage behavior within LD and ED programs. There simply are far too many programs, all of which are usually adapted to fit program parameters and student needs. However, since not all disruptive-behavior-disordered students are educated within the confines of exceptional education, it is necessary that educators understand basic behavior principles and practical management skills that are necessary to manage children presenting with disruptive behavior. Even if students are enrolled within an EEN program, they may be mainstreamed, and this would also require the regular education teacher to be familiar with response cost and other management principles. We would like to provide, then, an overview of the types of behavioral interventions that may prove helpful in the classroom management of these students.

A few basic assumptions must be discussed and their concepts applied before an effective behavior management program can prove successful:

1. Parents and teachers must have realistic academic goals and expectations for the child. Obviously, if their demands clearly exceed the child's capacity to perform, then the "system" is simply asking for some degree of disruptive reaction due to the stress of continued failure. The implication here is that if a management system were to be implemented because of the child's basic inability to attend, self-monitor, organize, or otherwise inhibit disruptive or interfering behavior, to add the element of academic frustration would be to jeopardize the potentially positive effect that such a management program could have upon behavior.

2. Certain extraneous variables must be accounted for. The seating arrangement for the child in question should be considered. To seat the child near other students who themselves present with similar behaviors (who are not being monitored) would seem to foster student noncompliance and thus potentiate failure. For example, a seventh-grade student diagnosed with Attention-deficit Hyperactivity Disorder/Oppositional Defiant Disorder was having

particular difficulty in his math class. This student was not in an EEN program, but was in the process of being referred for suspected emotional disturbance. It so happened that the math teacher had the student sitting in the back of his room with another ADHD student to his left and a student behind him who experienced a good deal of difficulty organizing herself and staying on-task (she was mainstreamed from an LD program). The teacher, at the M-Team meeting, actually said, "I don't understand why this student can't get his work done." In all fairness, there were other issues to be resolved by the M-Team, but it was somewhat naive to ask that question given the student's location and the interactive effect of his immediate neighbors.

3. Curricula specifically designed for an unstructured or independent approach to learning will probably enhance failure in students with Disruptive Behavior Disorders. Their need for structure and reasonably immediate reinforcement for desired behavior and consequences for inappropriate behavior is clear: An independent orientation would do little to foster the success of a management program.

4. There must be a certain "match" between the child's behavior and the teacher's temperament before suggesting the teacher provide "extra" time and assistance to the student. Clearly, most educators are very accommodating of their student's needs and provide additional services when asked to do so. However, at all levels of educational service one may encounter a teacher with either unusually rigid behavior or academic perspectives, biases that might interfere with managing disruptive-behavior-disordered or EEN students, or one who simply believes that, given the normal rigors of educating children, it is not necessary to provide "extra" time and effort. For example, one elementary school teacher was particularly intolerant of a student's inability to keep his desk and immediately surrounding area neat and picked up. The teacher's approach to providing a consequence to this was to, upon occasion, tip the desk upside down and empty the contents, subsequent to which the child was to pick up his belongings and keep his desk neat. This is the same teacher who would periodically, when the child remembered to go to the office and take his medication, have the class applaud. Perhaps the teacher felt these procedures were appropriate consequences and reinforcements, but his expectations and temperament were not a good match with those of the student. Thus, addressing the unique needs of this child specific to a behavior management program with this particular teacher was not an easy task. This is not to suggest that teachers and/or the educational system must always accommodate the student; clearly, students play a role in the interaction and need to show some accommodation of their own (as do their parents). We do suggest, however, that in developing a successful management program with disruptive-behavior-disordered students, certain factors should be considered prior to implementing the intervention. Obviously, the best conceptualized manage-

ment program is only as effective as the degree of cooperation displayed by parents and teachers.

With these assumptions, let us now address the literature supporting the use of behavior principles in managing disruptive behavior within the academic setting. Strategies such as teacher praise for appropriate behavior, ignoring inappropriate behavior, establishing clear rules, directions, and expectations, use of time-out, reprimands, and contingency contracting have all proven to be successful methods of improving disruptive behavior (Abramowitz, O'Leary, & Rosen, 1987; Acker & O'Leary, 1987; Barkley, 1981, 1983; Brantner & Doherty, 1983; Goldstein & Keller, 1987; Becker, Madsen, Arnold, & Thomas, 1967; Taylor, Cornwell, & Riley, 1984). The combination of one or more of these strategies results in even more improved behavior than when used alone. Token reinforcement programs have also been established as effective mediators in the management of disruptive behavior. Many children with Disruptive Behavior Disorders appear to have the capacity to consistently display appropriate social and academic behaviors. The use of external reinforcers often times is necessary in order to maintain an acceptable pattern of behavior.

One method of expanding upon the school based token program is to incorporate parents as the primary reinforcing agent, i.e., home-school behavior management program. Such home-based reinforcement programs have been useful in managing both within-home and within-school behaviors, ranging from productivity issues to more noncompliant and aggressive behavior (Ayllon, Garber, & Pisor, 1975; Barkley, 1981, 1983, 1989a; Lahey et al., 1977; O'Leary & Pelham, 1978; Safer & Allen, 1976). Basically, these programs involve a set of targeted behaviors that are monitored by means of a small rating card throughout the school day. As each targeted behavior is appropriately displayed, the student is then provided either a teacher signature, sticker, or some type of acknowledgment that the behavior was noted. These in turn are given a certain point value or poker chip value by the parents. Each teacher signature may, for example, be worth 5 chips. Parents then develop a list of potential reinforcers, each of which is given a chip value (e.g., 15 minutes additional of TV or some type of home video game might be purchased for 10 chips). Reinforcers range from those requiring but a few chips to those costing in excess of 80 to 100. The ratio between the number of chips that could possibly be earned in one day and number of chips required per reinforcer is an extremely important consideration, as to make chips too difficult or too easy in relation to the type of reinforcers that may be purchased can easily affect the success of this program. It is also a rather easy process to establish a few targeted behaviors within the home setting, arranged and reinforced in the same manner as those in the school environment. Parents have for example included such interactions as picking up the child's room, bedtime or mealtime behaviors, homework, etc. as targeted behaviors and assigned varying chip values to each upon their completion. This type of a management program can also assist in fostering direct and consistent communication between parents and teacher, which many times is necessary given the nature and severity of behavior displayed by disruptive-behavior-disordered children and adolescents.

Tables 4.2 and 4.3 present a psychometric profile of a first-grade student diagnosed with ADHD and the card we developed in monitoring a selected few behaviors that were interfering with classroom success. The teacher was more than willing to complete this card each school day. Prior to implementation, the teacher, parent, and clinician met to discuss definitions of targeted behaviors and general administrative procedures. The clinician had already met with the child's mother and developed an extensive list of reinforcers and chip values. The child was to receive a star for each category that met with specified compliance, i.e., behavior was not disproportionate to the classroom norm. We had discussed the possible need for medication, but we felt that this type of a management system should be attempted first. We also expanded the program into the home setting, though not before mother and clinician met to discuss other parenting-related issues that had surfaced during the evaluation.

Classroom management of interfering or disruptive behavior does not always require a lot of additional teacher time. As can be seen by the program outlined in Table 4.3, the teacher was not asked to spend much time completing forms. Of course, the form presented here was specific to the child: Other more- or less-detailed monitoring cards can be developed, depending upon the student's grade and need. The key is home–school communication and cooperation. Whether one employs token reinforcement, encouragement-reprimand, contingency contracting, or a home–school behavior management program, we suggest that such intervention be carefully developed and based upon results from a thorough evaluation of presenting behavior within the home and school setting. These programs may appear relatively simple on the surface (and to a degree they are), but many subtle factors must be addressed before they will prove successful. For these reasons, we believe they should not be implemented on a casual basis, only after appropriate assessment and consultation are provided.

PHARMACOLOGICAL TREATMENT

Many children identified as having one or more of the Disruptive Behavior Disorders are placed on medication. The most often used medications are

TABLE 4.2
Psychometric Profile of a 6½-year-old girl with diagnosis of Attention-deficit Hyperactivity Disorder

CBCL-T		*CBCL-P*	
Anxious	55	Depressed	55
Social Withdrawal	60	Social Withdrawal	55
Depressed	55	Somatic Complaints	55
Unpopular	57	Schizoid–Obsessive	55
Self-destructive	69	Hyperactive	85
Inattentive	68	Sex Problems	55
Nervous–Overactive	71	Delinquent	57
Aggressive	63	Aggressive	55
		Cruel	70
CTRS		*CPRS*	
Conduct	46	Conduct	58
Hyperactivity	88	Impulsive-Hyp.	55
Inattentive-Pass.	70	Hyp. Index	85
Hyp. Index	75		
SSQ		*HSQ*	
No. of Problems	7.0	No. of Problems	9.0
Mean Severity	5.9	Mean Severity	4.2
Unsupervised Setting	1.7	Nonfamily Transactions	1.5
Task Performance	4.2	Custodial Transactions	3.2
Special Events	2.5	Task-Perf. Transactions	5.0
		Isolate Play	0.0

In-clinic Restricted Academic Observation
Off task   80%; Fidgeting   67%; Out of seat   27%; Vocalizing   93%; Plays with objects   10%.

stimulants. There is little doubt that in the majority of children with such disorders medication facilitates a normalizing effect in their behavior that can be observed across several domains. Perhaps most common is the administration of stimulants to children with ADHD as the primary diagnosis. These pharmacologic agents are less commonly used with children primarily diagnosed with Oppositional-Defiant or Conduct Disorders, although they may have their place even within this population (O'Donnell, 1985; Rapoport,

TABLE 4.3
Home–School Behavior Monitoring Card

Name_____   **Day**_____

Subject	Raised Hand Before Talking	Stayed in Seat or Place	Work Done Correctly	Worked Quietly
Before Morning Recess				
After Morning Recess				
Afternoon				
Teacher Comments				

1983; Stewart, Myers, Burket, & Lyles, 1990). Because of the relatively wide-spread use of medication within this population, it is important to understand the variety of medicines available, their effects, and under what conditions they should be considered. Since the drugs most often prescribed to these children are stimulants, they will be the focus of our discussion. However, other types of medication used to treat these children will also receive attention.

Types and Characteristics

The efficacy of stimulant medication with children presenting with poor impulse control, inattention, motor restlessness, and noncompliant behaviors has long been established (Barkley, 1981, 1989a; Birmaher, et al., 1989; Campbell & Spencer, 1988; Campbell, Green, & Deutsch, 1985; Cantwell, 1980; Cantwell & Carlson, 1978; Conners & Wells, 1986; Donnelly & Rapoport, 1985; Klein & Abikoff, 1989; Schatzberg & Cole, 1986; Werry, 1982). It is beyond the scope of this section to discuss in detail the wealth of literature on this subject. However, it is necessary to highlight several related issues in order to describe the role pharmacotherapy has in the overall management of children with Disruptive Behavior Disorders.

Table 4.4 presents summary information regarding the three stimulant medications commonly used with these children: Ritalin, Dexedrine, and Cylert. We will make some general comments relevant to all three medications and then add specific comments about each medication. Research has indicated all three stimulant medications have value in reducing the primary and some secondary symptoms often associated with ADHD and are superior to placebo in reducing such behaviors and symptoms. While these medications tend to have similar effects upon the central nervous system (i.e., to stimulate, energize, and otherwise increase arousal), some individuals may have a more positive response to one agent versus another (Barkley, 1981; Donnelly & Rapoport, 1985). If a youngster does not respond well to Ritalin (or one of the others), it may be premature to conclude that pharmacotherapy is not an appropriate treatment. Assuming that proper drug monitoring had been conducted, a trial with a different stimulant might then be indicated. Given that one stimulant may have more or less effect than another, initial response to medication cannot be used to confirm the diagnosis or to decide to terminate therapy. Supporting this contention are data suggesting approximately 25% of ADHD children do not respond in a positive fashion to stimulants, and that this class of medication may also have the same effect on normal children: increased attention, reduced motor restlessness (Barkley, 1977; Rapoport, 1983; Werry, 1982). Thus, using initial response to stimulant medication as a diagnostic indicator or terminating drug therapy subsequent to an initial poor response would appear to be a naive, outdated practice.

Other general characteristics of stimulant medication are the side effects, also noted in Table 4.4. Side effects vary in frequency and intensity. We have found some children to be quite sensitive to stimulants and experience many adverse effects, while others tolerate the medicine quite well. For example, we have had some parents report their child sleeps better at night with a late afternoon dose, while other parents complain their child has great difficulty falling asleep even without the late afternoon dose. Similarly, some children experience diminished appetite during the noon and dinner hours while others eat well all the time. Some children will experience what is known as a "washout period," which may occur for about an hour or so after the medication has lost its primary therapeutic effect and begins to wash from the system. During this period, some children become particularly sensitive (emotionally), weepy, irritable, have little appetite, and may generally be "difficult to live with." Typically, after an hour or so the child returns to his/her "normal" self. This washout period may not be experienced, or not experienced to the same degree, by all children taking stimulants. Concern has also been expressed about the potential for height and weight suppression as a side effect of ingesting stimulants. Results of studies investigating this issue have not been consistent. For children in whom such effects have been observed, the dosage of Ritalin and particularly Dexedrine has been rather high. Barkley (1989a) noted that suppression may not be unusually severe or common if adequate diet control is observed. Nevertheless, children taking stimulants should be routinely monitored for height and weight, particularly if they are slight of

TABLE 4.4
Stimulant Medications, Side Effects, and Typical Dosage

Brand name (generic name) of medication	Preparation
Ritalin (methylphenidate)	5 mg tablet 10 mg tablet 20 mg tablet 20 mg sustained-release tablet
Dexedrine (*d*-amphetamine)	5 mg tablet 5 mg/5 ml elixir 5 mg spansule 10 mg spansule 15 mg spansule
Cylert (magnesium pemoline)	18.75 mg tablet 37.5 mg tablet 37.5 mg chewable tablet 75.0 mg tablet

Typical and potential side effects of stimulant medication as most commonly reported, in descending order

Insomnia, loss of appetite, irritability, headache, dizziness, abdominal discomfort, nervousness, heightened emotional sensitivity, skin rash, tics. (Cylert may also increase lip-licking/biting and/or finger-tip picking and may possibly be implicated in hepatocellular dysfunction.)

Typical dosage of stimulant medication

Medication	Extended Range/Average Range Per Day		Range mg/kg
Ritalin	5.0–60.0 mg	10.0–30.0 mg	0.2–1.0
Dexedrine	2.5–40.0 mg	5.0–15.0 mg	0.15–0.5
Cylert	37.5–112.5 mg	18.25–75.0 mg	0.5–2.0

Dose ranges by weight for Ritalin

Weight in pounds	Range[a] (mg/kg)					
	0.2	0.3	0.4	0.5	0.6	0.7
50	5 mg	7.5 mg	10.0 mg	12.5 mg	12.5 mg	15.0 mg
55	5	7.5	10.0	12.5	15.0	17.5
60	5	7.5	10.0	12.5	15.0	20.0
65	5	10.0	12.5	15.0	17.5	20.0
70	7.5	10.0	12.5	15.0	20.0	22.5
75	7.5	10.0	12.5	17.5	20.0	22.5
80	7.5	10.0	15.0	17.5	22.5	25.0
85	7.5	12.5	15.0	20.0	22.5	27.5

(Continued)

TABLE 4.4 (Continued)

Weight in pounds	Range[a] (mg/kg)					
	0.2	0.3	0.4	0.5	0.6	0.7
90	7.5	12.5	17.5	20.0	25.0	27.5
95	7.5	12.5	17.5	22.5	25.0	30.0
100	10.0	12.5	17.5	22.5	27.5	32.5
105	10.0	15.0	20.0	25.0	27.5	32.5
110	10.0	15.0	20.0	25.0	30.0	35.0
115	10.0	15.0	20.0	25.0	32.5	37.5
120	10.0	17.5	22.5	27.5	32.5	37.5

[a]Dosages are derived by dividing child's weight in pounds by 2.2 and multiplying by 0.2, 0.3, 0.4, 0.5, 0.6, and 0.7 to generate the number of milligrams of Ritalin per dose (rounded to the nearest 2.5 mg).

build and/or have already developed poor diet habits. The side effects presented in Table 4.4 are very often fairly mild, dissipate within the first week or two of administration, and/or reduce in intensity as the dosage is titrated downward. Both positive and adverse side effects of this class of medication, then, may be somewhat unique to the child. As a result, monitoring drug effects across home and school settings is an important facet in the overall treatment program.

The last characteristics to be discussed here are those conditions where stimulants do not appear warranted or are contraindicated. Specifically, stimulant medications should either not be provided or given under extreme care in those individuals with cardiovascular anomaly, hypersensitivity, hypertension, or, in the case of Cylert, renal dysfunction. Stimulants are also inappropriate for general use with individuals presenting with a Thought Disorder or an Anxiety Disorder, as the drug could exacerbate these conditions. It is not generally recommended to administer stimulants to preschool children, although under unusual situations this may be necessary. The success rate in the very young is less than for children age six and above. Last, administration of stimulants to individuals with a history of or current presentation of motor tics should be done with extreme caution. Of concern here are reports noting a high degree of ADHD symptomatology as well as conduct problems in children with Tourette's Disorder and some clinical reports that administering stimulants to some ADHD children has brought on tics or, more seriously, Tourette's Disorder (Barkley, 1981; Comings & Comings, 1984; Erenberg, Cruse, & Rothner, 1985; Golden, 1988; Lowe, Cohen, Detlor, Kremenitzer,

& Shaywitz, 1982; Mitchell & Matthews, 1980; Price, Leckman, Pauls, Cohen, & Kidd, 1986; Sverd, Curley, Jandorf, & Volkersz, 1988). On the other hand, others have suggested that stimulants may not play a direct role in the onset of or worsening of tics (Comings & Comings, 1984; Sverd, Gadow, & Paolicelli, 1989) and that Ritalin may be less likely to exacerbate tics than Cylert or Dexedrine (Sverd et al., 1989). Given that approximately 30–70% of children with Tourette's Disorder may present with conduct problems, learning disabilities, and/or ADHD (Barkley, 1988b; Young, Leven, Knott, Leckman, & Cohen, 1985) and less than consistent findings exist as to the efficacy of stimulants with this population, it would seem appropriate to proceed with a high degree of caution when considering medication for these children.

We would now like to address considerations specific to each of the stimulant medications. Probably the most studied of the three has been Ritalin. As Table 4.4 indicates, Ritalin is available in three tablet forms of varying dosage and one sustained-release (S-R) tablet. Regardless of whether regular or Ritalin S-R is used, positive behavior effects can usually be noted within 30–45 minutes. The regular tablet forms may be crushed or cut in half without altering the therapeutic effect. Each tablet's duration of action is approximately 4 hours, although instances may occur where the positive response will be closer to 3 hours. The S-R tablet has a primary duration of action lasting about 6–8 hours, although this too may vary from child to child. The advantage of Ritalin S-R is that it should have a consistent effect upon the system throughout the 6–8 hour time span. However, with some children the course of action varies. We have had experience with certain individuals where Ritalin S-R appears to lose much of its effect after about 4–5 hours. It may be that some children metabolize this medicine differently, and quite possible that a child may be getting far too much medication in the first few hours and not enough during midafternoon hours. These children may then need a regular Ritalin (5-mg) tablet around noon in order to maintain desired behavior. This process would, however, seem to call into question the efficacy of providing a S-R tablet in the first place.

The necessary dosage to facilitate the desired effect varies from behavior to behavior and from individual to individual. Some have suggested that less medication is necessary for optimal cognitive as opposed to social performance (Werry, 1982). In addition, some prefer to begin treatment with 5 mg twice daily and gradually titrate upward until the desired behavior consistently occurs. Others attempt to gauge the initial dose by means of the child's weight though this procedure has not been shown to be a consistent or precise method of administering stimulants. However, if adhering to this procedure, the typical range would be in the order of 0.3–1.0 mg/kg. If one were to follow this type of an approach strictly, a larger child could rather quickly be taking what we consider to be a hefty dose of stimulant medication (see Table 4.4). One can gain a perspective as to the amount of medication some children/adolescents must have been taking given literature reports of 0.7 mg/kg and above. We included these comparisons in Table 4.4 so the reader could gain an appreciation as to the range of medication children have been given for purposes of research (frequently reported in terms of mg/kg) and general clinical practice.

Dexedrine is available in a variety of forms. The lowest dose (5 mg) may be taken in a regular tablet form or as an elixir. While both have similar effects in duration of action and effect on behavior as Ritalin, Dexedrine is roughly twice as strong as Ritalin. Thus, 5 mg of Dexedrine may be considered equivalent to 10 mg of Ritalin. The 5 mg-tablet of Dexedrine may be crushed without losing its impact on behavior. Dexedrine spansules may be obtained in three forms: 5 mg, 10 mg, and 15 mg, and is to be taken orally. Spansules appear to be as consistent in action as Ritalin S-R. Other than the convenience of not having to take a noon dose, there does not appear to be clear evidence that the spansule has a pharmacologic advantage over the regular tablet (Brown, Ebert, Mikkelsen, & Hunt, 1980). In using the regular tablet, an initial dose for small children may be 2.5 mg and could be titrated upward by a similar increment. It is of course difficult to titrate a spansule or slow-release form of medication as they cannot be cut in half or crushed as one might need to do in a drug–placebo assessment (Barkley et al., 1988), nor can one simply increase the dose by a small amount.

Cylert is a stimulant medication that may be the drug of choice after a trial of Ritalin has proven ineffective (Barkley, 1981). It has a positive effect for approximaely 6–8 hours. Cylert has some advantages over the other two types of medicine in that the street value is less than that of Ritalin or Dexedrine, it is the least abusable, it can be prescribed by telephone (for parental convenience), and it can be crushed or cut in half in order to titrate to the most effective dose. Cylert may be purchased in two forms, a 37.5 mg chewable tablet or regular 18.75 mg, 37.5 mg, or 75 mg tablets. The initial dose is frequently 18.75 mg and titrated, if need be, by the same increment until desired effects are observed. The clinical action of Cylert is slower than Ritalin or Dexedrine, and sometimes optimal therapeutic effects are not well established for several weeks. This may largely be a function of titration, although the same could be noted for other stimulants, in that one may need to adjust dosage over a 2–3 week period before consistent and optimal effects are noted. In addition to the potential adverse side effects of stimulants listed earlier, some have suggested Cylert may cause hepatocellular damage in about 1–3% of children (Schatzberg & Cole, 1986). As a result of this potential risk factor, regular tests of liver function should be conducted during treatment with Cylert.

Several issues regarding administration of stimulants have recently been topics of debate (e.g., how often, drug holidays, etc.). Not long ago it was common for practitioners to suggest that the medication be given only during school hours and not on weekends, during prolonged vacation, or over the summer months (Cantwell, 1980). While it certainly makes good clinical and pharmacologic sense not to medicate unless necessary, current thinking suggests that medication should perhaps be given on weekends and other non-school days. These are situations that frequently pose problems for ADHD children, their caregivers, peers, and neighbors (Barkley, 1989a). Similarly, if an individual enjoys a positive response to medication in one setting (school), perhaps it is a relative injustice not to assist the child in the same manner across other settings. Where the child is taking a regular Ritalin or Dexedrine tablet, a third dose given during the late afternoon or on nonschool days can many times assist family members in managing the child and facilitate the child's capacity to conform to family rules and expectations. Should this be the routine, one must be careful to ensure that sleep patterns are not significantly disrupted. By the same token, it is equally important to give the child an opportunity to function without medicine. If the child can behave in a reasonably appropriate manner and one or more environments are better equipped to manage the child than another, then medication should not be given all the time. In this case, however, a careful system of monitoring behavior should be implemented to ensure the child should indeed be taken off medicine.

Normalizing Effects of Stimulant Medication

Stimulant medication has many short-term positive effects upon behavior. There is little doubt that, in the majority of situations, stimulants are helpful in reducing many of the primary and secondary behavior problems associated with Disruptive Behavior Disorders (e.g., inattention, task-irrelevant behavior, poor impulse control, aggression, and noncompliance) in children and adolescents (Barkley, 1989a,b; Brown & Borden, 1986; Coons, Klorman, & Borgstedt, 1987; Hinshaw, Buhrmester, & Heller, 1989; Klorman, Coons, & Borgstedt, 1987; Tannock et al., 1989). This positive effect or tendency to "normalize" behavior has been replicated across a number of domains. Parent–child interactions qualitatively improve when the child is taking an effective dose of stimulant medication (Barkley, 1985a,b, 1988d; Barkley & Cunningham, 1979; Barkley, Karlsson, Pollard, & Murphy, 1985; Barkley, Karlsson, Strzelecki, & Murphy, 1984; Schachar et al., 1987). Under such conditions, the child is more attentive and has a greater capacity to maintain a compliant manner, display appropriate behavior during task interactions, and initiate more positive behavior. In addition to, and perhaps as a partial result of, the child's behavior improvement, mothers tend to be less controlling and negative and they decrease the number of commands directed toward the child. The entire parent–child interaction may become more positive and rewarding, as opposed to the characteristically tense, stressful, and negative cycle of interaction.

Similar behavioral improvements have been noted for teacher–child interactions, peer interactions, and academic productivity (Abikoff & Gittelman, 1985; Barkley, 1981; Douglas, Barr, O'Neill, & Britton, 1986; Pelham et al., 1985; Pelham et al., 1988; Pelham, Milich, & Walker, 1986; Pelham, Walker, Sturges, & Hoza, 1989; Richardson et al., 1988; Speltz, Varley, Peterson, & Beilke, 1988; Stephens, Pelham, & Skinner, 1984; Whalen, Henker, & Dotemoto, 1981; Whalen et al., 1987). Although impressive evidence exists suggesting the positive effects stimulant medication has on behavior across settings in children with Disruptive Behavior Disorders, it is very presumptuous if not incorrect to believe medication alone will result in consistent and/or long-term positive effects. Some type of environmental management program and/or supportive service is necessary in order to attend to the child's vast array of presenting concerns. Since children diagnosed as having a Disruptive Behavior Disorder represent a heterogeneous group, it is reasonable to expect that their responses to medication will also vary. Positive effects are often not apparent to the same degree in all situations, or for all symptomatology: Specific responses patterns appear unique to the individual (Barkley, 1989a). In addition, stimulant medications apparently have little or no therapeutic effect in a significant minority (perhaps 20–25%) of these children.

One other important consideration in the normalizing effect of stimulants on the behavior of children with Disruptive Behavior Disorders is that of dosage. In reviewing the literature, it became quite obvious that children have required quite a dosage range to optimal effects. This ranged from as little as 0.1 mg/kg to as much as 1.0 mg/kg. Responsive behaviors differed across dosages and settings, with relatively little consistency. It has recently become more common to assess drug efficacy as a function of dosage (Barkley, 1981; Barkley et al., 1988; Evans, Gualtieri, & Amara, 1986; Pelham et al., 1985; Rapport et al., 1985, 1987, 1988). In general, improved academic productivity and social behaviors can be noted within a range of 0.3 mg/kg through 0.7 mg/kg (Ritalin) for most children. Given the varied response to medication previously noted and lack of consistent predictive indicators of responsivity (Halperin, Gittelman, Katz, & Struve, 1986; Taylor, 1988), it would seem questionable to prescribe medication without fully understanding the child's array of presenting problems or to fail to monitor drug effects across settings and behaviors. In addition, it would seem to be equally poor judgment to initiate medication therapy on a fixed-dose or a mg/kg ratio, note little behavioral improvement, and then conclude the child will not respond to medication. Clearly, the varied responses to stimulants require a comprehensive approach in monitoring drug effects.

Other Medications

In situations where stimulants are contraindicated, have proven ineffective, or where there are primary concerns relative to anxious and depressive features (in addition to inattention, poor impulse control, etc.), the use of tricyclic antidepressant medications may be appropriate (Barkley, 1989a; Donnelly & Rapoport, 1985; Schatzberg & Cole, 1986; Watter & Dreifuss, 1973; White, 1977). Evidence suggests that where antidepressants are a consideration, the drug of choice appears to be Imipramine. Pliszka (1987) reviewed a relatively large number of studies investigating the efficacy of this medication in treating children and adolescents with Attention-deficit Hyperactivity Disorders, concluding (in part) that tricyclics may be a suitable second choice to stimulants and may prove particularly helpful in treating these children when presenting with a concomitant mood disturbance. It would appear that low doses of tricyclics can result in improved behavior. More recently, Desipramine has been suggested as an alternative tricyclic medication for use with this population (Biederman et al., 1989a,b; Riddle, Hardin, Cho, Woolston, & Leckman, 1988), though due to the potential for cardiovascular side effects, those taking this medication need careful monitoring (Schroeder et al., 1989).

More common adverse side effects of Imipramine or Desipramine may include drowsiness, constipation, increased blood pressure, tachycardia, skin-rash, dry mouth, and nausea. We suggest where possible a physician specializing in child and adolescent psychiatry function as the medical consultant when prescribing and monitoring tricyclic medications for several reasons. First, by virtue of their biochemical action, tricyclics may be contraindicated more frequently and potentially have more adverse effects than stimulants. Second, in comparison to stimulants, use of tricyclics to treat children with Disruptive Behavior Disorders has been less well studied, thereby necessitating an even more judicious approach in their administration. Third, use of tricyclics would suggest additional affective concerns than are normally associated with these children and may therefore require more intense or varied treatment. Finally, it has been our experience that physicians specializing in pediatric or family practice medicine are generally less comfortable using tricyclics than stimulants and typically refer to a child psychiatrist if one is readily available.

When to Medicate

The issue of when to medicate can at times be controversial and delicate. We have encountered situations where agreement regarding the need to medicate occurs between parent, teacher, psychologist, and physician, which enhances the ease of administering medication and monitoring drug effects. Conversely, situations where one or more individuals are not in agreement require added care in sorting through the pros and cons of medication. These differences can be a function of belief system, poor information regarding rationale for and probable effects of medication, as well as poor communication between parents and professionals. We would like to offer a few suggestions to assist those involved in determining the need for pharmacotherapy, realizing the need to interpret and implement these suggestions in a judicious yet flexible manner. Within this context, we would like to expand somewhat and add to those issues already raised by Barkley (1981, 1989a).

1. The issue of whether to medicate should be decided based upon information gained from a thorough evaluation of behavior across home and school settings. We explained in earlier chapters the necessity for conducting a careful and thorough assessment and why a superficial or cursory evaluation is far from accommodating the breadth of problem behavior of children with Disruptive Behavior Disorders. Part of an evaluation is determining the severity, duration, and related implications of certain behaviors. If the stress level associated with the child's behavior is particularly high and/or the child is displaying behavior that could foster personal injury or injury to others, it may be advantageous to offer a trial dose of medication as one method of treatment. Thus, the decision to medicate should be based, in part, upon the severity of presenting problems, which would be difficult to ascertain without an extensive evaluation.

2. The child's age may be a factor in deciding whether to medicate. Stimulants (and certainly antidepressants) are generally not regarded as appropriate for preschool children. The effects on behavior tend not to be as positive below the age of 4 or 5 as they are for older children. However, there may be situations where a trial dose of medication followed by careful monitoring of effects may prove helpful in reducing certain stressful behaviors in very young children. An additional issue, one that appears more prominent with age, is the child's willingness to take medicine. Adolescents may simply refuse to take their medication and children of all ages may be less than reliable in taking their medication during the school day. The fear of or anxiety associated with being "singled out" due to being sent to the health room or office to take a pill fosters "forgetting" and general irresponsibility in taking medication. Such factors are frequently alleviated by administering a slow-acting or time-release medica-

tion. Children of varying ages and maturity may also have different views as to why they need to take the medicine, which would then affect their rate of compliance. Proper communication with the child is therefore critical.

3. With exceptions for unusual situations, medication should be attempted after other reasonable methods of treatment have proven unsuccessful in reducing problem behaviors. It is at times difficult to decide which interventions should be attempted, the relative level of success expected, and to what degree parents and teachers are willing to be inconvenienced (to say nothing of the child's perception of his interactions) by the child's behavior before medication is considered. Part of the difficulty with this line of reasoning is that it implies medication will be effective. We know that this is not going to be the case in all situations. Nevertheless, there should be some attempt to work with the child and related systems before expecting the focus of intervention to be medical.

4. Somewhat related to this issue is whether to first medicate or to enroll a child in exceptional education. Assuming the child's behavior is sufficient to warrant exceptional education and is consistent with the diagnosis of (for example) ADHD, an interesting dilemma may develop concerning whether medication should be viewed as the last treatment approach or attempted first in favor of the educational perspective of least restrictive learning environment. Part of the reason we addressed exceptional education earlier in the manner we did was to suggest that, from an educational perspective, an EEN program really should be the last form of intervention. This would suggest that medication might be an earlier choice of treatment. On the other hand, it would be just as easy to suggest that to "drug a child" without attempting all other avenues of treatment (including EEN services) is an injustice to the child. Both views, in our mind, are very legitimate and equally sensitive issues that need to be resolved in a professional manner. Due to a variety of interactions and unresolved issues, the child may find his way into an EEN program anyway (even with medication), but we have seen instances where, with proper medication and dosage, the child's capacity to function within acceptable parameters improves to the point that exceptional education is not necessary. We suggest a careful, sensitive, and realistic appraisal of child/parent needs before deciding on one approach over another.

5. There needs to be some degree of assurance that the child's parents will administer medication in a responsible manner, following physician recommendations. Parents should be told it is not permissible to alter the dosage as a function of child behavior, family activity, or parental mood without informing the physician. If one suspects parental irresponsibility, potential for child or parent to abuse the medication, or in some instances school irresponsibility in administering the noon dose, greater supervision may have to be exercised.

6. Prior to administering medication, we suggest a thorough physical be conducted in order to rule out medical complications in accounting for the presenting behavior profile. In addition, this allows the physician to gain a baseline relative to height, weight, blood pressure, etc., and other related factors that would enter into a medical monitoring process regarding the positive and negative side effects of medication. An important consideration is to ferret out any contraindications that would preclude the use of a particular type of medication, e.g., tics, excessive anxiety, depression.

7. Since children and adolescents may require dosage adjustment prior to establishing an optimal dose or perhaps a different stimulant if one proves ineffective, the administration and monitoring of medication is not a simple and quick process. It requires cooperation on the part of parents and teachers in documenting any behavior changes noted within their respective environments and reporting them to the attending physician. Without parents, teachers, and physician communicating effectively, medication could be inappropriately maintained, increased, or terminated. Clearly, when children are placed on a behavior-controlling medicine, there should be a systematic and well-designed method to monitor effects. We will suggest a protocol for this type of monitoring in Chapter 5.

8. The use of medication should not be viewed as a "cure-all": It should be used in conjunction with appropriate behavior-management strategies in the home and school settings as well as with curricular adjustments. To medicate and not address related social, emotional, academic, and/or familial issues just because the child seems better controlled is to work against the rationale behind conducting a thorough assessment and the offering of a complete treatment program. Drugs, after all, "teach" nothing to anyone. The child, family, and educational system require other methods of coping and adjusting to one another's needs and expectations. Medication may well assit this process, but individuals presenting with behaviors ranging from attention deficits to conduct deficits all too often have problems that medication by itself simply cannot address.

9. Parents and teachers should be given accurate information as to potential side effects and general information about the medication being prescribed.

PARENT TRAINING IN BEHAVIOR MANAGEMENT

Overview

Behavior Parent Training (BPT) refers to a set of procedures based upon respondent and operant learning principles and designed to alter the reciprocal interaction patterns that exist between parents and children. The goals of these procedures typically include increasing appropriate, proactive, competent parent child-management techniques and decreasing general child noncompliance and behavior problems. The literature examining parent training is extensive, and recently entire volumes have been concerned with its review and synthesis (e.g., Dangel & Polster, 1984; Schaefer & Briesmeister, 1989). Several comprehensive reviews of this literature are available (Berkowitz & Graziano, 1972; Dangel & Polster, 1984; Gordon & Davidson, 1981; Graziano, 1977; Moreland, Schwebel, Beck, & Wells, 1982; O'Dell, 1974, 1985; Sanders & James, 1983; Twardosz & Norquist, 1987; Wilson, Franks, Brownell, & Kendall, 1984), and the reader is referred to these for a more exhaustive discussion than will be presented here. Several programs have been designed specifically for use with parents of Disruptive Behavior Disordered children. Although these developments represent as much a natural evolution in theoretical and clinical endeavors as the activities of any particular individual, several major contributors in the area of parent training (Barkley, 1987; Eyberg, 1986; Forehand & McMahon, 1981) have noted the influence of Constance Hanf (1969) on their subsequent work. Our focus here will be to review the typical components of parent training programs and then discuss several that have demonstrated utility with Disruptive-Behavior-Disordered children.

Parent training involves teaching parents to implement systematically and consistently various techniques based on operant and respondent learning principles in order to manage their child(ren)'s behavior more effectively. The underlying assumption of this model is that parenting deficits, including ineffective child management methods, have been partly responsible for the development and maintenance of child noncompliance and behavior problems. For example, Patterson (1982, 1986) provided a detailed analysis of the manner in which the inadvertent use of negative reinforcement shapes and maintains coercive and noncompliant behaviors. The parent-training approach usually involves formal instruction regarding principles of positive and negative reinforcement, punishment, extinction, and so forth. In terms of specific techniques, at the rudimentary level, parents have been taught the use of differential reinforcement, often paired with mild forms of punishment (e.g., response cost or time-out contingencies) to manage various mild-to-moderate behavior problems, such as noncompliance, temper tantrums, bedtime crying, and similar behaviors (Berkowitz & Graziano, 1972). At more complex levels, parents have been taught intricate techniques, such as token reinforcement systems, negative practice, or relaxation training to manage such problems as firesetting (Welsh, 1968), improper toilet training (Azrin & Foxx, 1976; Walker, 1978; Walker, Milling, & Bonner, 1988), nocturnal enuresis (Azrin & Besalel, 1979), and severe nightmares and sleepwalking (Clement, 1970). Parent trainers (therapists) typically employ a variety of interventions through the course of a parent-training program, including didactic instruction, modeling, behavioral rehearsal, shaping, and structured homework assignments. Evidence suggests that use of parental positive reinforcements or reward systems for attending, participating, and employing the targeted skills enhances outcome and generalization of skills (see Bernal, 1984).

As a strategy for behavior change, parent training can impact the Disruptive-Behavior-Disordered child, parent, and broader family system in a variety of ways. *First* and foremost, interventions are implemented in natural settings, through the individuals who are most influential in the child's life, and making full use of existing sources of reinforcement. As a result, "therapy" is potentially available to the child 24 hours per day, 7 days a week, rather than (for example) 1 hour per week. Assuming a minimum degree of cooperation and consistency on the part of parents, this should yield interventions that are more potent than interventions delivered in more traditional models of therapy. *Second*, parent training offers the opportunity to disrupt the coercive interactive patterns maintained through negative reinforcement that often exist between parents and children. These are then replaced with noncoercive patterns based upon positive reinforcement and effective punishment strategies. As previously noted, if the contingencies that maintain coercive patterns are not altered, a continuation and escalation of aggressive behavior problems may result (Patterson, 1982, 1986). *Third*, as a consequence of developing effective behavior management skills through parent training, parents frequently experience an increase in their feelings of competence (Blechman, 1984). This often has additional positive effects in terms of enhancing parental self-esteem, reducing depression, and perhaps reducing marital conflict and discord. *Fourth*, through parent training, parents are taught a variety of behavior-management skills that are presumably more effective than the skills they employed previously. Parents will hopefully use these skills in future situations to manage their child's behavior more effectively, thereby minimizing or preventing further behavior problems. *Finally*, as a direct result of the increased use of positive reinforcement and the decrease in negative reinforcement and coercive interaction patterns, positive transactions will occur more frequently in the parent–child relationship (Eyberg & Robinson, 1982).

In assessing the efficacy of parent training, reviewers noted that initial studies showed somewhat mixed results. Conclusions were difficult to reach due to the mediocre quality of much of the research. More recently, data from better-designed research have become available. Overall, recent studies have demonstrated that parent training is an effective intervention for many childhood problems. Rincover, Koegel, & Russo (1978) reviewed the types of parenting skills required for successful outcome and concluded that most parents could master these skills with appropriate training and professional guidance. Graziano (1977) expressed the opinion that "utilizing parents as cooperative change agents and training them in therapeutic skills may be the single most important development in the child therapy area" (p. 257). Similarly, in assessing the strengths and weaknesses of parent training, Bijou (1984) concluded:

> Parent behavioral training currently ranks high among the achievements of behavior modification....Everything considered, parent training has as much validity as do other acceptable clinical and remedial practices. It is a feasible and effective way of dealing with children's behavior problems. It is relatively easy to train parents from a wide range of educational and social backgrounds in the essential behavioral techniques (p. 20).

Programs Designed Specifically for Use with Disruptive-Behavior-Disordered Children

Several parent training programs have been designed specifically for use with parents of children with Disruptive Behavior Disorders. We will review four programs that have been developed for use with preadolescents with Disruptive Behavior Disorders (typically ages 3–10) (Barkley, 1987; Eyberg & Robinson, 1982; Forehand & McMahon, 1981; Webster-Stratton, 1981a,b, 1987).

Barkley (1987) has developed an effective and empirically validated program for training parents in the management of behavior problem children. The program was intended for use with children between the ages of 2 and 11 years, although in certain circumstances it can be adapted to children as young as 18 months and as old as 12 years. It was designed primarily for parents of children who display noncompliant behaviors, whether alone or in concert with other childhood disorders, including ADHD, Conduct Disorder, and Oppositional Defiant Disorder. It can be implemented in either an individual family or group format, apparently with comparable effectiveness. Goals of the program include increasing parental knowledge of the causes of childhood misbehavior, improving parental behavior management skills and competence, and improving child compliance with parental rules and commands (Barkley, 1987). Several reasons for specifically targeting noncompliance were discussed in the manual. *First*, noncompliance appears to be the most frequent complaint of families who seek treatment for a child, regardless of formal diagnosis. Thus, the program addresses the concerns that prompted the parents to seek treatment. *Second*, noncompliance underlies a majority of negative interactions between the referred child and his family members, so that improvement in the child's compliance may lead to reduced stress in general family interactions. *Third*, research has demonstrated that noncompliance is a significant underlying factor in a variety of behavior problems. Thus, interventions that are successful in reducing noncompliance may also facilitate improvement in a wide range of behavior problems. *Fourth*, evidence suggests children who exhibit significant noncompliance are at higher risk for later adjustment difficulties, including conduct disorders, delinquency, and poor social adjustment. Again, interventions that reduce noncompliance may also minimize or prevent future difficulties. *Finally*, it is difficult to treat many other presenting problems successfully if the child's noncompliance is not first addressed.

The actual parent training program outlined by Barkley (1987) is organized into ten sequential steps or integrated instructional units. Each unit is comprised of didactic presentations, opportunities to learn and rehearse specific behavior management skills (e.g., methods to increase compliance, decrease disruptive behavior, appropriate use of time-out, etc.), and homework assignments. Each unit can be covered in one session, and the entire program can be completed in approximately 10 weeks. However, the presentation of the program can be adjusted (i.e., more quickly or more slowly) to meet the specific needs of clients, particularly if the program is being presented in an individual rather than group format.

A brief summary of each unit is as follows: *Step 1* is primarily didactic, concerned with teaching parents typical causes of child misbehavior and helping them begin to identify relevant causes operative in their family situation. *Step 2* is intended to sensitize parents to the manner in which they attend to their children, train them to reduce or eliminate their ineffective attending behaviors, and begin to increase more effective forms of attending. *Step 3* is concerned with teaching parents to increase child compliance by contingently responding to compliance with positive social reinforcement (e.g., attention, appreciation, and praise). *Step 4* builds upon the previous step, teaching parents how to attend to a child effectively who is *not interrupting or bothering the parent*. Thus, the parent is taught how to begin shaping child behaviors that are positive, appropriate, and not bothersome to the parent.

It is recognized that socially mediated positive reinforcement is often not potent enough to reduce noncompliance, particularly in clinic-referred children, who may have an extensive history of reinforced noncompliance. Thus, the next several steps focus on comprehensive behavior management programs and punishment procedures.

Step 5 teaches parents how to design and implement effective motivational programs, such as poker chip or token programs, to increase child compliance with parental directives, general rules, chores, etc. In *Step 6*, parents are taught basic forms of punishment, including response cost and time out from reinforcement procedures. The response cost is tied to the program developed in Step 5, such that penalties (e.g., loss of some poker chips) are assessed for inappropriate behaviors. The suggested time-out procedure involves *immediate* isolation of the child to a chair or a corner contingent upon the occurrence of noncompliant or unacceptable behavior. *Step 7* extends information provided in Step 6, to allow for an extension of basic time-out procedures to other forms of noncompliance and/or misbehavior. *Step 8* is concerned with teaching parents how to manage child noncompliance in public settings, such as restaurants, stores, etc. Previous methods (positive reinforcement, response cost, time out) are utilized with some adaptations made depending on the setting. In addition, parents are taught to "think aloud—think ahead," a method of orally rehearsing with the child relevant rules immediately prior to entering the public setting and reminding the child of what positive and negative consequences will accrue from the child's behavior. *Step 9* is concerned with reviewing previous material and helping parents explore how they might use the skills which have been learned to handle future incidents of noncompliance. *Step 10* is a booster session, typically held 1 month after the previous session. Some effort is made to assess the parents' own compliance to the treatment methods, ability to troubleshoot current problems, and make modifications as needed. Parents are warned about the common tendency to slip back into old, less-effective behavior management practices and encouraged to persevere. An additional follow-up session is typically scheduled about 3 months later to monitor their progress.

Forehand and McMahon (1981) provided a detailed description of a parent training program they have developed through their research at the University of Georgia. The program is intended for use with children between the ages of 3 and 8 years, although it can be adapted to children as old as 10 to 12 years. It was designed primarily for parents of children who display noncompliant behaviors, whether alone or in concert with other childhood disorders. The program was built upon the assumption that "the child's noncompliant, deviant behavior is shaped and maintained through maladaptive patterns of family interaction, which reinforce coercive behaviors" (Forehand & McMahon, 1981, p. 46.). Thus, the focus of the program involves teaching parents to change their parenting behaviors, thereby facilitating more appropriate styles of family interaction. Goals of the program include: increasing parental knowledge regarding causes of childhood misbehavior, particularly the coercive patterns of interaction maintained through negative reinforcement; improving proactive parenting skills that utilize positive reinforcement, such as attending and socially reinforcing behaviors; improving the effectiveness of parental disciplinary behaviors; and improving child compliance to parental rules and commands (Forehand & McMahon, 1981).

The parent training program was designed for use with individual families rather than groups. The actual program is organized into two phases, Differential Attention and Compliance Training, with several subcomponents in each phase. The program attempts to teach five skills: two types of reinforcement skills (appropriate attending behaviors and use of rewards), an extinction procedure (ignoring), giving appropriate commands, and a response cost procedure (time out from reinforcement). Each subcomponent has specific objectives relating to the acquisition of one of the skills, a sequence of activities designed to reach the objective, and behavioral performance criteria to ensure that the parent has obtained an acceptable degree of competence in the particular skill. The first three skills are taught in Phase One (Differential Attention), and the last two skills are taught in Phase Two (Compliance Training). Several methods are used to teach parents these skills, including didactic presentations, modeling, role playing, and home practice exercises. The treatment model has been designed to facilitate a gradual shaping and strengthening of various parenting skills. A standardized sequence of treatment activities, organized in a 10-session format, as well as relevant Parent Handouts are provided. The actual number of sessions required to reach all objectives varies from family to family. Thus, while the treatment program is well standardized, it is flexible enough that it can be individualized to meet the needs of each family.

Eyberg (Eyberg, 1986; Eyberg & Matarazzo, 1980; Eyberg & Robinson, 1982) developed the "Parent-Child Interaction Training" program, which teaches parents and children a global set of positive interaction skills that can readily be applied to their unique problem situations. The program consists of two phases: the Child-Directed Interaction (CDI) phase and the Parent-Directed Interaction (PDI) phase. During the CDI phase, parents are taught several "Dos" and "Don'ts" of interacting with their child through didactic instruction, modeling, and live coaching. These interactions can lead to mutually positive interactions between parents and children (Eyberg & Robinson, 1982). During the subsequent PDI phase, parents are taught behaviors and techniques to increase child compliance in a manner that is fair and noncoercive for the child. For example, parents are taught to give clear, direct commands that are stated positively and that require developmentally appropriate responses from the child. Additionally, parents are taught methods, such as time out, to manage episodes of noncompliance.

Webster-Stratton (1981a, 1981b, 1982a, 1987) developed a parent training program for use with children between the ages of 3 and 8 who exhibit noncompliant and conduct-disordered type behavior. It is generally implemented in group format, though can be adapted for individual use. The program is built around 10 videotapes which are commercially available with an accompanying therapist manual (Webster-Stratton, 1987). The 10 videotapes contain 250 2-minute vignettes. Each vignette depicts parents interacting with children and attempting to manage various child behaviors. The vignettes illustrate concepts such as nurturance, sensitivity, individual differences in children, and behavioral management skills. Some of the vignettes include both appropriate and inappropriate parental interventions or behaviors. After viewing each vignette, the therapist facilitates a discussion about the interactions. Parents are given homework assignments to practice various parenting skills between sessions. Through this process, parents discuss their attitudes and beliefs about the depicted parental behaviors, benefit from the modeling of effective parenting behavior, have opportunities to practice behavioral strategies learned, and are provided with considerable didactic information from the therapist in a format which minimizes defensiveness. Several outcome studies have demonstrated that parents report high levels of satisfaction with the program and that it produced positive changes in both parent-child interactions and parental perceptions of child behaviors. Significant improvements were evident in ratings of child compliance and the reduction of deviant behavior, many of which were maintained through a one year follow-up (Webster-Stratton, 1981a, 1981b, 1982a, 1982b; 1984b).

Issues of Patient Selection and Enhancing Program Effectiveness

The programs reviewed above have been designed for use with disruptive-behavior-disordered children and obviously have many similarities. Several of the manuals and other references in the literature addressed issues relating to patient selection and enhancing program effectiveness. These issues will be reviewed here briefly. First, it is recognized that not all families with disruptive-behavior-disordered children benefit from parent training programs. Some families may terminate training prematurely, while others may even deteriorate with this form of treatment. Factors identified as contraindicating parent training include significant parental psychopathology, including moderate to severe depression and/or psychosis, substance abuse, and marital discord, a strong tendency for the mother to insulate herself from social support systems, and whether treatment is mandated or based upon self-referral. Bernal (1984) also noted that many of the current parent training programs are best suited for white, middle- and upper-class families and may be inappropriate (or at least require substantial modification) when used with families of significantly different social, cultural, or ethnic backgrounds.

Second, families of children with Disruptive Behavior Disorders may have other difficulties as well, and it is very often necessary to coordinate parent training with other forms of intervention. For example, either or both parents may be in need of one or more other forms of treatment, such as marital therapy or treatment for moderate to severe depression or substance abuse. Similarly, the child may be in need of other types of intervention, such as medication, special educational programming, cognitive-behavioral or social skills training, or even treatment for substance abuse. Thus, based upon the evaluation, consideration may be given to prioritizing multiple clinical needs and coordinating various interventions. If conditions exist that would severely limit the effectiveness of parent training, these issues must be addressed and better resolved *before* undertaking parent training. In other circumstances, where such difficulties exist but are not severe enough to limit the effectiveness of parent training (e.g., mild depression, or some marital discord, with agreement between the partners that improved child management is needed), it may be best to proceed with the parent training first and subsequently address other issues. In such cases, the gains made through parent training may even reduce maternal depression or stress associated with the marital discord. Finally, in many circumstances it is best to provide parent training and one or more additional interventions *concurrently*. For example, if stimulant medication is warranted, medicine intervention and parent training can commence simultaneously. Even in circumstances where medication provides a dramatic improvement in the child's behavior, its effect often fades in the evenings. Medicine may not be administered during weekends or prolonged holidays. These are times when parents need to engage in effective behavior management, skills that would be taught during a parent training program. Thus, parent training is often very beneficial in providing improved behavior management skills that can result in enhanced child compliance and improved family interaction.

Third, the programs reviewed above have been designed for implementation in a relatively time-limited manner (e.g., 10 sessions). However, there is often a need to take a long-term view of the behavior or other problems presented by disruptive-behavior-disordered children and their families. Barkley (1981) suggested these types of disorders are often not "curable," but require long-term management to minimize negative effects and enhance prognosis. For example, it is not uncommon for such children to present new and different behavior management problems as they mature into a new developmental phase, such as from preschool to primary school, or from primary school to preadolescence, etc. In addition, some parents are less able to generalize the skills learned through a parent training program to novel situations or to deal with the various crises that may develop with each new phase of development. Thus, some parents often need intermittent, short-term "booster" sessions or may even need to replicate the entire program periodically in order to enhance long-term effectiveness. Finally, some evidence suggests that duration of treatment influences the short-term and long-term outcome (Kazdin, 1985, 1987). Based upon these data, it may often be beneficial to extend the length of treatment beyond that recommended in the manuals so as to guarantee sufficient opportunities for extensive modeling and behavioral practices. On the other hand, one need be sensitive to parental commitment, as extending treatment may reduce parental motivation and compliance.

Fourth, there has been much discussion in the literature concerning whether the effects of clinic-based parent training programs generalize to other settings or circumstances, whether the effects are maintained over time, and what if anything might be done to enhance generality. Forehand and Atkeson (1977) provided a review of this information. They indicated several types of generalization are relevant to the parent training paradigm: (1) generalization across settings (e.g., from the clinic setting to the home and school settings), (2) generalization across time (i.e., long-term maintenance of effects), (3) generalization across behaviors (i.e., from targeted behaviors to other behaviors), and (4) generalization to siblings (i.e., the skills learned through parent training were also appropriately used with the identified child's siblings). Several recent reviews of the parent training literature have examined studies that addressed one or more of these types of generalization (Forehand & McMahon, 1981; McMahon & Forehand, 1984; McMahon & Wells, 1989). Briefly, conclusions reached by reviewers are that: (1) parent training is an effective method of increasing child compliance, increasing positive parental child-management behaviors, and improving the quality of parent–child interactions, (2) when parent training is conducted in the clinic, effects generalize from the clinic to the home setting, but apparently not to the school setting, (3) in most cases these effects are maintained over time, with follow-up assessments ranging from several months to $4\frac{1}{2}$ years after treatment, (4) effects generalize to untreated or nontargeted child behaviors, such that there is also a decrease in nontargeted noncompliant behavior, (5) these effects generalize to *untreated* siblings of the referred child, with parents displaying an increased use of these behaviors with untreated siblings, and untreated siblings increasing their compliance with parents, and (6) parent training appears to enhance long-term decreases in aggression, destructiveness, and inappropriate verbal behaviors. Finally, some evidence suggests that maternal depression and marital discord may improve as a consequence of parent training. While methods that might enhance generalization have been examined in several studies, not enough evidence is available to allow for definitive conclusions. Tentatively, evidence suggests that generalization may be enhanced if the program provides parents with in-depth knowledge of social learning principles, ample in-session opportunities for modeling and behavioral practice, and considerable feedback and reinforcement for the acquisition and appropriate use of the targeted skills.

Conclusions

The following conclusions may be drawn from the foregoing discussion. *First*, parent training is immediately concerned with reducing coercive family interaction patterns, improving specific communication and disciplinary skills in parents, and improving child compliance. Evidence suggests that parent training is a practical, effective method of dealing with noncompliance and a wide variety of externalizing behavior problems commonly found in children with Disruptive Behavior Disorders. *Second*, parent training can be provided in either a group or individual family format, apparently with equal effectiveness. *Third*, parent training provides several advantages over alternative models of intervention, as it can be implemented in a relatively brief time frame and by the individuals most influential in a child's life, thereby reducing the "artificial" aspects of alternative models. *Fourth*, some evidence suggests that parent training may have considerable long-term preventive effects, depending on the degree of generalization that occurs either spontaneously or as a result of a deliberate process. This suggests that in addition to improving the current behavior management problems, parent training may contribute to an improved long-term prognosis. *Finally*, although preliminary in nature, some evidence suggests that generalization can be enhanced by providing in-depth knowledge of social learning principles, opportunities for modeling and behavioral practice, as well as feedback and reinforcement for the acquisition and appropriate use of targeted skills.

COGNITIVE–BEHAVIORAL SELF-CONTROL TRAINING

Overview

During the late 1960s and 1970s significant advances were made in the field of cognitive science. These advances have been regarded by some as a major paradigmatic shift in the science of psychology (Craighead, Meyers, & Craighead, 1985). As part of these advances, attempts have been made to apply cognitive theory to the conceptualization and treatment of various clinical conditions. Major innovators in this effort included: Bandura (1977), who articulated the theory of reciprocal determinism; Beck and his colleagues (Beck, 1976; Beck et al., 1979), who developed a cognitive model of conceptualizing and treating depression; Meichenbaum (1977), who developed a series of self-instructional therapy procedures designed to modify internal dialogues and self-guiding statements; and D'Zurillia (D'Zurillia, 1986; D'Zurillia, 1988; D'Zurrilia & Goldfried, 1971), who extended cognitive principles to develop clinical applications in the area of cognitive problem solving. In many instances, the theoretical advances and therapeutic techniques were incorporated by those who had previously endorsed a behavioral framework, leading to therapeutic approaches that have collectively been identified as "Cognitive–Behavioral."

Cognitive–Behavioral Therapy (CBT) refers to a group of related strategies and procedures that emphasize "the learning process and the influence of the contingencies and models in the environment while . . . underscoring the centrality of mediating/information-processing factors in . . . the development and remediation of . . . disorders" (Kendall, 1985, p. 359). As originally proposed by Bandura (1977), the individual exists in an environmental context such that individual and contextual variables reciprocally influence one another. Thus, the CBT approach focuses upon the reciprocal interaction between the individual and his environmental variables. Individual-level variables of interest have included overt behavior, cognition (processes and products), and, to a lesser degree, physiology. More recently, there has been a movement to account for the individual variables of emotion (Craighead, 1983; Craighead et al., 1985) and developmental level (Achenbach, 1982; Craighead et al., 1985). Environmental level variables of interest initially included immediate contextual antecedents and consequences of targeted behaviors. More recently, there has been an effort to also account for more complex reciprocal influences that exist at various systematic levels (e.g., familial, community, societal) (Bronfenbrenner, 1979).

Currently, the CBT literature is well developed and somewhat diverse. Various modifications have been developed to deal with a wide range of adult and childhood disorders. From the CBT perspective, somewhat different assumptions are made concerning the development and maintenance of maladaptive behaviors or negative emotional experiences of adults and children. With adults, perhaps the most fundamental assumption of CBT is that maladaptive behaviors and negative emotional experiences are largely the result of cognitive distortions that lead to faulty perceptions and/or inaccurate attributions about the external world (Beck, 1976; Beck et al., 1979). However, with childhood problems, particularly externalizing or Disruptive Behavior Disorders, the fundamental assumption is that such disorders result from deficiencies in effective cognitive mediating strategies for controlling behavior (Braswell & Kendall, 1988). In other words, it is assumed that the child is deficient in, or completely lacking, the necessary cognitive skills needed to control and monitor his behavior. The goal of cognitive–behavioral approaches with children displaying disruptive behavior problems is to train the child in various cognitively mediated strategies, such as self-control and response-delay strategies, problem-solving skills, self-instructional training, anticipation of consequences, etc. It is then assumed that the development and strengthening of such cognitive skills will lead to an increase in self-control and a corresponding decrease in impulsive and disruptive behaviors.

The literature examining CBT with children is extensive. Several recent comprehensive reviews of this literature are available (Abikoff, 1985, 1987; Braswell & Kendall, 1988; Harris, Wong, & Keogh, 1985; Kendall, 1985; Kendall & Braswell, 1985; Meyers & Craighead, 1984) and the reader is referred to these for a more exhaustive discussion than will be presented here. In general, there is support suggesting CBT interventions are effective for many childhood disorders (Meyers & Craighead, 1984). However, when examining the efficacy of CBT with disruptive-behavior-disordered children, there are many inconsistencies. Several recent studies have not found cognitive therapy techniques to be effective, have documented statistically significant but clinically insignificant effects, or have noted that the effects were no longer evident at follow-up (e.g., Abikoff, 1985, 1987; Abikoff & Gittelman, 1985; Brown et al., 1986; Brown, Wynne, & Medenis, 1985). In a recent review of studies that evaluated various cognitive–behavioral interventions in children diagnosed as having ADHD, Whalen, Henker, and Hinshaw (1985) concluded that "the results of CBT are not very strong, somewhat inconsistent, difficult to replicate, and decidedly disappointing" (p. 393). Similar conclusions were reached by Abikoff (1985, 1987), who concluded that the efficacy of such interventions remains unproven. Similarly, in a review of studies that evaluated cognitive problem-solving skills training with cliniically aggressive and conduct disordered children, Kazdin (1987) noted that cognitively based interventions generally led to positive changes that are maintained for at least one year. However, while many of these changes were statistically significant, they were of marginal clinical significance.

Despite these disappointing trends, methodological difficulties in many of the studies preclude the possibility of reaching definitive conclusions at this time. Perhaps the greatest concerns include the following. *First*, while generally tied to cognitive and developmental theories, the exact nature of cognitive deficits associated with various disorders needs further clarification (cf. Dodge, 1985). *Second*, in many of the reported studies selection criteria and sample characteristics have not been adequately specified, limiting both the implications of and generalization of results. For example, it may be that the cognitive interventions produce clinically meaningful changes in a subgroup of children (e.g., nonaggressive hyperactive children, or oppositional-defiant children without significant hyperactivity) and not in other subgroups. Statistical evidence for these differences may have been lost in some studies due to samples that were too homogeneous. *Third*, the majority of studies assessed the impact of training on various cognitive processes, often in laboratory or controlled situations, rather than on deviant child behavior in real-life circumstances (Kazdin, 1987). *Finally*, few studies attempted to alter contingencies in the children's natural environment to facilitate the shaping and maintenance of targeted behaviors. It is quite likely that the failure to attend to altering such contingencies may lead to relatively rapid extinction of recently acquired behaviors or skills (Braswell & Kendall, 1988).

Given these and other methodological difficulties, and evidence from some studies suggesting that cognitive interventions prove effective with some children who exhibit impulsivity and disruptive behavior problems, there is a need for additional research that further examines the efficacy of cognitive therapy. Until sufficient evidence is available to allow for more definitive conclusions, it does not seem reasonable to consider cognitive-behavioral training as a primary treatment modality with Disruptive-Behavior-Disordered children. However, there may be situations in which including CBT in a comprehensive treatment package is warranted. Thus, for illustrative purposes, we will briefly examine a typical CBT program.

Programs Designed For Children with Disruptive Behavior Disorders

Much of the information currently available concerning child CBT programs is contained in research articles reporting on the development and efficacy of the programs or summarized in various edited texts. For example, programs have been devised and adapted in efforts to increase self-control skills in impulsive and hyperactive children (Bornstein & Quevillon, 1976; Goodwin & Mahoney, 1975; Hinshaw, Henker, & Whalen, 1984a; Kendall & Urbain, 1981; Kendall & Wilcox, 1980; Kendall & Zupan, 1981), improve academic performance in hyperactive and impulsive emotionally disturbed children (Kendall & Finch, 1978; Varni & Henker, 1979), and to control anger in aggressive children (Lochman, Burch, Curry, & Lampron, 1984). The research reports generally contain brief descriptions of the particular CBT program but not sufficient detail to allow a clinician to adapt the program for clinical use. In addition, despite obvious similarities in the interventions across published reports, many differences were evident.

Currently, only a few comprehensive treatment manuals are available that have been specifically designed for use with impulsive, disruptive children or that can readily be adapted for such children (e.g., Camp & Bash, 1985; Kendall & Braswell, 1985; Spivack, Platt, & Shure, 1976). Recently, Kendall and Braswell (1985) provided a detailed, standardized CBT treatment manual designed for use with impulsive children. The manual represents the culmination of more than a decade of empirical research and clinical application by Kendall and colleagues. We found their manual representative of the current literature and written in sufficient detail that clinicians can easily adapt the program for clinical use. In addition, the model proposed by Kendall and Braswell has evolved through their research program, so that it is perhaps the most thoroughly investigated and empirically supported program currently available. Thus, we will limit our discussion to an overview of the program articulated by Kendall and Braswell (1985), while acknowledging that other cognitive-oriented programs for use with children have been reported.

The approach outlined by Kendall and Braswell (1985) was designed for use with children who exhibit cognitive impulsivity, behavioral impulsivity, hyperactivity, and aggression. Although specific age limitations were not stipulated, the program was generally intended for elementary school children (ages 7 through 12) who have average or above-average intelligence. The program includes training in cognitive and behavioral self-control, utilizing strategies of problem-solving, self-instructional training, behavioral contingencies, modeling, affective education, and role playing. The standardized treatment program was designed to be implemented in 12 50-minute sessions. It is recommended that sessions occur twice per week for 6 weeks, although the actual number and frequency of sessions can be modified to fit individual need. Goals of the program include fostering the development of cognitively mediated self-instructions in children, enabling them to "stop and think," and providing the structure to help children learn to consider various response alternatives and their consequences.

The actual treatment program outlined by Kendall and Braswell (1985) is organized into four sequential and integrated instructional units. Throughout the program, modeling, self- and social rewards, and response cost procedures are employed by the therapist to shape child behavior. In addition, various homework assignments are utilized to minimize learning decay and enhance generalization. The first unit (sessions 1–3) focuses on orienting the child to the therapeutic program and fostering the acquisition of self-instructional procedures. The child is presented with a series of relatively simple, impersonal, and nonthreatening problem-solving tasks. While working jointly on these tasks, self-statements designed to help the child "stop and think," follow the stated directions, examine the particular task demands, consider response alternatives, and evaluate the response consequences are modeled by the therapist. These skills are then shaped through reinforcement and response cost. Throughout the second unit (sessions 4–6) the same self-instructional skills that were previously modeled continue to be shaped through reinforcement and response cost procedures. However the nature of the task shifts from impersonal and nonthreatening problem-solving tasks to grade-appropriate mathematical equations and problems and more-abstract puzzles. The goals of this phase are to shape the previously acquired skills and to begin to generalize these to other problem-solving situations where the child's impulsivity may lead to incorrect responding and perhaps behavior problems. Also during this phase, the therapist begins to fade his/her verbal promptings so that the child gradually begins to emit self-instructional behaviors without prompting.

Throughout the third unit (sessions 7–10) the same self-instructional skills previously modeled continue to be shaped through reinforcement and response cost procedures. The nature of the task shifts from grade-appropriate equations and problems to various social and interpersonal situations. During sessions 7 and 8, the therapist engages the child in common childhood games, continuing to shape appropriate use of self-instructional skills. These sessions are intended to further generalize the use of self-instructional skills to various social situations, help the child learn to inhibit impulsive responding, and learn greater adherence to rules. During sessions 9 and 10, the therapist poses hypothetical social and interpersonal situations, many of which are problematic or conflictual. The child is expected to generalize the use of the previously acquired self-instructional skills to these conflictual social situations. Typically, these situations involve exploration of emotional responses. The child then begins to generalize self-instructional methods to inhibit impulsive emotional responding.

The final unit (sessions 11–12) involves further generalization of self-instructional skills to social situations through the use of role playing. In the 11th session, the therapist poses additional hypothetical situations that involve more realistic interpersonal situations, such as waiting in line, or problems encountered while playing games with other children. In the 12th session, the therapist poses hypothetical social situations designed to approximate the types of situations the particular child has experienced. In both cases, the child is expected to employ the previously acquired self-instructional skills and to physically act-out or role-play what he/she might do in the situation.

Issues Related to Patient Selection and Enhancing Program Effectiveness

Cognitive–behavioral interventions have shown some degree of effectiveness with a variety of childhood disorders and have yielded positive results in some studies with children exhibiting poor impulse control and/or Disruptive Behavior Disorders. At the same time, the general trend with children exhibiting such disorders suggests these results are not very strong, somewhat inconsistent across studies, and difficult to replicate. One conclusion is that not all children exhibiting poor impulse control and/or a disruptive behavior respond the same way to cognitive–behavioral interventions. Some appear to derive significant benefit, while others seem to derive little or none. Given these findings, it seems worthwhile to examine the outcome literature to determine what if any child or situational variables serve to moderate the effectiveness. A limited number of studies yield data addressing the issue of differential effects. Therefore, the following conclusions should be considered tentative. First, several interrelated child variables appear to moderate the effectiveness of CBT. Younger children, those with lower general intelligence, and those who are cognitively less mature all seem to benefit less from CBT than children with more mature qualities. In terms of specific levels of cognitive functioning, it appears that the child must exhibit some functional use of logic characteristic of Piaget's period of Concrete Operations. In children of normal intelligence and normal cognitive development, these characteristics begin to emerge in the age range of 7–8 years. Additionally, functional use of more developed reasoning and logic skills characteristic of Piaget's period of Formal Operations (ages 11–15) would seem to allow the child to derive even more benefit from such interventions.

Concerning other potential moderating variables, there is no evidence that gender produces a differential effect. The issues of whether race or socio-economic backgrounds are moderating variables have not been sufficiently examined to allow for tentative conclusions. There is some evidence that the level of child aggression is a potential moderator, with a tendency for more aggressive children to derive less benefit from CBT interventions than less-aggressive children. However, these conclusions are preliminary and sufficient research has not been undertaken to determine whether these interventions may be modified in some manner to produce better outcome with more aggressive children.

Next, it appears that several treatment variables also contribute to effective outcomes. First, evidence suggests that active modeling by the therapist is a very potent means of conveying targeted skills and coping methods. In addition, outcome is enhanced to a greater degree when the therapist vocalizes his or her thoughts while modeling targeted skills than when the therapist does not vocalize thoughts. Second, treatment packages which have provided sufficient opportunities for role playing, or performance-based learning experiences, have generally produced better outcome. Studies have allowed children to participate in role-playing exercises with the therapist and child or with children of other ages. In general, both have proven effective, with peer role-playing situations showing slightly better outcome. Third, utilizing various contingency management procedures as a formal part of the treatment package to shape and maintain appropriate skills appears to contribute to better outcome. Methods that have been utilized successfully include: social reinforcement delivered by the therapist and self-reinforcing self-statements contingent upon emitting the correct behavior or skill; contingency management programs, which typically include tokens (intermittently redeemed from a menu of rewards) for emitting the correct response or targeted behavior; and mild punishments, in the form of response-cost (e.g., loss of token) contingencies. Finally, the intervention program must be of sufficient duration to ensure that the newly trained skills or behaviors become firmly established in the child's repetoire, and if possible that ongoing contingencies are arranged in the natural setting to facilitate generalization and guard against extinction once the program is terminated.

Conclusions

The following conclusions may be drawn from the foregoing discussion. The fundamental assumption of cognitive–behavioral treatment, when applied to childhood problems such as externalizing or disruptive behavior disorders, is that such disorders result from deficiencies in effective cognitive mediating strategies for controlling behavior (Braswell & Kendall, 1988). The goal of cognitive–behavioral approaches with these children is to train them in various cognitively mediated strategies, such as self-control and response-delay strategies, problem-solving skills, self-instructional training, anticipation of consequences, etc. It is assumed that the development and strengthening of such cognitive skills will lead to an increase in self-control and a corresponding decrease in impulsive and disruptive behaviors. Some evidence suggests that cognitive–behavioral treatment has demonstrated effectiveness for a variety of childhood disorders, including disorders characterized by impulsivity and disruptive behaviors. At the same time, there are inconsistencies in the outcome research. It appears that not all children exhibiting impulsivity and/or disruptive behavior disorders benefit equally from cognitive–behavioral interventions, and some seem to derive no benefit.

The following tentative guidelines for the application of CBT with children exhibiting poor impulse control and/or a disruptive behavior disorder seem warranted. *First*, such programs seem to have little effect in most children prior to the age of about 7. Beyond this age, interventions will probably prove more effective if the child has average or above-average intelligence *and* displays evidence of Concrete Operational thinking. In clinical practice, it has been our experience that older children with strong verbal skills respond most positively to this type of training. *Second*, CBT interventions are less effective with more intense levels of child aggression. Children with a primary diagnosis of ADHD who exhibit relatively low levels of aggression may benefit more from this type of treatment than, for example, an aggressive conduct-disordered child. *Third*, the therapist should make use of modeling, with active vocalization of thought processes, as a means of conveying targeted skills and coping methods. *Fourth*, the therapist should provide ample opportunities to role-play targeted skills and behaviors. *Fifth*, the treatment program should include various contingency management procedures as a formal part of the treatment package to shape and maintain appropriate skills and behaviors. *Sixth*, the intervention program should be of sufficient duration to ensure that the newly trained skills or behaviors become firmly established in the child's repertoire. *Seventh*, the therapist should give some consideration to implementing interventions designed to maintain and generalize results outside of the treatment setting, such as arranging contingencies that will maintain and reinforce the targeted skills in the home and school settings. In clinical practice, it has been our experience that when such arrangements can be worked out with the parent(s) and/or teacher(s), the generalization and maintenance of skills is generally enhanced considerably. *Finally*, there is no evidence available that gender, race, or socioeconomic background lead to differential treatment effects, although none of these has been sufficiently examined to allow for definitive conclusions to be reached.

FAMILY SYSTEM THERAPY

Overview

Recently, there have been several interesting efforts to conceptualize Disruptive Behavior Disorders in terms of ecosystems concepts (Buchanan, 1987; Smith, Smith, & L'Abate, 1985; Robin & Foster, 1989). A thorough review of these recent developments is beyond the focus of this text. At the same time, a brief overview is worthwhile. Much of this literature on children with Disruptive Behavior Disorders tends to focus upon understanding patterns of behavior or relationships which exist between various family members as well as between the family system and other systems that might serve to develop, maintain, or exacerbate the child's behavior problems. The focus has generally not been upon replacing existing modes of treatment (e.g., pharmacological, contingency management, educational, etc.) with an alternative focus, (i.e., family therapy).

Within the family system framework, disruptive behavior disorders are viewed as complex and multifaceted in their development, maintenance, and treatment. The family system model does not attempt to replace other modes of intervention, but rather to augment them. Smith et al. (1985) indicated "the most intensive form of treatment of families of hyperactive children combines medical and educational interventions with family therapy" (p. 1170). The systems of concern might include the child's biological (e.g., neurochemical) system, the familial system (e.g., sibling, marital, child–parent), and the relevant social systems (e.g., school, mental health, medical, juvenile courts) that make up the contexts in which the child and family interact. Dysfunctional family interaction patterns, such as ongoing marital conflicts, parent–child conflicts, or conflicts between the nuclear family and extended family (three-generational conflicts), may serve to maintain and exacerbate disruptive behavior in children. Family system treatment interventions are then targeted to the hypothesized relational conflicts. An oversimplified example (which most child mental health professionals have probably seen in the course of their professional work) involves a family system in which parents have basic disagreements about child management which are in part causd by and fueled by ongoing marital tensions. In such a context, the child may routinely be given inconsistent limits by the parental subsystem as well as inconsistent consequences for misbehaviors. It may even evolve to the point where one parent prompts the child to misbehave as a means of aggravating or indirectly fighting with the other parent. Systems therapists would suggest that, in such cases, stimulant medication may reduce the level of overt behavioral overactivity but would not address the contextual influences that maintain the child's maladaptive behavior. The focus of family intervention would be to alter the relationship patterns that maintain the child's maladaptive behaviors (Gurman & Kniskern, 1978).

We have found recent efforts by Robin and Foster (1989) very much in line with the focus of the present text. They have provided a synthesis of behavioral and family system concepts as applied to the conceptualization and treatment of parent–adolescent conflicts. With the exception of pharmacological and perhaps exceptional education interventions for children with Disruptive Behavior Disorders, most treatment approaches (in certain respects) seem to have diminishing usefulness as the child reaches and moves through adolescence. For example, as the child moves through adolescence he/she begins to deal with the developmental tasks of separating from the family of origin, developing an independent identity, and asserting independence. In our clinical experience, utilizing a structured parent training program such as those developed by Barkley (1987) or Forehand and McMahon (1981) with families of adolescents may not only prove ineffective but may trigger a complementary escalation in the parent–adolescent conflicts. An alternative approach such as the one articulated by Robin and Foster (1989) seems to offer greater promise in these circumstances.

The model proposed by Robin and Foster (1989) makes several assumptions about the state of affairs in families with adolescent–parent conflict. It is hypothesized that each of these factors is more or less present in dysfunctional families and that difficulties in any of the dimensions may lead to heightened conflict. These assumptions are as follows: *First*, the family is a homeostatic system that is disrupted by the adolescent's emerging and changing developmental needs for independence. *Second*, the parent(s) and/or adolescent may have some deficits in problem-solving and communication skills. *Third*, some cognitive distortions may occur that contribute to the emergence of misunderstanding and conflicts involving the parent(s) and/or adolescent. Cognitive distortions may include arbitrary inferences, overgeneralizations, absolutist or dichotomous reasoning, perfectionism, etc. *Fourth*, each individual's behavior may serve some function in the larger context of the family interaction. For example, coalitions, triangulations, excessive enmeshment, or excessive disengagement may occur. In particular, the adolescent's rebellious behavior may serve some function within the marital relationship, such as detracting from or preventing the overt expression of marital conflicts. Again, in a given family, one or more of these factors may contribute to the development and maintenance of a clinically significant adolescent–parent conflict.

The treatment program combines problem solving, communication training, cognitive restructuring, and functional/structural interventions in a goal-oriented treatment sequence. Treatment involves four distinct phases: engagement, skill-building, resolution of intense problems, and disengagement or termination. Robins and Foster (1989) provide an outline of a standardized treatment format, designed for ten sessions. In clinical applications, treatment typically runs from 7 to 20 sessions, with adjustments made within each phase to meet the individual needs of each family. In the standardized format, the first phase, *engagement*, requires two sessions. During this phase, the therapist assesses presenting problems within the context of both current interaction patterns and family history, attempts to build rapport with the family, provides a rationale to the family for treatment as a unit, rather than treating an individual, and negotiates a treatment contract. Once the family has been adequately engaged, and a treatment contract been negotiated, treatment moves into the second phase, *skill building*. This phase requires three sessions. During the skill-building phase, the therapist engages the family in discussions and provides some training in problem-solving, communication, and cognitive restructuring. The problem-solving model consists of five steps: problem definition, generation of alternative solutions, decision making, planning solution implementation, and if needed, renegotiation. Families are taught to proceed sequentially through the five steps to arrive at a negotiated solution that accommodates everyone's perspective. Communication training proceeds more informally, as determined by the degree of negative patterns evident in the family's spontaneous communications. As negative or inappropriate communication patterns occur, the therapist interrupts the discussion, points out the negative pattern, models and/or prompts a more appropriate response, and then requires the family to "replay the scene." Cognitive restructuring occurs in two forms. The first simply involves reframing or relabeling negative comments one family member may make about another family member's behavior. The second form involves a more systematic process of attempting to alter relatively entrenched cognitive distortions in one or more of the family members, as in the model outlined by Beck et al. (1979). Various exercises and homework assignments are utilized to foster acquisition and generalization of the skills covered during this phase. Families with relatively circumscribed problems and reasonably intact skills may proceed through this phase in three or four sessions. Obviously, those with more pervasive conflicts, or significant skill deficits, may require much longer to master the skills.

Once family members exhibit mastery of skills covered in the second phase, treatment progresses to the third phase, *conflict resolution*. This phase requires four sessions. During the conflict resolution phase, the therapist sequentially selects existing adolescent–parent conflicts for discussion, problem solving, and resolution. The therapist actively intervenes to assist the family in utilizing recently acquired problem-solving, communication, and cognitive restructuring skills to negotiate and resolve existing conflicts. Typically, conflicts dealt with during this phase are those that initiated family contact as well as those that may have surfaced during the course of treatment. As in the previous stages, exercises and homework assignments are utilized to promote continued discussions and negotiations and to foster generalization of skills. Again, families with relatively circumscribed problems and reasonably intact skills may proceed through this phase in about four sessions. However, those with more pervasive conflicts may require much longer to negotiate suitable resolutions. For example, it may be common that a family presents with major conflicts in three or four areas, each requiring several sessions to negotiate resolution.

The fourth phase, *disengagement*, requires two sessions. This phase is entered once the major conflicts between the adolescent and the parents have been adequately negotiated and resolved. During this phase, the family conducts a final problem-solving discussion and the therapist gradually takes the role of an observer, decreasing the number of prompts and the amount of feedback provided. Then the therapist facilitates a review of the therapy process and attempts to help the family recognize progress made to date as well as where continued problems exist. Therapy terminates with some active planning for future maintenance of the skills developed and the progress made.

To date there are only a handful of studies examining the efficacy of the approach summarized by Robin and Foster (1989). Most of these studies were undertaken by Robin, Foster, or their colleagues, and are reviewed in some detail in the text by Robin and Foster (1989). The literature, while preliminary in nature, offers encouraging results. Several studies have indicated problem-solving communication training has produced statistically significant improvements in problem-solving and communication behaviors as well as indices of family conflict. Most improvements have been maintained at 6–8 week follow-ups. However, data from longer follow-up investigations have not been reported. Similarly, studies comparing the relative efficacy of this approach with alternative approaches have not been reported. We have found the approach to be effective in our clinical practice, particularly in families with adolescents who have ADHD or Oppositional Defiant Disorder. It has proven relatively less effective in families with adolescents who exhibit a more entrenched, longstanding Conduct Disorder. In most cases, however, the program has required a longer course of treatment, typically 20–25 sessions. It is our impression that this approach offers considerable promise. However, further studies are needed to document immediate and long-term efficacy and demonstrate whether it is more effective than alternative approaches.

SUMMARY

In this chapter we have summarized the primary treatments commonly used with disruptive-behavior-disordered children. In addition, we provided a brief review of the literature examining the effectiveness of clinical application of each treatment. We presented issues relating to identifying exceptional education needs in these children. In this context, we examined differences between current mental health and educational criteria, focusing on how they could contribute to identification and treatment inconsistencies as well as potential communication problems among professionals and between professionals and parents. We also discussed the concepts of a least-restrictive learning environment and the recently espoused at-risk initiative. Classroom management of disruptive behavior was also reviewed in the context of the at-risk process. We then provided a brief review of pharmacological therapies, focusing primarily upon the stimulants Ritalin, Dexedrine, and Cylert. Consideration was also given to the tricyclic antidepressants Imipramine and Desipramine. We noted that substantial evidence indicates these medications provide positive improvements in the behaviors and other symptoms of children identified as having a Disruptive Behavior Disorder. At the same time, many individual differences are evident in the degree of therapeutic benefit produced by medications. For example, the dosage required for optimal effect, and the presence and severity of adverse side-effects, and even whether the agents will prove effective appear to vary from child to child.

We then turned to individual and family interventions designed to help the child and family better manage behavior and other issues common to Disruptive Behavior Disorders. First we briefly reviewed the parent-training literature, highlighting several programs designed specifically for use with children with these disorders, noting support for their efficacy. Next, we reviewed and discussed individual cognitive–behavioral training, focusing primarily upon Kendall and Braswell's (1985) program designed for use with children who exhibit problems with impulse control. We noted that while studies examining the efficacy of this approch on children with Disruptive Behavior Disorders have so far produced inconclusive results, the approach has potential usefulness with some children. Finally, we reviewed recent developments in the family systems literature that have focused on conceptualizing the development and maintenance of disruptive behavior disorders in terms of ecosystem influences. We highlighted a recently developed program by Robin and Foster (1989) designed to help families exhibiting adolescent–parent conflicts to negotiate and resolve these conflicts. Although sufficient empirical evidence of this program's effectiveness with families of children/adolescents exhibiting Disruptive Behavior Disorders has not yet accumulated, the approach offers considerable promise.

Our intent was to overview those treatments found most effective with disruptive-behavior-disordered children and their families. The importance of understanding not only the variety of treatments available but being able to select them as appropriate specific to information generated from the evaluation cannot be underscored enough. Clearly, the purpose of conducting a comprehensive assessment is to utilize that information in properly guiding if not providing treatment specific to presenting needs. It may well be that, in providing a comprehensive treatment program, one or more of these approaches will be necessary.

5

DISRUPTIVE BEHAVIOR DISORDERS:
Integrating Assessment

This chapter will focus on issues that need to be addressed prior to the clinician formulating a diagnostic impression and then developing a set of meaningful treatment/management recommendations to parents and teachers. We will suggest an assessment protocol based upon information presented earlier, such that a more standardized approach to assessing Disruptive Behavior Disorders may be utilized. We will then propose a method of integrating this information in a manner conducive to differential diagnosis and the development of appropriate treatment strategies. A comprehensive treatment program for children identified as having a Disruptive Behavior Disorder often includes pharmacologic, psychotherapeutic, behavioral, and educational interventions. We will discuss integrating these approaches, as well as issues involved in integrating and monitoring these strategies. Case examples will also be presented in an effort to highlight certain procedures.

A FUNCTIONAL ASSESSMENT PROTOCOL

An attempt was made in Chapters 2 and 3 to identify methods of data collection that are necessary for a comprehensive evaluation of children presenting with disruptive behavior problems. Subsequent to collecting information from parents, teacher, and child, the clinician must be able to sort through all data

164

in a systematic fashion in order to arrive at an accurate differentially based diagnosis. This is not a quick or simple process, as the clinician's data base will typically include information from several interviews, review of prior records, review of parent and teacher completed behavior questionnaires, observations, and perhaps current psychometric test results.

There are a number of issues to be considered in synthesizing these data and arriving at a diagnostic impression. *First*, those individuals responsible for conducting an evaluation and discussing results and related implications with parents should be thoroughly familiar with psychiatric nomenclature, particularly childhood and adolescent disorders. This we cannot stress enough. Children can present any given behavior profile for a variety of reasons. The clinician needs to be in the position of considering all possible motives and reasons for the child's behavior in order to arrive at an appropriate diagnosis. This suggests that in addition to understanding guidelines, characteristics, and the behavioral implications of children with Disruptive Behavior Disorders and Specific Developmental Disorders, one must also be cognizant of other psychiatric anomalies such as Affective Disorders, Anxiety Disorders, Pervasive Developmental Disorders, and Thought Disorders. With many of these disorders, the individual can present with some degree of inattention, difficulty following and adhering to rules, and generally disruptive behavior. If the clinician does little more than view a behavior rating scale and gain information from a parent, he/she certainly stands to not only misdiagnose the condition but also to miss the wealth of information necessary to provide helpful treatment recommendations and follow-up services. Thus, the clinician has to be in the position of ruling out other psychiatric disorders that could account for the presenting behavior profile. For example, we have been involved in situations where parents were given the impression from another source (e.g., classroom teacher, the news media, family members) that their child might be "hyperactive" due to the child's excessive activity level and noncompliance. After a comprehensive evaluation the diagnostic impression formed was that the child did not have ADHD but some other disorder, such as an Adjustment Reaction or an Anxiety Disorder. There have even been cases where a young child was relatively normal, but the parent did not have a realistic understanding of normal behavior for the child's age. In some of these cases, parents would not have accepted the feedback if it could not be made clear to them *why the child did not have ADHD*, and/or *why it was felt the child had some other disorder* (or no disorder). We feel strongly that, if a mental health professional cannot provide this type of in-depth feedback to parents, either due to a lack of time to complete a comprehensive evaluation or a lack of appropriate clinical background, such a clinician should not be conducting the assessment.

Second, we suggest that in conducting an assessment the clinician follow a relatively standard protocol that will generate relevant information. By this, we do not mean to suggest that one must have a predetermined protocol from which there can be no deviation or modification. There will be situations in which child and/or family needs may not surface until well into the evaluation, and in such cases the clinician needs to have the flexibility to incorporate additional interviews, specialized psychometrics, and/or additional specialized parental/child self-report rating scales. However, we do believe that an initial (minimum) standard protocol is necessary to guarantee that a comprehensive, reliable, and valid assessment is conducted. The minimum protocol we recommend is outlined in Table 5.1. As noted, the protocol should include interviews conducted with parents, child, and, where appropriate, the teacher. In addition, the developmental questionnaire presented in Chapter 2 should be completed prior to the interview. While we reviewed many child behavior questionnaires that have potential use with children diagnosed as disruptive-behavior-disordered, we suggest one or more of the following scales be in-

TABLE 5.1
Suggested Minimum Standard Protocol for Assessing Disruptive Behavior Disorders

1. Review of Developmental Questionnaire.

2. Parent, child, and teacher, interview.

3. Review of child behavior questionnaires completed by parents and teachers.

   a. Questionnaires must be well standardized, multifaceted by design, and allow for statistical and normative comparisons, ideally by age and gender.

   b. While many such scales are available, we recommend that the parents complete the Child Behavior Checklist (CBCL), the Revised Conners Parent Rating Scale (CPRS-R), and the Home Situations Questionnaire (HSQ). If possible, teachers should complete the Teacher Report Form of the Child Behavior Checklist (TRF), the ADD-H Comprehensive Teacher Rating Scale (ACTeRS), and the School Situations Questionnaire (SSQ).

4. If possible, in-clinic and/or in-school observations.

5. Where available, use measures specifically designed to assess impulse control and attention. We do not suggest their use unless they are well developed and standardized and normed by age.

6. Where appropriate, use measures designed to assess general cognitive (e.g., Wechsler Intelligence Scale for Children-Revised, Wechsler Preschool and Primary Scale of Intelligence-Revised) and academic (e.g., Peabody Individual Achievement Test-Revised, Woodcock-Johnson-Revised) skills.

7. Where appropriate, use specialized self-report questionnaires (e.g., Children's Depression Inventory, Child Behavior Checklist Youth Report Form, Reynolds Adolescent Depression Scale, Beck Depression Scale, Parent Stress Index, Issues Checklist, etc.).

corporated in a standard assessment protocol: Child Behavior Checklist (CBCL), Revised Conners Parent Rating Scale (CPRS-R), Home Situations Questionnaire (HSQ), Teacher Report Form of the Child Behavior Checklist (TRF), ADD-H Comprehensive Teacher Rating Scale (ACTeRS), and School Situations Questionnaire (SSQ). Each questionnaire was selected because of its adequate psychometric properties and evidence suggesting each discriminates children with Disruptive Behavior Disorders from normal children and non-disordered clinic samples. In addition, these measures provide an objective baseline against which to assess treatment. It should take most parents and teachers approximately 30 minutes to complete each questionnaire.

There are of course many other questionnaires that may provide useful information concerning dimensions of the child's behavior and parental/family functioning. In situations where the referral or other preliminary information suggests additional data would be useful, the clinician may choose more specialized questionnaires (e.g., Beck, RADS, PSI) than those routinely used. Given normal developmental deviations and situational variability in behavior (as discussed in Chapter 1) it is recommended that additional questionnaires selected meet the following minimum requirements. *First*, the questionnaire should allow for normative statistical comparisons, preferably by age and gender. *Second*, behaviors should be assessed across multiple settings, such as home and school settings. *Third*, the questionnaires should be used to augment, rather than replace, the previously recommended methods of data gathering (e.g., behavioral specificity on the CBCL and situational variability of parent/teacher–child interaction on the HSQ/SSQ). Where the clinician has reason to believe that additional information is needed concerning parent/child affective or family-related stress issues, we suggest using the Beck Depression Inventory, the Child Depression Inventory, Reynolds Adolescent Depression Scale, Parent Stress Index, or the Issues Checklist. Given the array of well-developed questionnaires, clinicians must to be careful to avoid becoming "carried away" and inundating parents and teachers with too many questionnaires.

The last section of our protocol includes psychometric tests and behavior observations. Measures of general intellectual functioning (e.g., WISC-R, KABC) and academic achievement (e.g., WJ-R, PIAT-R) are frequently needed to augment the general behavioral assessment and should be readily available. On the other hand, measures of impulse control and attention (as mentioned earlier) are typically not as available. Since well-developed measures of impulse control and attention are not yet commercially available (other than the GDS), it seems premature to suggest such measures be included as part of a routine protocol. Where they are available, appropriately developed, and normed, such measures would seem to have merit with elementary-school children. We are also hesitant to suggest that behavior observations be included in a routine protocol. There is little doubt as to their efficacy. However, it is likely that most clinicians working with children are not in a setting that has the physical capacity for providing adequate in-clinic observations. A series of observations conducted in the school setting would appear the most reasonable alternative to gathering this type of information, particularly using an instrument such as the one offered in Chapter 3. While most clinicians working privately or in a mental health agency may not be able to conduct observations in the school setting, it may be appropriate to request a school mental health professional (e.g., school psychologist, counselor, social worker) to conduct observations and forward results to the attending clinician. It would, on the other hand, appear reasonable that, if the evaluation itself were to be conducted by school personnel and results forwarded to the child's physician, classroom observations be conducted as a routine part of the assessment.

The *third* consideration involves interpreting and synthesizing information gained through various sources during the evaluation. Table 5.2 may assist in this process. We suggest the outline be used as a "mental guide" in processing and integrating information gained through the assessment. In using this guide, the clinician should note whether patterns of behavior are consistent across categories and informants. For example, similar reports of motor restlessness, impulsivity, as well as inattention across informants and settings (e.g., several teachers, mother, father) might suggest a diagnosis of ADHD. However, similar reports within the home setting and reports of relatively normal behaviors within the school might suggest a family-based problem, such as inconsistent parenting practices, significant marital discord, or child abuse. In addition, relevant historical factors, the pervasiveness and intensity of behavior problems or other concerns, and prior attempts to deal with the problems (and their outcomes) need also be noted. The clinician is in the position, then, to determine whether further testing, completion of additional self-report questionnaires, or some means of gathering supplementary data should be pursued.

At this point a word of caution seems in order concerning interpretation of child behavior questionnaires. We recognize the benefits of their use within a clinical protocol. However, as we suggested in Table 5.2, their interpretation should be viewed from statistical and functional perspectives. From a statistical viewpoint, before a given behavior or cluster of behaviors can be interpreted as either inappropriate or of clinical significance, the behavior must be significantly deviant from the norm for age and gender. This is particularly important as many behaviors in question change through the course of normal development, such as the level of motor activity, attention span, etc. Typically, "significant" deviation is represented in a T-score greater than or equal to 70 (top 2% of the distribution, or two standard deviations above the normative mean). In addition, a score falling one to two standard deviations above the mean merits consideration as atypical. One may view this range as borderline

TABLE 5.2
Integrating Information Gained from the Evaluation

1. Review of developmental questionnaire

   a. Primary concerns
   b. Noteworthy factors in the child's development

2. Clinical interview

   a. Parent: primary complaints
   historical significance
   pervasiveness
   b. Teacher: primary complaints
   historical significance
   pervasiveness
   c. Child: primary complaints
   behavior of child during interview and testing

3. Review of child behavior questionnaires

   a. Parent: factors at or above a T score of 70
   functional or item analysis of factors
   b. Teacher: factors at or above a T score of 70
   functional or item analysis of factors

4. Review of Parent and or Child Self-report Questionnaires
   factors or total test score of significance
   functional or item analysis of scale

5. Review of existing records: psychological/educational/medical (Primary concerns, unusual findings, etc.)

6. Results of psychometric measures currently administered

   a. General cognitive ability
   b. Academic achievement levels
   c. Attention and impulse control

7. Impressions from behavior observations

8. Review effects of previous treatment interventions: Educational, psycholog   ical, medical, behavioral

9. Noteworthy stressors or family/school dynamics issues

or perhaps indicating a mild form of the disorder, depending upon (in part) other information gained through the evaluation and the types of items checked by the informant as being of concern. Generally speaking then, a score falling within the clinically significant range on an Aggressive, Delinquent, Hyperactive, and/or Inattentive subtest or factor may be necessary before rendering a diagnosis of a Disruptive Behavior Disorder. Ideally, such deviations would be evident across several questionnaires (e.g., CBCL and CPRS-R) and across multiple informants (e.g., parent and teacher). Clinicians should, however, be cautioned against hastily making such a diagnosis based solely upon a significant elevation on a factor or ruling out the disorder because none of the relevant factors reached the "cutoff" of two standard deviations above the normal mean. Indeed, such a view would be overly simplistic and clinically naive.

This suggests a more "functional" approach (in addition to a statistical approach) in interpreting questionnaires. Most currently used child behavior questionnaires were developed, in part, utilizing multivariate statistical procedures, particularly factor analysis. Such procedures derive groups of items that are significantly intercorrelated in the normative sample. Clusters or factor groupings are then given a name that is seemingly consistent with the clustering of behaviors, e.g., Hyperactive, Aggressive, Inattentive, etc. However, one should not assume that since an item loaded on a particular factor, the item content is directly or necessarily related to the construct represented by the factor name. For example, on the CPRS-R, item #39 ("basically an unhappy child") loads on the "Conduct Problem" factor. Certainly, conduct-disordered children can be unhappy, but such behavior is not necessary for a DSM-III-R diagnosis of Conduct Disorder or Oppositional Defiant Disorder. Thus, the item may be representative of some children with conduct problems, but it could also be representative of many other types of difficulties, e.g., learning problems, mood disorders, etc. A second example is found on the parent-completed CBCL. For boys aged 6–11, "speech problem" loads under the Hyperactive factor. We are unaware of criteria for the identification of ADHD that include speech problems. Given that a raw score of 10 approximates two standard deviations above the mean on the Hyperactive factor, a rating of 2 on this particular item would account for a rather sizeable percentage of the numerical value needed to attain clinical significance, even though the item itself is not particularly important to the diagnosis. The point of these two examples is by no means to be critical of either questionnaire, but rather to illustrate the need for clinicians to exercise a functional approach to interpreting questionnaire profiles. Indeed, names or titles of factors or subtests from any questionnaire should never be interpreted as synonomous with diagnosis.

Thus, a child who earns a T-score of 70 or greater on the CBCL Hyperactive or Inattentive factor should not automatically be viewed as having an ADHD. It is necessary for the clinician to go beyond interpreting the statistical deviation (T-score) and examine those items or behaviors that loaded on that factor. Items comprising each factor may of course be consistent with the direction of a potential diagnosis (e.g., hyperactive, impulsive, can't concentrate behaviors for the CBCL Boys aged 6–11 Hyperactive factor). On the other hand, some items loading on the factor have little clinical relevance to the given factoral dimension (or presumed associated diagnosis). The point is that the simplistic interpretation of factorally derived clusters of items may result in erroneous conclusions, and the clinician may miss a wealth of information (item content) if he/she does not consider the manner in which the child earned a significantly elevated score. Thus, appropriate interpretation should incorporate *both* the statistical deviation of the given factor, *and* a functional consideration of what items led to such elevation. Table 5.3 illustrates this point. The two girls highlighted in this example were both 10 years old and referred for evaluation due to a variety of disruptive behavior problems. They presented as being fairly similar across many of CBCL factors and HSQ/SSQ summary scores. However, they were given quite different diagnoses. One was diagnosed as having ADD/H and the other as having Childhood Onset Pervasive Developmental Disorder (COPDD). Had the clinician simply given these questionnaires, based diagnostic impressions upon questionnaire data, and then proceeded to suggest treatment, it is quite possible the youngster with COPDD would have been misdiagnosed as ADD/H. Clearly, questionnaires have the potential to be abused (as do all other aspects of assessment strategies) or misinterpreted, and as a result, clinicians must approach their analyses from a responsible and functional or clinical perspective.

The *fourth* and final concern is to view patterns of behavior in terms of potential alternative primary diagnoses. Implicit within this process is the tentative formulation of possible etiologies for the existing profile. We do not mean to suggest that in all cases one will be able to identify an etiology. However, the clinician does need to consider possible reasons or contributing factors for the child's behavior other than "simply" identifying a Disruptive Behavior Disorder (e.g., family/school dynamics issues, medical factors, dysfunctional family, psychiatric anomaly other than a Disruptive Behavior Disorder, etc.). Doing so not only facilitates the process of arriving at a differential diagnosis but also allows for more individualized and sophisticated rationale for treatment.

A fairly simple example is as follows. A fourth-grade student presents with some degree of lethargy and motor restlessness in school, noncompliant behavior, difficulty following directions, poor academic achievement and productivity, daydreaming, and forgetting assignments. This pattern also occurs within the home setting (particularly as applied to schoolwork), although it is more intense due to parental needs to have this child perform well in school and their tendency to "come down hard" on the child for his shortcomings. While this general pattern has been of concern over the past few academic school years, it has steadily become more intense in both settings during the fourth grade. The teacher has become very tired of the child's antics, and parents have come to the realization that perhaps their child will not simply "outgrow" these tendencies. Their previous perception that he is "all boy" is no

TABLE 5.3
**Comparison of CBCL, HSQ, and SSQ Data for Two Girls Given Diagnoses of
Attention Deficit Disorder with Hyperactivity (ADD/H) and Childhood Onset
Pervasive Developmental Disorder (COPDD)**

Factor	T score		Factor	T score	
	ADD/H	COPDD		ADD/H	COPDD
Child Behavior Checklist–Teacher			*Child Behavior Checklist–Parent*		
Anxious	62	73	Depressed	76	80
Social Withdrawal	57	75	Social Withdrawal	76	78
Depressed	85	85	Somatic Complaints	72	72
Unpopular	77	75	Schizoid–Obsessive	68	68
Self-destructive	73	65	Hyperactive	83	84
Inattentive	77	98	Sex problems	70	55
Nervous–Overactive	81	81	Delinquent	76	76
Aggressive	80	71	Aggressive	83	81
			Cruel	77	66
Home Situations Questionnaire			*School Situations Questionnaire*		
Number of problems	7	8	Number of problems	11	14
Mean severity	4.4	4.1	Mean severity	5.0	4.1

Note: Diagnostic categories were based upon the DSM-III. Both girls in this comparison were 10 years old.

longer amusing or acceptable. As curricular demands became sophisticated in nature and required greater independence on the part of the child for completing assignments, this student became increasingly frustrated and experienced more failure. Prior to the referral, parents and teachers believed that the presenting profile was a function of attitude and that an acceptable academic/behavior profile could be attained if only the student would "apply himself." In the initial interview, parents indicated he was a youngster in good general health and had no prior medical complications. He had always appeared somewhat more active and rougher than peers, but parents did not view such behavior as being a "real problem." Conduct grades prior to this school year were usually below average but not significantly deficient. Academic skills were immature. On parent- and teacher-completed behavior questionnaires, Inattentive/Hyperactive and Aggressive factors to fell within 1 to 2 standard deviations above the mean, based upon age and gender norms. Psychometric testing indicated average general intelligence, but basic spelling and particularly reading skills approximated a two-year deficit, certainly enough to create functional problems within the classroom. The child was placed in a program for the learning-disabled and mainstreamed for those academic areas in which he could be successful. He was enrolled within the exceptional education program due to the academic deficits, which appeared of primary concern, and not because of behavior. The M-Team viewed the presenting nonacademic behaviors as secondary in nature and in part due to the frustration experienced and a sense of being overwhelmed. It was not felt that the child had an ADHD. By no means did the inappropriate social and oppositional behaviors simply disappear subsequent to being enrolled in the learning disabilities program, but parents and teachers were better able view this child's behavior from a more developmental perspective, and from the context of frustration secondary to the learning disability. This allowed them to develop more appropriate goals and expectations for this child. A behavior management program was then implemented in an attempt to deal more effectively with the presenting nonacademic behaviors. The point of this rather simple example is to suggest that behaviors can occur for a variety of reasons, and if the clinician is to provide an appropriate diagnosis by virtue of, in part, ruling out other problems, alternative explanations for behavior must be considered. Parenthetically, these parents initiated the evaluation because they thought their child had "ADD" based upon information gained from listening to a television talk show. One could apply this scenario to many different clinical situations in which there exist, for example, two forms of a Disruptive Behavior Disorder (one secondary to the other), or disruptive behavior secondary to a Psychoactive Substance Use Disorder, an Adjustment Disorder, an Anxiety Disorder, etc. Thus, the process of identifying and ruling out psychiatric problems is far from a simple, quick, and unifaceted process.

Once information gained through the clinical assessment is synthesized and differential diagnostic conclusions are reached, the focus shifts to discussing and implementing appropriate treatment. As noted in Chapter 1, evidence suggests that most children with one or more Disruptive Behavior Disorders exhibit a variety of problems throughout childhood, adolescence, and perhaps well into adulthood. It is not uncommon for new and different problems to emerge as the child develops and matures. In addition, some evidence suggests that the child's problems may contribute to or exacerbate intrapersonal and/or interpersonal dynamics issues with other family members, such as maternal depression, or marital conflicts. Thus, a realistic approach to intervention with most of these children and their families should necessarily have a long-term, multidisciplinary focus. It should be obvious that no one professional can hope to treat the myriad of problems that may develop with most of these children and their families. A fair degree of interdisciplinary cooperation will be required for effective management. In general, the goal of treatment should be to assist parents and child (and teacher) to manage the disorder, rather than holding onto unrealistic hopes for a "cure." Intervention should be designed to minimize current problems, improve the general quality of the child's and family's lives, and attempt to alter factors in such a manner that long-term prognosis may be improved. In addition, emphasis should be on developing treatment that addresses the unique features or characteristics of the child and family. For example, a clinician may be working with two ADHD children of the same age who present with nearly identical behavior profiles. In one family the parents may be reasonably supportive of one another and very amenable to a parent-training program as well as other treatment. In this family, intervention would probably be undertaken with some success. In the other family, there may be longstanding marital conflicts and some evidence that the adults undermine each other in their parenting efforts. In this family, it would be unlikely that the parent-training program would have much success, at least without attempting to resolve certain marital dynamics, and so the specific intervention of parent training would probably not be an initial suggestion.

The most common treatment approaches utilized with children exhibiting Disruptive Behavior Disorders were reviewed in Chapter 4 and fall into three broad categories: pharmacological, psychosocial, and educational. This implies that, for most situations, effective management may require interdisciplinary cooperation involving mental health professionals, physicians, and school personnel. The process of progressing from initial presentation, through a comprehensive evaluation, culminating in appropriate treatment and management of behavior is summarized in Figure 5.1. Each category of treatment involves an ongoing series of choice points, including an initial determination of which interventions are perhaps most critical to begin with. If several types of interventions are indicated, it must be determined whether they could be undertaken simultaneously or whether they need to be prioritized and undertaken sequentially. Several specific issues must then be addressed relative to each category or type of intervention. These would include selecting the specific intervention to be used, monitoring and assessing effectiveness, and reevaluating whether the intervention needs to be continued or altered. Again, the focus should remain on long-term management of the disorder and not simply on an immediate "fix" to the problem. Ideally, the comprehensive evaluation will provide enough relevant data to allow some meaningful consideration of which forms of intervention would be most responsive to the child's and family's needs as well as provide a data base by which treatment efficacy and long-term progress may be assessed.

While much of this seems straightforward, we have seen too many situations in which a clear, treatment-focused assessment of Disruptive Behavior Disorders has not been followed. For example, we have seen situations where the child and family could probably have derived substantial benefit from all three types of interventions (e.g., medication, psychosocial, educational). However, once medication was initiated and some improvements were noted in the child's behaviors, other modes of intervention were not undertaken, and no

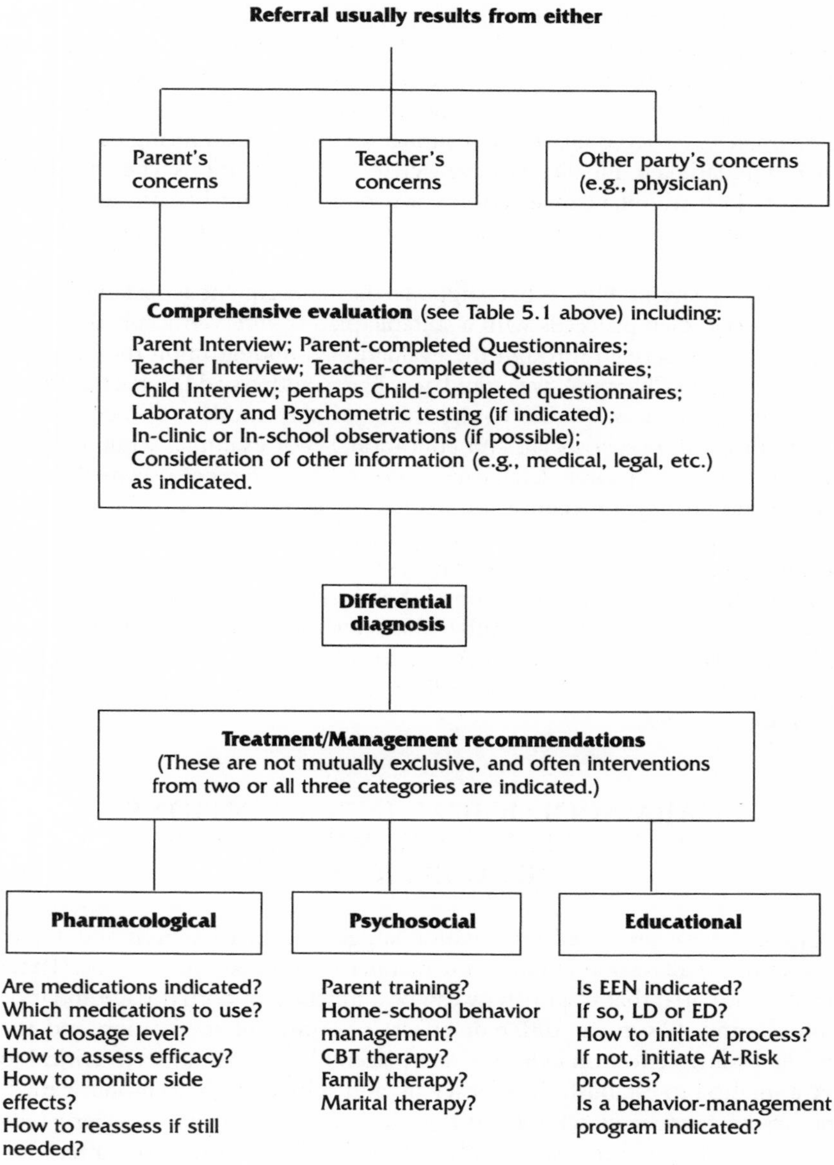

Referral usually results from either

| Parent's concerns | Teacher's concerns | Other party's concerns (e.g., physician) |

Comprehensive evaluation (see Table 5.1 above) including:

Parent Interview; Parent-completed Questionnaires;
Teacher Interview; Teacher-completed Questionnaires;
Child Interview; perhaps Child-completed questionnaires;
Laboratory and Psychometric testing (if indicated);
In-clinic or In-school observations (if possible);
Consideration of other information (e.g., medical, legal, etc.)
as indicated.

Differential diagnosis

Treatment/Management recommendations
(These are not mutually exclusive, and often interventions
from two or all three categories are indicated.)

Pharmacological	**Psychosocial**	**Educational**
Are medications indicated?	Parent training?	Is EEN indicated?
Which medications to use?	Home-school behavior	If so, LD or ED?
What dosage level?	management?	How to initiate process?
How to assess efficacy?	CBT therapy?	If not, initiate At-Risk
How to monitor side	Family therapy?	process?
effects?	Marital therapy?	Is a behavior-management
How to reassess if still		program indicated?
needed?		

FIGURE 5.1. Flow chart depicting major phases in a treatment-focused assessment of a child presenting with disruptive behavior problems.

one continued to monitor the child's or family's ongoing adjustment. Similarly, we have observed situations where the child had academic delays and did not (yet?) qualify for an EEN program. Student's have then been left in a relative state of educational limbo, as no one seems to know quite what to do. Unfortunately, At-Risk initiatives or similar long-term monitoring procedures were not undertaken. Finally, we have seen too many situations where the child was started on stimulant medication with some apparent benefit, and maintained for several years with no systematic reassessment to determine the need for medication.

The flow chart in Figure 5.1 suggests that subsequent to establishing a diagnosis, one then proceeds with a suitable plan of intervention based upon the many needs derived through the evaluation. Building upon the information presented in Chapter 4, we would now like to address additional treatment issues and procedures specific to the three primary modes of intervention: pharmacological, psychosocial, and educational. For example, while medication was discussed in some detail earlier, no specific reference was made to an effective monitoring procedure. Similarly, while we discussed the need for improved and increased behavior-management skills for parents and teachers when interacting with disruptive-behavior-disordered children, we would now like to suggest how to implement a basic behavior-management program. The sequence *thus* far has been to offer characteristics, intervention, and now methods of integrating or implementing treatment. We close this chapter by presenting two case studies we believe exemplify the processes offered throughout this text.

PHARMACOLOGICAL INTERVENTIONS: ESTABLISHING AND MONITORING DRUG EFFICACY

In Chapter 4 we presented information suggesting that children and adolescents may not all respond in the same manner to stimulant medication. These data also indicated that responsivity can be a function of both dosage and type of medication. Given the different effects of stimulant medication and the periodic positive effect on behavior that placebo has, it would seem critical to have a method to establish the efficacy of, and subsequently to monitor medicine across home and school settings. It is relatively naive to query only parents as to drug effects, particularly if the child is not taking a late-afternoon dose. Unless parents discuss changes in their son or daughter's behavior with the classroom teacher, they may not be in the best position to provide feedback to the attending physician. We suspect many parents of children taking stimulant medication do not understand the types of questions to ask a teacher. Also, we are not certain that teachers necessarily understand the types of behaviors they should be observing. That is, global impressions of child behavior (e.g., she seemed to be better this week or nothing has really changed this week) may be insensitive to the types of changes that could occur as a result of pharmacotherapy. It is therefore necessary to have in place a consistent method or protocol to monitor behavior and the side effects of medication typically given to children with Disruptive Behavior Disorders.

In developing such a protocol, a number of factors should be considered. *First*, different settings may have more or less opportunity to implement such a protocol. Obviously, settings that specialize in identifying and treating Disruptive Behavior Disorders may be in the position of having observation rooms with one-way mirrors, finances that might allow for an instrument such as the Gordon Diagnostic System, and other physical accommodations that would facilitate implementing a most impressive protocol. Others, however, simply will not have these luxuries, though they may still have to offer some type of protocol to their clients. We would like to present both a detailed protocol and one that, at minimum, could easily be implemented by any individual in the position of monitoring drug effects. *Second*, initial procedures involving a placebo would have to use the regular Ritalin or Dexedrine tablet and not a timed-release or slow-acting stimulant. Drug–placebo protocols typically call for the drug to be crushed, and these are the only two stimulants that may be crushed without losing their pharmacologic impact upon the central nervous system. While Cylert may be crushed without losing its effect, it is a slower-acting medicine and its use within this type of a format is not recommended. This is not to suggest, however, that one could not use Cylert with a placebo, only that it may be easier and quicker to establish efficacy (initially) using one of the other stimulants. *Third*, part of the protocol involves monitoring side effects through a questionnaire. We will present two such questionnaires for clinical use, one for stimulants and one for antidepressants. These should be viewed as a general but suitable overview of possible side effects for either medication. Certain medications (particularly the antidepressants) may require the clinician to develop a more detailed account of side effects to aid informants. Given these considerations, we would now like to discuss the development and implementation of a protocol that could be used in establishing drug efficacy and subsequent monitoring procedures.

Rationale and Development of a Drug–Placebo Protocol

Most protocols designed to assess the differential dosage effects of Ritalin employ multiple measures across a variety of settings. Clinics specializing in child psychology and psychiatry are becoming more common, and these settings likely have the physical accommodations to conduct a detailed assessment of drug responsiveness. Although measures chosen for inclusion may vary from clinic to clinic, they typically focus upon child behavior within the home and school settings, drug side effects, academic productivity, as well as impulse control and attention span (Barkley, Fischer, Newby, & Breen, 1988; Barkley, McMurray, Edelbrock, & Robbins, 1989; Pelham & Hoza, 1987). Since Barkley and his colleagues have developed one of the more thorough methods of establishing drug efficacy, we would like to review their approach as a prototype drug–placebo evaluation protocol. The outline of their multimethod assessment for establishing drug efficacy is presented in Appendix C. As can be seen, the procedure includes measures assessing elements of behavior within the home, school, and clinic, attention span, impulse control, verbal memory, as well as potential drug side effects. These measures are appropriate for use in that they adequately provide data regarding the core behaviors of children with Disruptive Behavior Disorders, account for the pervasive and situational varied nature of problem behavior with these children, and have generally been shown to be sensitive to drug effects. Their protocol also suggests using, at least to some degree, the same measures during an initial evaluation as during the drug–placebo evaluation. One could, of course, expand the data base for purposes of an initial evaluation, but the drug–placebo protocol should include as many of the same measures used earlier as possible. This would allow for the acquisition of unbiased baseline information. If such initial data are not available, a one-week baseline may need to be established before implementing the drug–placebo evaluation. However, there may be situations where the need for establishing drug efficacy is at a premium and an additional week to gather unbiased information (just for the sake of the evaluation) may prove cumbersome if not annoying to parents and teachers. Thus we suggest, where possible, including measures in the initial evaluation for a suspected Disruptive Behavior Disorder that would probably be used in conducting a drug–placebo assessment, should this be one potential recommendation to result from the evaluation.

Not all clinicians providing services to disruptive-behavior-disordered children and their families have the physical accommodations, time, or administrative assistance to conduct a drug–placebo assessment in the manner just described. It may become necessary to establish a protocol that is somewhat less comprehensive yet at the same time provides sufficient information necessary to establish drug efficacy. Afterall, the primary rationale for conducting such an assessment is to permit structured observations of behavior during drug conditions in a method conducive to determining whether medication was more effective than placebo (or baseline) in improving behavior, and if so, in which settings was behavior change noted and to what degree was improvement a function of dosage. In providing this information we believe that, at minimum, information should be obtained from the home and school regarding changes in behavior as well as the degree to which side effects are present. This would entail completion of questionnaires sensitive to such behavior.

In so doing, we suggest the HSQ, SSQ, CPRS-R, ACTeRS, and a Side Effects Questionnaire would nicely suffice in these situations. The HSQ and SSQ are presented in Appendix B, information on obtaining the CPRS-R and ACTeRS are also in Appendix B, and the side effects questionnaire is located in Appendix C. We chose these measures because of their acceptable psychometric characteristics, item content, factoral dimensions, and ease of administration/scoring. Admittedly, there are other questionnaires suitable for this type of protocol and they could be substituted in place of those presented here, providing they too met with acceptable psychometric and clinical standards. Tables 5.4 and 5.5 present an outline of a protocol and summary chart we have found to provide appropriate information regarding behavior change; these are of practical utility insofar as they do not require an inordinate amount of time to complete or implement. (Appendix C contains a more extensive suggested protocol for those with more time and resources.) If behavior observations can be completed and/or well-developed computerized tests of attention span and impulse are available, they too may be added as they would only enhance the comprehensiveness of the drug–placebo protocol.

Table 5.6 illustrates a completed drug–placebo protocol that had been conducted with a 14-year-old student diagnosed as having an ADD without Hyperactivity. Parenthetically, certain measures used in this protocol were different from those proposed in this text. The discrepancy was a function of clinic policy and availability of questionnaire. In any case, the general format

---

TABLE 5.4
Protocol for Establishing Efficacy of Stimulant Medication

1. Parent-completed Questionnaire

    a. Conners Parent Rating Scale-Revised
    b. Home Situations Questionnaire
    c. Home Side Effects Questionnaire

2. Teacher-completed Questionnaire

    a. ACTeRS
    b. School Situations Questionnaire
    c. School Side Effects Questionnaire

3. Clinic Measures

    a. Gordon Diagnostic System
    b. Observations within a Restricted Academic Situation format

TABLE 5.5
Drug–Placebo Summary Chart

Child's Name_____ Age_____ Parents_____
Drug Conditions: Week 1_____ Week 2_____ Week 3_____

	Condition			
Variable	Baseline	Week 1	Week 2	Week 3

Parent-completed Section

Side Effects Questionnaire
  Number of side effects
  Mean rating

Home Situations Questionnaire
  Number of problem situations
  Mean rating
  Factor raw scores
    Nonfamily transactions
    Custodial transactions
    Task-performance transactions
    Isolate play

Conners Parent Questionnaire

  Factor raw scores
    Conduct problems
    Impulsive-hyperactive
    Hyperactive index

Teacher-completed Section

Side Effects Questionnaire
  Number of side effects
  Mean rating

School Situations Questionnaire
  Number of problem situations
  Mean rating
  Factor raw scores
    Unsupervised settings
    Task performance
    Special events

ACTeRS raw scores
  Attention
  Hyperactivity
  Social skills
  Oppositional

is consistent with our proposal. The primary reason for the referral was to determine the effectiveness of his current Ritalin therapy. Results indicated that medication had a positive effect upon many aspects of his behavior. It was ultimately decided that 10 mg, tid, was the most effective dosage to sustain the type of attention necessary to aid in academic productivity in the school setting and during the evening hours. However, it is also clear that all measures did not show improvement, an observation that is not uncommon in a protocol assessing multiple behaviors. It would be rather difficult to find consistent behavior change across all variables and conditions. Nevertheless, it is important to note both specific aspects of behavior change and any general trends. That is, while one particular measure may suggest limited improvement, the joint effect of the other measures may be to suggest a consistent level of improvement. This approach along, with subjective analyses by parents, teachers, and child would typically be sufficient to determine whether enough behavior change had occurred across conditions to warrant continued use.

Procedure for Implementing a Drug–Placebo Assessment

After developing a set of measures conducive to establising drug efficacy, the clinician then must begin designing a method by which the assessment will be implemented. We suggest the following procedures be considered in conducting a drug–placebo evaluation.

1. An overview of design is discussed with physician and parents. This will ensure that all participants understand the rationale, goals, and procedures. Data collection should be as consistent as possible, i.e., home, school, and clinic data should be completed on the same day each week by the same informant. It should also be made clear at this point that parents and teachers will be kept blind to the child's drug condition. In situations where undergraduate or graduate-level students or clinic employees are conducting observations and/or psychometric assessments and then reporting data to the supervising clinician, they also should be kept blind to drug conditions. The child's teachers may then be provided the same information. Parents need to be assured that, if adverse side effects occur, they may call the physician and/or clinician and have the procedure terminated. Upon completion a report will then be provided outlining the basic procedure, dosage of medicine used, order of administration, changes noted across settings and/or dosages, and suggestions for continued use or rationale for discontinuing medication.

2. Parent and teacher questionnaires appropriate for use in monitoring behavior must be gathered, stapled together, and identified as week 1, week 2,

TABLE 5.6
Drug–Placebo Summary Chart on a 14-Year-Old Student

Child's Name_____ Age_____ Parents_____			
Drug Conditions: Week 1___Low___ **Week 2**_Placebo_ **Week 3**___High___			

Variable	Baseline	Week 1	Week 2	Week 3
Parent-completed Section				
Side Effects Questionnaire				
Number of side effects	8	2	6	1
Mean rating	3.1	5.0	4.8	7.0
Home Situations Questionnaire				
Number of problem situations	5	0	4	1
Mean rating	2.8	0	4.8	1.0
Conners Abbreviated Parent				
Questionnaire raw score	9	1	6	1
Teacher-completed Section				
Side Effects Questionnaire				
Number of side effects	2	0	1	2
Mean rating	3.0	0	2.0	2.0
School Situations Questionnaire				
Number of problem situations	8	9	7	7
Mean rating	6.0	4.2	5.4	2.9
Conners Abbreviated Teacher				
Questionnaire raw score	11	7	5	3
Kagan Matching Familiar Figures Test				
Mean time to response	19.8	20.4	15.0	6.6
Number of errors	2	6	5	2

and week 3, along with the date each is to be completed. While parents may be given their packed upon each new appointment, teachers could be sent their three packets together with a request that each be sent to the clinician upon completion.

3. The physician must determine the low and high doses of methylphenidate (e.g., 0.2 mg/kg and 0.4 mg/kg) and whether medication will be given two or three times per day. Each drug condition is to last one 7-day week.

4. The prescription is then filled by the local pharmacist. Medication is

crushed and placed in a gelatin capsule. The placebo may consist of a lactose powder and is also placed in the same type of gelatin capsule as was the medication. The pharmacist should provide extra capsules for each drug condition. This will reduce potential problems if the child becomes ill or an appointment needs to be rescheduled. Unused capsules should then be returned to the clinician at the end of each condition. The pharmacist should not identify the bottle in a manner that parents or child can realize contents. It is usually sufficient to label the three bottles week 1, week 2, and week 3. The pharmacist's and clinician's records should reflect the actual order of administration.

5. Parents may need to seek a statement from the physician authorizing the school to dispense a noon dose of medication. To ensure that the school has an adequate supply of medication for noon administration, we suggest that the parents provide the school office or nurse with a bottle of 5 capsules each week or that a school official obtains each bottle from the parents prior to the new drug condition. In no situation should the child or adolescent be expected to deliver medication.

6. Three appointments must be scheduled at 1-week intervals. For children participating in a more comprehensive evaluation that might involve in-clinic observation and/or administration of psychometric tests, parents should be asked to give their child medication approximately 1 hour before each clinic visit. This ensures that an optimal drug effect will be observed. During each appointment, each clinician completes the appropriate section of the protocol outlined in Table 5.4. Parent, teacher, and child comments regarding behavior over the past week should be documented. At end of each session, parents may be given the new medicine.

7. Upon completion of the entire protocol, parents should be told of drug conditions, dosages, and a general overview of results. Results, along with a discussion of data, are forwarded to the physician. In following the design of this or a similar protocol, the physician would then be in a good position to decide whether a positive response to medication has occurred and, if so, what dosage might be of most therapeutic value.

There may be situations mitigated by time, financial, or administrative factors that prevent the use of a placebo and two doses of medication. Perhaps the clinician, physician, and parents feel that a single dose of medication with careful monitoring of drug effects is most appropriate given the current set of conditions. In this instance, we suggest the measures purposed in Table 5.4 would remain appropriate for monitoring single-dose drug effects. Once the child is appropriately medicated, periodic completion of these questionnaires may prove helpful indicators relative to need for subsequent adjustment of medication.

SELECTING AND IMPLEMENTING PSYCHOSOCIAL INTERVENTIONS

Of everything reviewed and discussed in this text, perhaps no area has been more hotly debated in the literature than the question of whether various psychosocial interventions have demonstrated efficacy with disruptive-behavior-disordered children. The brief review of cognitive interventions contained in Chapter 4 is perhaps characteristic of much of this literature. Some studies have clearly documented positive outcome, while others have not. Regardless of outcome, however, most studies have methodological flaws, including inadequate specification of subject characteristics, insufficient attention to individual differences in children (e.g., particular skill deficits in hyperactive children), insufficient attention to possible mediating variables (age, level of cognitive development and intelligence level), limited overlap between the training demands and the outcome task demands, and limited follow-up data. Perhaps the only reasonable conclusion that can be reached is that the literature is inconclusive and that the clinical utility of cognitive training procedures in the treatment of Disruptive Behavior Disorders has yet to be established (Abikoff, 1985, 1987). Similar concerns can be raised about the efficacy or appropriateness of social skills programs, dietary, and nutritional treatments.

Despite the inconsistencies in the research literature, it has been our clinical experience that most children with Disruptive Behavior Disorders and/or their family members are in need of and derive some benefit from various psychosocial interventions. It is not possible here to provide a detailed analysis of how to determine which if any psychosocial interventions offer the most promise for success with a particular child and family. The development of this type of critical analysis and decision making accrues primarily from extensive supervised clinical training with many diverse clients and perhaps partly from an intuitive sense of what would work best with this given child and family. However, a few salient issues can be mentioned.

1. As previously noted, in determining which types of interventions to pursue, consideration must be given to the unique features of *this* child and family. Many individual child and family characteristics affect the efficacy of a particular treatment program. For example, while the research literature suggests that parent training in behavioral management is generally an effective intervention in families with children diagnosed as having a Disruptive Behavior Disorder, specific characteristics of this family, such as the presence or absence of significant marital discord, parental depression, or other psychopathology, alcohol, or drug abuse, will determine whether this intervention will prove helpful.

2. It has been strongly recommended that a long-term view of treatment be adopted when working with disruptive-behavior-disordered children. It is not

sufficient merely to intervene to reduce the current level of disruptive behavior or other difficulties. Once this has been accomplished, some effort should also be directed at improving the quality of the family interactions, the parenting skills, the social skills of the child, etc., with the goal of attempting to improve the long-term prognosis for the child. This may involve a wide variety of more traditional forms of therapy, such as marital or family therapy, communication training, social skills training, etc.

3. It has been our experience that due to low self-esteem, mild depression, or other adjustment difficulties, many children and adolescents with Disruptive Behavior Disorders benefit from individual therapy. This mode of intervention may need to focus upon a variety of issues, including intra- and interpersonal dynamics.

4. Although we have found that standard components of typical parent-training programs as discussed in Chapter 4 (e.g., differential attention, social praise, brief time-out procedures, etc.) are of benefit to a significant number of children with Disruptive Behavior Disorders and their families, we have found that such programs are not sufficient to bring about the desired improvements in some families. In many of these situations, we have found that the family environments were reasonably inconsistent, unstructured, and perhaps chaotic, and that the parent–child interaction patterns could be characterized as involving a high degree of negative reinforcement. For various reasons, parents have had considerable difficulty maintaining clear and consistent communication of their expectations for the child, and/or providing reasonably consistent consequences. Or, a cycle may have evolved wherein the child is often noncompliant with parental requests and engages in considerable talking back or verbal arguing. The parent then, rather than argue, completes the task. For example, a mother may ask the child to pick up some toys. The child does not comply and engages the parent in a verbal argument and the mother stops asking and picks up the toys herself. Often, there is a fairly consistent degree of verbal arguing over rules, chores, or other parental expectations. In such circumstances, parents have often made comments to the effect that "it is easier just to do it myself than to continue to argue about it." We have found that developing and implementing a structured Contingency Management Program is an approach that has been effective with many of these families.

Contingency Management Programs (also referred to as "point systems" and "token systems") involve a structured format wherein rewards and punishments are presented or withdrawn contingent upon the occurrence of certain specified or targeted behaviors. The programs seem to have several advantages over other methods, and potentially facilitate several positive changes in the parent–child interactions. There are many variations of such programs, and they have been included as components of some standardized parent training programs (e.g., Barkley, 1987). A brief outline of the model which we have used with success in our clinical practices is contained in Table 5.7. We have found that some parents are able to progress through these steps and successfully implement a program in only two or three sessions, whereas others require a bit longer. We will discuss each of the steps. A case history will be presented later in the chapter.

Since positive results obviously require the cooperation of the parents, one essential ingredient in a positive outcome is a strong conviction on the part of the parents that the program will work with their child. Consequently, we do not begin to develop a specific program with parents until they understand the concept of Contingency Management Programs, what generally will be expected of them, and how this type of intervention might benefit them and their child. Rationale and explanations we have often discussed with parents include the following points.

1. Parental expectations and the potential consequences (both positive and negative) are articulated in a clear manner. This often involves making covert parental expectations more overt, so that everyone knows exactly what is

TABLE 5.7
Steps in Developing a Contingency Management Program

Step 1	Discuss the general nature of the program with parents, and facilitate their interest and motivation to cooperate.
Step 2	Specify the targeted behaviors with parents (and child?).
Step 3	Develop reward menu with parents (and child?).
Step 4	Assign point values for targeted behaviors and rewards.
Step 5	Implement.
Step 6	Trouble-shoot.
Step 7	Discuss Response Cost for misbehaviors with parents, decide on targeted behaviors and consequences (optional).
Step 8	Implement Response Cost (optional).
Step 9	Trouble-shoot Response Cost (optional).
Step 10	Discuss with parents how to amend the program to adjust to changing circumstances, including adding new targeted behaviors, new rewards, etc.
Step 11	Follow up.

expected. Ambiguities, inconsistencies, and arbitrariness in parental expectations are then minimized, reducing misunderstandings and opportunities for conflict. Similarly, the program may minimize parental punitiveness, as parents are less able to withhold or deny earned rewards simply because the child has misbehaved earlier in the day.

2. Contingency Management Programs often increase the parent's awareness of the child's appropriate, positive, and compliant behaviors. We have seen situations in which the child behaves in an appropriate, compliant manner most of the time, and is negative or noncompliant infrequently. However, for various reasons the parents have been less aware of the positive behaviors and more aware of the negative behaviors, creating the impression in the parents that the child has a greater frequency of misbehaviors than is actually the case. The Contingency Management Program requires the parents to be more aware of the child's appropriate, positive, and compliant behaviors, which otherwise may be overlooked.

3. It has been our experience that such programs provide added structure for some children who have deficits with (internalized) rule-governed behavior. As part of the implementation of the program, the targeted behaviors are typically written in a checklist format and posted in one or more places, such as on the family refrigerator and/or on the child's bedroom door. These posted checklists serve as visual reminders and discriminative stimuli for the child, and thereby provide the child with greater external structure.

4. Although we have not seen any empirical evidence of this reported in the literature, it has been our clinical experience that in families where there has been a fair degree of arguing over rules, responsibilities, and chores, the program may have the effect of objectifying and impersonalizing some of the rules and expectations. Once the targeted behaviors are posted in a checklist format, the rules and expectations exist "out there," in reality. Some children then seem to associate the rules less directly with the parent, and accept them as part of their environment. Thus, the child may argue *less with the parent* about the chores, responsibilities, and expectations. Complaints may continue, but often they take the form of generalized complaints about rules, with less arguing *directly with* the parent. Some parents, too, seem less defensive and have an easier time ignoring the child's complaints.

5. Contingency Management Programs allow parents to utilize a range of positive and negative consequences to manage the targeted child behaviors. Rewards are typically dispensed on both immediate (chips, points) and delayed (cashing in chips or points for rewards) reinforcement schedules. In addition, the child is given the flexibility to choose the reward that is of greatest interest or value to him at that time, increasing the incentive value of the reward. Finally, since there is a menu of potent reinforcers, it is less likely that a child will quickly satiate, as may happen with other forms of tangible rewards, such

as stickers, food, etc. As a result, improvements in child compliance often accrue more rapidly and are maintained better over time, than what would be accomplished through other methods.

6. Once implemented, Contingency Management Programs are a very flexible and convenient method of managing child behaviors. The programs allow for consistent implementation of consequences across situations and across individuals. For example, in cases where parents work different shifts, or a single parent utilizes a grandmother or babysitter to help with the children, the targeted behaviors and reinforcement schedules can remain constant across supervising adults and settings. Similarly, with minimal cooperation from the school personnel, the program can be expanded to incorporate various behaviors in the school setting, such as talking out or being disruptive in class, noncompliance with rules, and completing and turning in assignments.

7. Contingency Management Programs provide a useful mechanism to teach children the manner in which their behavior will be consequated by society. Occasionally we have parents who initially indicate that they do not like the concept of the program, that they think it is too artificial, or that it is unnecessary. We then explain to them that it is not artificial, but rather that it is a useful mechanism to teach their children how to be responsible in the real world. We point out that while some individuals enjoy their work and others do not, very few (if any) would work for free. Essentially, we note the similarities between the Contingency Management Program and the parent's employment circumstances: the parents would be unlikely to arrive at their employment setting on time, and meet their job responsibilities, if they did not receive a regular paycheck. The paycheck, obviously, is analogous to the points a child can earn in the program and use to purchase objects or experiences which they need or want. We also point out that most tend to enjoy their work more (or dislike it less) if they have a very clear sense of what is expected of them (i.e., a clear job description). Most parents readily understand these comments and begin to understand that, in addition to providing a method to manage the child's behaviors, the program provides a useful socialization experience for their child.

After sufficient discussion of these issues, we also try to elicit from parents their impression of whether this type of program might work with their child. If the parent expresses the opinion that it might not work, we take this very seriously, and spend some time with them exploring concerns or reservations. Occasionally, parents have misunderstood the nature of the program and some clarification is in order. At other times, the parents may note certain circumstances that may make the implementation more difficult, such as strong disagreements between parents about what is expected of the child. Here, additional discussion of opposing parental expectations, and perhaps underlying marital discord, may be needed. Finally, parents may not be motivated to implement the program and may express this in terms of doubts that it would work. In either case, it has been our experience that unless parents indicate that they generally understand the program, think it might work with their child, and express some motivation to cooperate with the development and implementation of the program, the program will probably not be effective with the child.

Once these issues have been successfully discussed and negotiated, the focus turns toward helping the parents specify the targeted behaviors. We have found it best if older children (ages 8 and up) are initially included in this discussion. Such children are at times better able to identify what is expected of them, and any areas of inconsistent expectations, than are the parents. In addition, inclusion of the children may facilitate their cooperation later, once the program is implemented. On the other hand, there has not been much benefit to including younger children, although there is no reason to exclude them. We have found it best to start by having the parents (and child) specify what is already expected of the child, and to write these expectations down as the discussion progresses. Occasionally, the existing expectations are not even clear for the parent: more often, the parent has some expectations, but communicates these in an unclear, inconsistent manner. For example, parents may state that they expect the child to make the bed. However, the actual pattern of behavior is somewhat different. Once or twice per week the child makes the bed appropriately without a response from the parent; a few times per week the child "forgets" to make the bed, and the parent then makes it; and, a few times per week the child "forgets," and no one makes it. In such as situation, the parent has not communicated clearly, in words or behavior, that making the bed is the child's responsibility. Thus, the focus of the discussion here is in helping the parents clarify for themselves such exact chores, responsibilities, or rules. Generally, typical household chores and responsibilities (making the bed, picking up toys, setting or clearing the table for a meal, helping to wash or dry the dishes, taking out the garbage, etc.) are the main focus of this initial discussion. Typically it is helpful if the expectations can be specified as precisely as possible. For example, if the child is expected to make the bed, by what time should this be accomplished? Do the parents' expectations concerning the targeted time to make the bed change with circumstances (e.g., before going to school on school days, but when on weekends?). There may be other social–behavioral expectations as well, such as no yelling, swearing, or hitting in the house.

Once the *existing* expectations are sufficiently clear, the discussion may turn to additional expectations, if any, the parents would like to include. Here, it seems best if the child is not present. For example, it may be that the parents have not yet expected the child to help with the dishes, but given the child's age, the parents would now like to begin expecting this of the child. We have found better success if the program initially targets *only* the existing expectations, and gradually incorporates additional expectations once the program has been successfully implemented. Identifying an additional expectation or two at this point will provide an opportunity to work with parents in later modifying the program.

Next, the discussion should turn toward developing a list or menu of rewards and privileges. In most cases, the eventual success or failure of the program will depend upon whether a list of rewards can be generated *that the child finds reinforcing.* The eventual list should contain a wide range of rewards the child will like or want to do, to reduce the probability of satiation. Ordinarily, the child (regardless of age) is included in this process, and allowed to suggest activities, privileges or items for inclusion in the list. This ensures that the list includes items that are desirable or of value to the child. At a minimum, the list should contain 10 or 12 items. We have found that larger lists, of 25 or 30 items, work even better. About one third of the list should include short-term rewards that can be made available to the child every day. These might include activities or privileges such as a special treat or dessert after dinner or in the evening; playing a video game or stereo; watching TV; or 15–30 minutes of individual time with the parent to do something special, like playing ball in the yard, playing a board game, or reading a book. For example, if the child likes video games, a game or game cartridge can be "rented." About one third of the list should include intermediate activities or privileges that can be made available several times per week. These might include being allowed to stay up a bit past the regular bedtime (e.g., 30 minutes); having a friend over for dinner, or to play; accompanying the parent alone on a special trip, such as shopping; visiting grandparents (depending upon family finances); accompanying the parent for a special small treat, like getting an ice-cream cone; or purchasing a small, cheap toy. About one third of the list should include long-term activities or privileges that can be made available to the child infrequently. These might include going out to eat with a parent, going to a movie (at a theater) with a parent, spending the night at a friend's home or having a friend spend the night in the home, getting a highly desired toy or object, or going on a special trip.

Often, children suggest only a few activities or items, and parents are hard-pressed to come up with a wide variety of activities or privileges that would be highly motivating to the child. There are several ways to facilitate this process. First, over the ensuing week or so, have the parents observe what the child spontaneously enjoys doing when allowed to do whatever he/she wants to do. Often, these activities can be included in the reward list. Second, pay attention to what the child wants. Perhaps the child wants a new toy, a new baseball glove, etc. These objects can be included in the reward list. Third, build upon the already-identified interests of the child. For example, if the child enjoys sports, then being allowed to stay up late to watch a particular game, receiving sports-oriented objects (e.g., baseball cards, magazines, etc.), or attending a college or professional game with a parent would likely be very appealing.

The next step is to assist the parents in assigning point values for the targeted behaviors and rewards. We have found that it is generally best for the parents to assign all values, within general parameters suggested by the therapist. This seems to facilitate the parents' sense of ownership or responsibility for the program. The suggestions we typically make are as follows. "Points" can be accumulated and exchanged in a number of ways; with younger children (ages 8 and below) actual poker chips or other tangible tokens seem to work best. These are then given for the successful accomplishment of the targeted behaviors and exchanged for the various rewards on the menu. Some older children also enjoy this method as well, whereas other older children view this as "childish" and prefer a point system recorded on paper. The parents should assign a point value (whether in the form of number of chips or points recorded on paper) for each targeted behavior. The number of points assigned is arbitrary. However, most children prefer to earn more points rather than less, so it is often best to assign 10, 20, and 30 points rather than 1, 2, and 3. The number of points assigned for each targeted behavior should be determined by the parent and be relative to the amount of time and effort involved. For example, if it requires 5 minutes to set the table and 20 minutes to help dry the dishes, drying dishes should be given about 4 times as many points as setting the table. In addition, modifications may be made depending upon the subjective appeal or distaste that the child displays for the activity or behavior. For example, if setting the table and taking out the garbage require about the same amount of time and effort, but the child dislikes taking out the garbage more than setting the table, taking out the garbage may be given a greater point value.

Point values should then be assigned to the items on the reward menu based upon the total number of possible points that can be accumulated per day, and the amount of time, inconvenience, and expense that are involved in providing the reward for the child. For example, if the arbitrary assignment of points to targeted behaviors works out so that the child can earn up to 50 points per day, then short-term rewards on the menu that can be made available to the child several times per day may be assigned point values between 10 and 30 points. This would allow the child who has perfect compliance with the targeted behaviors to "purchase" several short-term rewards per day, if he/she prefers. Intermediate rewards, that can be provided once per day to several times per week, may be assigned point values between 50 and 200 points. This would allow the child who has perfect compliance with the targeted behaviors to "purchase" several intermediate rewards per week, if he/she prefers, or to combine a number of short-term and intermediate rewards. Long-term rewards that can be provided infrequently may be assigned correspondingly greater point values. A suggested guide to follow here is as follows: Assume the child has perfect compliance all of the time (earns all possible points) and saves all points to purchase this particular reward as often as possible. Considering the time, expense, and inconvenience involved in providing the reward for the child, how often could the parents provide the reward to the child? Then assign a corresponding point value. For example, if the reward could be given once per month, and perfect compliance yields 50 points per day, the item would be worth 1,500 points.

Once the point values have been worked out, the next step is to implement the program. This process is often facilitated if lists of targeted behaviors (with their assigned point values) and rewards (with their assigned point values) are written or typed on paper. (Examples are provided later in the chapter in Tables 5.13 through 5.16.) Barkley (1987) has suggested that with young prereading children it may help if the list of targeted behaviors or tasks has pictures depicting each of the various activities (e.g., making the bed). In preparing the list, parents may want to cut pictures depicting the various tasks from magazines and glue these onto the list. In addition, the chosen mechanism of assigning and exchanging points, whether through poker chips or checklists with points alotted, should be identified and explained. We have found that it is usually best if the program is presented and discussed with the child in its entirety with the therapist present, rather than having the parents implement it on their own at home. Often the child's receptivity to the program, and subsequent cooperation with it, depends largely on how it is initially presented to them. If the child has had an opportunity to participate in identifying potential rewards, and the program is presented in a positive manner, focusing upon the potential benefits (i.e., rewards) for the child, children are often agreeable and even enthusiastic about the program. On the other hand, if the program is presented in a punitive manner, with more focus on the expectations and responsibilities than the potential benefits, children are often negative about the program. Some parents inadvertently present the program in a more punitive than positive manner, but this approach can be interrupted or minimized if the therapist is present. In addition, children inevitably raise questions about various expectations, often in an effort to clarify and perhaps test the limits; this is particularly likely if parents have been inconsistent with the child in the past. Occasionally, a potential problem or loophole that was not anticipated by the parents or therapist will be identified and perhaps exploited by the child. Again, if the therapist is present many difficulties can be averted.

Once the program has been discussed, and everyone involved understands what is expected, it should be implemented. In our experience, two patterns of child response are common. If not forewarned, each pattern may lead parents to prematurely abandon the program; if forewarned, they often persevere, and the program has a positive effect. A small percentage of the children we have worked with have been negative about the program from the outset and are quite resistant to complying with the expectations. Typically, in the past these children were not required to do much (or were able to extinguish parental expectations through ignoring, noncompliance, or arguing), and/or had easy access to many desired activities and privileges. These children are generally unhappy about the expectations placed upon them and express this through noncompliance, perhaps through verbal arguing as well. Parents can become very disillusioned here and conclude that the program will not work with their child. If parents can persevere and implement the program consistently for several weeks, most of these children will gradually begin to comply. Other children are initially very enthusiastic about the program and exhibit nearly perfect compliance with the program for the first week or two. Then they become habituated to the program, begin testing the limits, and their compliance drops off. Parents can become disillusioned here and conclude the program has failed. Typically, however, if they persevere and maintain a consist attitude, the children gradually begin to comply once again.

Very often, some unanticipated difficulties develop with the implementation of the program. Many of these result from insufficient specificity when identifying the targeted behaviors at the outset. For example, the behavioral target may have been to make the bed, and no consideration was given to time factors. Then on a school day the child does not make the bed until after returning from school. The child believes that he has earned the points because the bed is made, whereas the parent believes he has not earned the points because the bed was not made before going to school. It is impossible to anticipate every possible scenario, and so some difficulties inevitably develop. Generally these can be resolved rather quickly by negotiating compro- mises between the parent and child and then more clearly specifying the relevant issues. However, if the family does not return so that these can be negotiated, the disagreements may lead to the breakdown of the program.

If a child exhibits some infrequent negative behaviors the parents would like to reduce, such as occasional yelling, hitting, swearing, etc., there may be some benefit in developing a parallel program utilizing positive rewards and response cost procedures, or even incorporating a response cost procedure for these behaviors into the existing program. Generally we find that such a component works best only after the child has fully accepted the program and has come to view it as a way he can get the rewards that he wants. Consequently, we do not include such a component until the program has been implemented and has run smoothly for at least several weeks. Then, we might discuss with the parents the possibility of expanding the program to include the negative behavior. For example, it may be decided that the child will be penalized a certain number of points or chips for engaging in negative behavior, such as 10 points for swearing. One must be very careful here, however, that the response cost procedures is not set up in such a way that it undermines the existing reward-oriented program. It is possible to assign too high a penalty for the behavior, with the result that everything the child earns is then taken away through penalties. This would only frustrate the child and probably lead to his noncompliance with the existing, previously successful, program. Consequently, we have found it more beneficial in some situations to develop a second, parallel program that includes both response costs and positive reinforcements for a negative behavior. An example of such a parallel program is included in the case history discussed later in this Chapter (see Table 5.16).

Most children do not like response cost procedures designed to reduce their negative behaviors, and occasionally parents implement these inappropriately, combining the response cost contingency with verbal reprimands, arguing, or some other negative consequence. Thus, many difficulties can develop with response cost procedures, and the implementation and effectiveness of these should always be monitored closely. There is almost always a need to discuss and trouble-shoot the implementation of response cost procedures with parents. This should be anticipated by the therapist.

After the program (with or without a response cost component) has been implemented and has run smoothly for at least several weeks, some discussion should be undertaken with the parents concerning the ongoing monitoring and management of the program. Unfortunately, we have seen several situations in which a program was initially very successful, and then the parents unilaterally decided that it was no longer needed. Within several weeks the child's noncompliance and other behavioral problems had returned to the level that existed before the program was implemented. Consequently, we are of the view that, particularly with children who exhibit Disruptive Behavior Disorders, a reasonably successful contingency management program should be maintained (or modified to accommodate new behaviors and interests) for a relatively long period of time. This type of program generally has diminishing effectiveness as the child matures into adolescence, and so it may be realistic to think in terms of continuing the program (with modifications as needed) into early adolescence, as long as it seems to be running smoothly. A program that has proven successful in the short term is probably contributing some necessary dimension in the child–family interaction. With an ADHD child, for example, the program may increase external structure, compensating somewhat for the child's deficits in rule-governed behavior, or heighten the child's motivation through tangible, desirable reward systems. For a child with Conduct Disorder or Oppositional Defiant Disorder, the program may lead to a reduction in the negative, coercive interaction pattern in the family, increase structure and predictability in the child's environment, and facilitate positive social and other reinforcements that would otherwise be less forthcoming. Parents often initially balk at the prospect of continuing the program indefinitely. However, when they are reminded of the analogy between the program and their employment situation, and it is pointed out that they would be unlikely to continue working for no pay, most understand the value of the program and agree to continue.

Finally, the discussion should shift to focus on how parents might independently amend or modify the program to accommodate changing circumstances and needs. This might include adding new target behaviors, new rewards, accommodating the child's new developmental needs and interests in the future, or adapting to new situational circumstances. The goal here is to ensure that the parents can independently modify and manage the program as needed. It is helpful, here, if one or two additional target behaviors were previously identified. This allows for a more concrete, practical discussion of these issues and an opportunity for the parents to make some changes in the program under the observation and guidance of the therapist. The process is similar to the one followed previously. In the case of new behavioral targets, the behaviors should be clearly identified and specified, and appropriate point values assigned. In the case of new rewards, the parent should assign costs (in points) depending upon the daily total of possible points, and the actual relative costs (in terms of time, money, inconvenience, etc.) of making the reward available to the child. The therapist's efforts should be focused upon phasing out of the active management of the program and facilitating the parent's appropriate management of the program. Most often parents will demonstrate that they can make these changes with no difficulty whatever. However, occasionally, some parents will have trouble managing this. In our experience, parents who have trouble at this phase may also be at risk for ongoing problems with parenting, and should be instructed to return for assistance if some modifications in the program seem indicated. If a more comprehensive parent-training program has not previously been conducted, it may be appropriate to undertake this type of intervention at this time. They should also be seen periodically for follow-up sessions to monitor the parent–child relationships and the parenting process. In any case, it is always a good idea to follow up with a phone call or office visit 3 months after the last session to monitor the status of the program and the general parent–child interactions.

Table 5.8 lists practical suggestions we often provide to parents of children with Disruptive Behavior Disorders to be used in conjunction with any type of psychosocial or parent-training intervention. These ideas have been adapted from Schmitt (1977), and from our own experience. Often, we present these ideas to parents in a written, handout form during our feedback session. Alternatively, with some parents we present the handout somewhat later, in conjunction with a parent-training program.

EDUCATIONAL INTERVENTIONS

We have mentioned that children with Disruptive Behavior Disorders frequently present with exceptional education needs. It is not the intent of this text to overview the many types of management programs EEN teachers develop and implement with their students. However, since some of these children with (perhaps) proper medication, psychosocial treatment, and behavior monitoring may not require exceptional education, it will be necessary for the regular education teacher to have established some type of management and monitoring system. We would like to present an example of how a relatively simple behavior management program could be implemented within the regular education system. The overall planning of such a program might prove an easier task if part of the At-Risk process. These types of management programs do not always result in desired behavior improvement, yet they have proven successful with certain children. In addition, many times it will be necessary to document clearly that management strategies have been attempted and failed before a student may be considered an appropriate candidate for exceptional education. We have also included a number of fairly routine but basic suggestions that any teacher may find helpful in managing disruptive behavior in children.

We have found that modifying the standard Contingency Management Program discussed above to include one or more behavioral targets in the school setting can produce a very effective and efficient home–school behavior management program for some children. For example, the program might inlcude behaviors that occur in the school setting, such as completing all assignments, turning in homework, working quietly, participating in class, etc. (Behaviors could be taken from the SSQ and then more behaviorally refined.) These behaviors may then be rated on a daily basis by the teacher, and chips/points awarded for appropriate behaviors. The chips/points can then be redeemed by the child to purchase activities or privileges on the reward list maintained at home by the parents. Developing and implementing the program requires some involvement on the part of the teacher, particularly to help identify appropriate behavior targets, to monitor the child's behavior, and to assign points for appropriate behaviors. Once the program has been developed through the cooperative efforts of the parents and teacher and appropriate rating cards or record sheets developed, the program requires limited time

TABLE 5.8
Parent Handout: Suggestions for Parenting the Disruptive-Behavior-Disordered Child

1. **Accept your child's strengths and limitations**. Every child needs to be accepted, loved, and nurtured by his/her parents. Most parents have inner expectations for their child. Parents may expect that their child will be well behaved, cooperative, friendly, and pleasant. Parents then have difficulties accepting the child when the child does not live up to these expectations. Parents of disruptive-behavior-disordered children must accept the fact that the child is active and energetic, probably more so than the parent expected. Parents should not expect to eliminate the overactive behavior completely, but just to keep it under reasonable control. Undue criticism or attempts to change the energetic child into a quiet, "model" child will cause more harm than good. Nothing is more helpful to the child than having a tolerant, patient, low-key parent.

2. **Establish and maintain a household routine**. All children have a need for structure, order, and predictability in their environment. When their environment is reasonably structured and predictable, they feel more secure and safe. They have a better idea of what is expected of them and what they can expect from others. Children with Disruptive Behavior Disorders have an even greater need for order and predictability. As much as possible, the normal family pattern should follow a consistent routine. If possible, the child should have the same "wake-up" time each morning. Meals should be at the same time every day. The child should also have a set routine for doing chores, homework, taking baths, etc. Finally, there should be a well-defined bed time. Sometimes the routine must be broken for reasons that you cannot control. For example, the dinner time may be changed because of a doctor's appointment. When this happens, help the child to "think ahead." Explain to the child why the routine is different, and what the child can expect. Be prepared to explain this more than once.

3. **Communicate clearly**. All children have simpler ideas and shorter attention spans than adults. If adults communicate with children the way they communicate with other adults, many children will not understand. For example, a child may not seem to hear you when you ask him to do something. Parents may then assume that the child is being stubborn or noncompliant. However, it may be that the child is unable to process the information as quickly as it is being presented to him. This is particularly true if you make more than one request at a time. When communicating with children it is important to talk in a clear, simple manner so they can understand. Try not to make two or more requests at the same time. Rather, break it up into one directive at a time. Be clear, direct, and to the point.

4. **Give the child responsibilities**. All children should have responsibilities in the household. The responsibilities should be appropriate to their age, and should increase as they grow. This is an important part of childhood development, helping them develop a sense of responsibility and grow toward independence. It is not good for children to have too few or too many responsibilities for their age. Be careful that what you expect of your child is within his abilities.

5. **Be consistent.** The child's world revolves around the parents. All children need consistency in their parents in order to feel safe and secure. If the parents are not consistent, the child will likely develop feelings of confusion, uncertainty, and insecurity. Each parent should work to provide the child with a consistent, dependable environment. Most of all, this means a consistent relationship with each parent. It is easy to

respond inconsistently to the child. If today you are rested and relaxed, you may find the child's behavior playful and respond approvingly and positively. If tomorrow you are tired and irritable, you find the same behavior annoying and respond disapprovingly. This does not help the child feel secure. In relating to your child, you should try to be consistent across various situations. You should try to make your behavior, manner, actions, tone of voice, etc., consistent. You should also try to be consistent in what you expect of your child, what is acceptable, and what is unacceptable to you. In addition, it is very helpful to the child if the home environment is consistent, regardless of which parent is home. This requires the parents to work together to develop similar expectations for the child.

6. **Be decisive**. Every day, there are situations in which parents must make decisions about what the child and the larger family will do. It is the parents' responsibility to make these decisions. It does not help the child if the parents are indecisive. Many children try to negotiate with or manipulate the parents. For example, they may try to talk the parents into an extra treat (taking the bath later, going to bed later, etc.). Parents should not be indecisive in such situations: The child should not be able to manipulate the parents. The parents should make the decisions, and then stick with what they have decided. It is better for the child to learn that you mean what you say. It also minimizes the number of arguments that can develop when parents are indecisive.

7. **Be firm**. Children with Disruptive Behavior Disorders are generally difficult to manage. Typically, they need more structured and planned discipline than other children. At the same time, they may have more difficulty than other children remembering rules or controlling themselves to conform to rules. Thus, unncessary rules should be avoided. Rather, the parents should have a few rules and limits for the child which are communicated clearly and then consistently maintained. Aggressive behavior toward the parents, siblings, or other children should not be tolerated. Parents should also respond immediately to excessive overactivity or noncompliance. For example, the parents should not allow the child to become loud, disruptive, or uncooperative in public settings. When the child misbehaves, the parent should intervene immediately in a clear, firm manner. The parent should also avoid threats that they cannot or will not carry out.

8. **Be patient**. Children typically do not process information as quickly or communicate their thoughts as clearly as adults. Also, children are often more impulsive than adults; for example, they may frequently interrupt others in discussion. As a result parents can become frustrated when talking with their children. It is important that the parent be patient with the child when communicating and not become too frustrated with the child for the child's impulsiveness.

9. **Provide outlets for the child's energy**. Most children have considerably more energy than adults. Children with Disruptive Behavior Disorders often have more energy than most children and are also more impulsive than most children. Thus, the child probably has difficulty containing the energy. The child will need regular, daily opportunities to release the energy, such as playing sports, running, walking, or riding a bike. At the same time, the children should be expected to expend their energy within acceptable limits; they should not be allowed to become overly rough in their play or to run wild in the home. Particularly during the winter months or in bad weather, parents often must think ahead and plan opportunities for the child to release energy.

10. **Avoid fatigue in the child**. When children with disruptive behavior disorders become tired, their self-control often deteriorates. They may become more impulsive, more restless and overactive, and less cooperative. In brief, it is harder for them to control their behavior. Many behavioral problems can be avoided if the parent ensures that fatigue is avoided and the child regularly gets sufficient sleep.

11. **Provide opportunities for the child to pursue interests**. One way in which children learn to feel good about themselves is through following their interests and enjoying or succeeding in some area of interest. Due to their restlessness, impulsivity, and perhaps other reasons, children with Disruptive Behavior Disorders often find common childhood situations, such as school, group, or team activities frustrating. Parents should help these children identify activities that the child finds interesting and rewarding and then provide opportunities to engage in these activities. Often, the child will experience satisfaction and increased feelings of self-esteem through such activities.

12. **Minimize extended formal gatherings or public settings**. Children with Disruptive Behavior Disorders often have difficulty controlling themselves in public settings. Behavior problems that develop in these settings can often be stressful and embarrassing for the parents as well as the child. Examples of this would include church, stores, restaurants, etc. While some of these situations cannot easily be avoided, many of them can. If these situations are routinely very stressful for the parents and/or child, it makes sense to limit how often the child is in public settings. After the child develops more adequate self-control at home, these public settings can be gradually introduced.

13. **Buffer the child from the overreaction of others**. Children with Disruptive Behavior Disorders often receive negative attention from neighbors or others in the community. The child may develop a reputation of being a "bad kid" or a "troublemaker." This type of reputation can lead the child to think poorly of himself, and to develop low self-esteem. It is extremely important for the child that the parents do not also develop such attitudes toward the child. Rather, parents should think of their child as a good child with excess energy. Parents should try to identify positive qualities in the child and to communicate their pride and affection to the child. A child must always feel accepted by the family for his/her self-esteem and self-confidence to survive.

14. **Discipline requires providing a positive environment, rich with positive consequences and feedback**. Often parents think about discipline only in terms of punishing negative or inappropriate behaviors. This is only a small part of disciplining a child. Discipline also involves providing a positive environment for the child. The child must have many opportunities to learn appropriate, positive behaviors, and sufficient motivation (in terms of positive attention and feedback from the parents) to engage in appropriate, positive behaviors. The environment should provide many social incentives for behaving positively and appropriately. Many negative behaviors can be reduced or eliminated if the child is provided with an environment which is very rich in terms of positive attention, consequences, and feedback for appropriate behaviors.

15. **Enforce discipline with nonphysical consequences (response costs, time-outs, etc.).** Physical punishment (e.g., spanking) often increases the degree of anger the child experiences toward the parent and can increase the child's noncompliance. Often physical punishment only increases the child's behavioral problems and the amount of his aggressive behavior, particularly with children who have Disruptive Behavior Disorders. Parents should attempt to develop nonphysical methods of punishment.

Many parents have found that using a brief time-out or some loss of privileges for misbehaviors has worked well with their child.

16. **Punish the behavior, not the child**. Whenever you punish your child, you should provide a specific consequence for a specific behavior. The consequence or punishment should be in proportion to the seriousness of the behavior. And the punishment should be individualized to fit the child (what is effective for one child many not be effective for another child). It wouldn't be fair to punish a child severely for a relatively minor, infrequent misbehavior. The parent should try to communicate clearly to the child what behavior has been inappropriate and what would be an alternative positive or appropriate behavior. And, the punishment should follow immediately after the misbehavior. In this way, the child is more likely to understand that he is being disciplined for his misbehavior and not unfairly picked on by the parent. Providing general verbal threats should be avoided. Also, providing delayed consequences (punishing the child in the evening for some misbehavior earlier in the day) should also be avoided. Finally, once the child has been punished, the parent should "start fresh" with the child and not continue to reprimand or punish the child for the earlier misbehavior.

17. **Nurture yourself and your marriage**. Parenting is usually stressful. It is often much more stressful with children who have Disruptive Behavior Disorders. Parents need time away from the child in order to rest, relax, and nurture themselves and their marriage. Being with some of these children 24 hours a day would be stressful for any parent. Parents should attempt to arrange regular breaks from their child. A babysitter two afternoons a week and an occasional evening out with the husband can go a long way to rejuvenate an exhausted mother. Involvement of the child in a pre-school nursery or headstart class often helps as well.

---

involvement on the part of the teacher. The teacher must simply indicate (typically through initialing or signing) whether the child completed the targeted task or engaged in the targeted behavior. Most teachers agree to cooperate with the program and often find that they spend very little time monitoring and rewarding the targeted behaviors. Tables 5.9 and 5.10 contain examples of daily record sheets we have used with home–school behavior management programs. A record such as the one shown in Table 5.9 has typically been used with children who are in the same classroom with the same teacher through most of the day. A record such as the one in Table 5.10 has typically been used with children who have several teachers throughout the day.

We have found that three problems may develop with home–school programs such as these. First, children may initially "forget" (whether intentionally or accidentally) to have the teacher initial the card. Most of the time this can be easily overcome in a few days if the teacher asks for the card at the end of the class period. Second, children may "forget" (whether intentionally or accidentally) to bring the card home. Typically this can be overcome by in-

TABLE 5.9
Daily Student Behavior Rating Record: Form A

Name_____ Date_____

Today . . . . .

SUBJECT	I finished my assignments in class	I paid attention	I worked quietly	I did not disturb others	I have homework tonight
Reading					
Math					
Language					
Spelling					
Science					

Note. The behavioral targets and classes are typical examples and can be modified to fit individual needs. This record can be copied or modified for clinical use without further permission.

cluding points for bringing the card home, and perhaps some response cost (e.g., loss of points) for failing to bring the card home. Third, occasionally we have found that children forge the teacher's initials, particularly at the initiation of the program. Often this is obvious and stops when the parents confront the child with the situation. When less obvious, this can be brought into the open if the parents and teacher agree to talk briefly by telephone once per week or so to discuss the program, *and they make the child aware* that the conversations will take place. During such conversations, the actual record can then be reviewed and discrepancies noted.

In Table 5.11 is a list of practical suggestions that many teachers of children with Disruptive Behavior Disorders have found useful. Often, we simply mail these ideas to the teachers in a written handout form after the parents are given feedback concerning the diagnostic impressions. If the evaluation has been completed in a clinic setting, we ensure that parents have signed a release of information, allowing us to discuss the child with the teacher. Typically, we have found that parents are willing to provide such consent and that teachers

TABLE 5.10
Daily Student Behavior Rating Record: Form B

Name_____   Date_____

Please rate this child in each of the areas listed below as to how he performed in school today, on a scale of 1 to 5.   5 = Excellent, 4 = Good, 3 = Fair, 2 = Poor, and 1 = Terrible or did not work.

	Class/Periods/Subjects							
Area	1	2	3	4	5	6	7	8
Handed in assigned homework								
Participation								
Classwork								
Followed rules								
Interaction with other children								
Teacher's initials								

Note. From *Hyperactive Children: A Handbook for Diagnosis and Treatment* by R. A. Barkley, 1981 New York: Guilford. Copyright 1981 by The Guilford Press. Adapted by permission.

are open to suggestions and perhaps further consultation concerning behavior management.

CASE EXAMPLES

Now that we have overviewed assessment, treatment, and integrative issues, we would like to present two fairly detailed cases that highlight each of these major processes. We realize that these examples are not indicative of the more complicated or severe cases that practitioners will encounter. However, in most instances the basic procedures noted here will generally be appropriate for even the more severe children and adolescents.

TABLE 5.11
Teacher Handout: Suggestions for Teaching the Disruptive-behavior-disordered Child

1. **Develop a positive individual relationship**. A child with Disruptive Behavior Disorders will often be better behaved if he/she feels that the teacher has taken a personal interest. If the child comes to value your friendship, your positive attention will be more reinforcing and your reprimands will be taken more seriously. Take a few moments each day to foster a positive, individual relationship with the child. It often goes a long way in improving the child's behavior in the classroom.

2. **Communicate clearly**. Tell the child exactly what you expect. Be clear and straightforward. Give directives or instructions one at a time. Try to avoid giving multiple directives. Talk in simple sentences.

3. **Individualize teaching**. As part of developing an individual relationship with the child, try to individualize the teaching process as much as possible. This might involve developing a daily written contract with the child. It might involve prompt, brief rewards (such as a hug or pat on the back, or some formal reward like a chip or token) when the child completes his work.

4. **Be consistent**. Be as consistent as possible in what you expect from the child. Try to avoid overreacting when you are tired or stressed out and being overly agreeable when you are relaxed. Try to provide the same expectations and limits all day, every day.

5. **Be firm**. Maintain a firm, yet pleasant manner with the child. Make sure that the child realizes that when you say no, you mean no.

6. **Seat the child**. Seat him in a place that will minimize distractions and help the child focus his attention. If possible, seat the child close to the teacher and away from distractions, such as the door or windows. Also, if possible, seat the child at an individual study carrel for part of the day. Give some consideration to which students are seated near the child. Other children with a tendency to be inattentive or impulsive will only worsen the presenting problem.

7. **Reward the child frequently**. Try to reward effort and improvement, not just achievement. The child may benefit if you reward normal, compliant, or cooperative behavior as well. Also, reward classmates for ignoring the child's disruptive behavior.

8. **Give suitable work**. Try to pace the work to accommodate the child's strengths and weaknesses. The child with a Disruptive Behavior Disorder may have a shorter attention span than his peers and be less able to sustain his attention during longer assignments or projects.

9. **Provide extra help**. Children with Disruptive Behavior Disorders often benefit from extra, individualized teaching. If there is some way in which this child could be given such help (e.g., teacher's aide, resource person, etc.), arrange this for the child.

10. **Repeat directions**. Children with Disruptive Behavior Disorders are often easily distracted and have attentional deficits. They often do not initially attend to or fully comprehend directions. Try to go over directions more than once, to make sure that the child understands what is expected. This can be done several ways. You may give the directions first, and then ask one of the children to summarize the directions. Then you

can paraphrase (correct if necessary) the child's summary. This facilitates the child's appropriate attending the first time, and causes the other children to realize that they may be called on to summarize the directions. It also allows the directions to be repeated three times. Or, you can try to give directions using a multisensory (auditory and visual) approach. For example, try to give the instruction verbally, then write it on the blackboard, and then say it again.

11. **Slow down**. Children with Disruptive Behavior Disorders are often easily distracted. If you move around a lot in the classroom, they may become distracted by the shifting visual stimuli and you may lose their attention. Try to slow down your physical movements and your speech, particularly when giving directions or making important points.

12. **Allow outlets for the child's energy**. Most children have considerable energy. Children with Disruptive Behavior Disorders often have more energy than most children and are also more impulsive than most children. Thus, the child probably has difficulty containing the energy. The child will need regular, daily opportunities to release the energy, such as at recess time. Try to avoid punishing the child by keeping him in from recess. Also, try to provide as much opportunity for physical activity as possible. For example, try to give the chilkd frequent errands, such as help with the audiovisual equipment, erasing blackboards, emptying the wastebaskets, watering plants, etc.

Case Example 1: Jim

Jim was a 9-year-old boy who was referred by his pediatrician after the mother complained of a variety of noncompliant and disruptive behavior problems. The mother had expressed the opinion to the pediatrician that Jim was hyperactive and had sought some medication to help control his behavior. In referring the child, the pediatrician indicated that he did not view the child as hyperactive but considered the problem to be one of family system difficulties with inadequate behavior management.

Evaluation

Relevant background information obtained in the initial interview included the following. Jim was the product of a full-term, uncomplicated pregnancy and normal delivery. He reached early developmental milestones appropriately, and in some cases even a bit early. Jim's medical history was unremarkable. He had never been hospitalized, had no chronic illnesses, and currently took no prescription medications. He was the product of an earlier relationship and had never met his biological father. Jim was currently a fourth-grade student, enrolled in a regular education classroom. He had never been left back. He consistently earned above-average grades (predominantly A), and there had never been any report from his teachers of social or behavioral problems. He had many friends at school and in the neighborhood, and he appeared to be well liked by his peers. He was active in a variety of extracurricular activities, such as team sports and Boy Scouts.

The mother married Bill, the stepfather, when Jim was 3 years old. The only father figure that Jim had ever known was Bill, and Jim related to Bill as "Father." The mother and Bill also had a son who was then 4 years old. The mother and Bill had separated about 3 months prior to the initial interview, and Jim had irregular and inconsistent contact with Bill. Thus, the current family constellation included the mother, Jim, and his four-year-old brother. The mother noted that there was considerable marital conflict, including frequent oral arguments, for about 6 to 8 months prior to the separation.

Concerning the reason for referral, the mother reported that she had had difficulty managing Jim's behavior since he was a small child. For example, she could vividly recall many difficulties with toilet training. However, difficulties appeared to be intermittent, and there were clearly periods lasting weeks or months when there were no significant behavior problems. Currently, problems included general noncompliance with her requests, considerable inconsistency in completing his chores or other household responsibilities, talking back and yelling at the mother, and occasional aggressive behavior (e.g., hitting, kicking, and/or biting the mother and the younger brother). She noted that the behavior problems had become much worse over the past 6 months or so but did not spontaneously associate these changes with the marital conflicts or separation. She expressed the opinion that she had more difficulty managing Jim than did Bill or her parents; then, when reflecting on these questions, she mentioned that it seemed as if Jim generally only misbehaved when he was with her.

In a brief interview, the child indicated that he was uncertain why they were seeing the clinician but expressed the opinion that it was a punishment for his misbehavior. He stated that he was generally happy and did not perceive any problems in his behavior. He acknowledged that his mother often yelled at him or punished him, but he expressed the opinion that much of this was unfair. He stated that the mother was at times mean to him and punished him for no reason. He readily identified his chores and responsibilities in the home but then indicated that his mom often did these for him. The impression formed based upon the child interview was one of inconsistent expectations placed upon the child, aversive parent–child interactions, and some arbitrariness on the mother's part in consequating his behavior.

Other stressors currently impacting upon the family and Jim included financial strain, which had increased since the marital separation. The mother was currently unemployed, and Bill worked as a construction laborer. It was obvious in the initial interview that the mother was intellectually bright; brief exploration revealed that she had employable skills and had previously been productively employed. In addition, the mother had generally withdrawn and isolated herself from various social supports. For example, she quit attending church several years prior and had infrequent contact with her family of origin, although her parents and several siblings lived in the immediate area. Finally, although this was not thoroughly assessed in the initial interview, there was evidence of mild depression in the mother.

At the conclusion of the initial interview, permission was obtained to contact the teacher, and the mother agreed to complete the CBCL, the CPRS-R, the HSQ, and the BDI. A brief interview was then conducted with the teacher. She indicated that Jim was a good student, evidenced no behavior problems in the school setting, and was generally well liked by his peers. She expressed surprise to learn that his mother wanted him to be evaluated, noting that in her opinion he was a normal, well-adjusted fourth-grader. She agreed to complete the ACTeRS and the SSQ, and these were mailed to her. The results of the parent- and teacher-completed questionnaires are reported in Table 5.12.

The profile on the CBCL suggests that the mother viewed Jim as displaying aggressive behaviors, some motor restlessness, and some behaviors suggestive of mild anxiety and depression. The factor loadings on the CPRS-R suggest that the mother viewed the child as displaying moderate conduct problems, with some behaviors suggestive of anxiety. Notably, there were no significant elevations on the CBCL or CPRS-R factors that purport to tap hyperactivity. A review of the individual item loadings on the CBCL and CPRS-R factors (i.e., a functional analysis) did not alter the interpretation of these factor scores. The items endorsed on the HSQ primarily involve situations wherein Jim is required to comply and cooperate with various parental directives and expectations. For example, moderate to high scores were given for item 1 (at mealtime), item 2 (while getting dressed), item 3 (while washing/bathing), item 8 (when asked to do chores at home), and item 9 (at bedtime). The teacher-completed questionnaires produced results consistent with the verbal report during the interview, showing a relatively normal 9-year-old who did not display significant behavioral problems in the school setting. Finally, on the BDI the mother earned a score of 23, which is within the moderately depressed range.

Summary and Treatment

In view of this database, combined with the interview information, the diagnostic impression formed was one of an Oppositional Defiant Disorder. The developmental history, teacher report, some of the mother's report, and the mother- and teacher-completed questionnaires were all inconsistent with a diagnosis of ADHD. Similarly, the pattern of behavior problems was incon-

TABLE 5.12
Results of Parent- and Teacher-completed Questionnaires for Jim

Factor	T Score	Factor	T score
CBCL-P		*CPRS-R*	
Schizoid/Anxious	58	Conduct Problem	74
Depressed	65	Learning Problem	45
Uncommunicative	55	Psychosomatic	62
Obsessive-Compulsive	55	Impulsive-Hyperactive	53
Somatic Complaints	57	Anxiety	68
Social Withdrawal	55	Hyperactivity Index	46
Hyperactive	65		
Aggressive	70		
Delinquent	61		
HSQ		*SSQ*	
Number of problems	7	Number of problems	2
Mean severity	4.6	Mean severity	2.5

Factor	Raw score	Percentile rank
ACTeRS		
Attention	24	60
Hyperactivity	5	85
Social Skills	32	79
Oppositional	7	49

Note. The ACTeRS is scored in such a manner that higher percentile ranks present the more desirable, less problematic direction.

sistent with a diagnosis of a Conduct Disorder. Problems were seen as relatively mild, largely limited to the home setting (specifically the mother–child relationship), and there was no evidence of more serious behavior problems, such as stealing, running away, fire-setting, truancy, etc. Several alternative formulations were also considered but ruled out. First, given the obvious recent stressor of the marital conflicts and separation, an Adjustment Reaction with mixed disturbances of emotions and conduct was considered. However, there was evidence that the behavior problems were relatively longstanding and preceded the recent marital conflicts, although the problems were perhaps exacerbated by the marital situation. In addition, the evidence suggested that the behavioral problems were largely limited to the home setting and were not pervasive across other settings, such as the school. Second, given the evidence of depressive and anxious affect, mood disorder (dysthymia or mild depression) and anxiety disorder were also considered. However, the ratings for depressive and anxious affect were both relatively mild, the teacher did not report any evidence of these difficulties, and mild depressive and anxious difficulties often coexist with Oppositional Defiant Disorder. Finally, it was concluded that the mother was experiencing a mild depressive syndrome, and there were ongoing marital difficulties.

The focus then shifted to developing appropriate treatment interventions. There was no reason to believe that pharmacological therapy or changes in Jim's educational program were indicated. The most pressing issue was reducing the degree of oppositional behavior which was displayed by Jim in the home setting. Some consideration was given to undertaking a standard Parent-Training Program, such as the one proposed by Barkley (1987) and reviewed in Chapter 4. However, given the marital concerns, the mother's depression, and evidence that the expectations for the child were quite inconsistent, it was decided to intervene more rapidly to assist the mother in developing a standardized Contingency Management Program. Thus, over the next three sessions a program similar to the one discussed above was developed with Jim and his mother. The goals in developing the program were to clarify for the mother and Jim exactly what was expected of him, to develop a structure in which his compliant, appropriate behaviors would be recognized and reinforced, and to minimize the degree of daily arguing and yelling about basic household chores and responsibilities. The situations endorsed on the HSQ were once again reviewed and discussed in more detail with the mother, and in several cases these became specific targets in the Contingency Management Program. In order to facilitate consistency on the mother's part concerning her expectations of Jim, and to foster clearer communication between Jim and his mother about the mother's expectations and the contingencies surrounding his behaviors, it was decided that each aspect of the program would be formally written up and provided to both Jim and his mother. The program included four parts: the list of expected behaviors, the weekly point sheet, the reward menu, and an additional response cost program for aggressive behaviors. These are presented in Tables 5.13 through 5.16.

As noted above, the program was developed over the three sessions following the initial interview and implemented after the fourth contact with the family. During the first week the program was not successful, and some minor modifications were required. In particular, it was determined that the mother continued to hassle and threaten the child *prior* to the time deadline, and orally criticize and punish him *after* the time deadlines if he did not comply. These behaviors on her part appeared to increase his anger and his tendency toward noncompliance and oppositionality. The mother was again instructed to re-frain from saying anything to him prior to the time deadline, to provide verbal praise and acknowledgement of the points earned if the chores were completed on time, and to say nothing if the chores were not completed. Subsequently, she generally complied with these instructions. There was modest improve-ment in the second week, and substantial improvements over the third and fourth weeks. After the fourth week the mother commented that Jim had not been this cooperative in years. The mother was then instructed to keep the program operating in its current form and to discuss any suggested alterations with the therapist *prior* to implementing changes.

The focus of treatment then shifted to the marital issues. The mother agreed

---

TABLE 5.13
Jim's Contingency Management Program—Part I: Responsibilities

---

General rules

Jim will do these chores by the given time. It is Jim's job to do these things, and he will not earn points if the chores are not *completed* on time. He will complete these chores whether or not his mom reminds him. Mom can change the times when the behaviors must be completed, if necessary. For example, if he spends the day at a friend's house, he would not be able to fill the dogs' water dishes on time. Then, his mom could change the time. If Jim does his chores by the right time, he will earn points.

Behaviors

1. *Feed and water the dogs in the morning*: Jim will put out food for the dogs and fill their water dishes in the morning before school, or by 9 AM when he does not go to school (weekends, holidays). (8 points per day)
2. *Make bed*: Jim will make his bed before he leaves for school or by 9 AM on days when he does not go to school (weekends, holidays). (4 points per day)
3. *Dress*: Jim will dress himself in the morning by 7 AM on school days, or by 9 AM on days when he does not go to school (weekends, holidays). (4 points per day)
4. *Make breakfast*: Jim will make his own breakfast (such as cereal) unless his mom is making a bigger breakfast (such as eggs, pancakes, etc.). Jim will clean up the mess that he makes while eating. This includes putting his dishes in the sink, putting away food (milk, juice, cereal boxes) and wiping off the table. (8 points per day)
5. *Get ready for school*: On school days, Jim will be ready for school by 7:30 AM. He will be dressed, finished with breakfast, and have his books and school supplies ready. (4 points per day)
6. *Water the dogs in the afternoon*: Jim will fill the animals' water dishes in the afternoon, before dinner. (4 points per day)
7. *Bathe*: Jim will take his bath every evening before 7:30 PM. (6 points per day)
8. *Pick up toys*: Jim will pick up his toys and put them away in the evening before he goes to bed. To earn the points, all of his toys must be put away by the time he is required to be in bed; the time that he is required to be in bed may change, depending upon his behavior. (See aggressive behaviors, below.) (5 points per day)

TABLE 5.14
Jim's Contingency Management Program—Part II: Weekly Point Sheet

	Total points possible	Mon	Tues	Wed	Thur	Fri	Sat	Sun
Jim's Point Sheet for Responsible Behaviors								
1. Feed and water dogs in the morning	8							
2. Make bed	4							
3. Dress	4							
4. Make breakfast	8							
5. Get ready for school	4							
6. Water dogs in the afternoon	4							
7. Bathe	6							
8. Pick up toys	5							
Daily totals	43							
Weekly total _____								

to arrange a conjoint meeting with Bill, the stepfather. During the subsequent week Bill informed the mother that he intended to follow through with the divorce. He did accompany her to the next interview, and he informed the therapist at the beginning of the session of his intentions. (The divorce became final about 1 year later.) Consequently, the focus of the treatment shifted to individual therapy with the mother, to address the depression, the impending divorce, and associated concerns. The mother was then followed intermittently

TABLE 5.15
Jim's Contingency Management Program—Part III: Reward Menu

Redeeming Points

Jim can buy various activities, privileges, etc., with the points he earns by completing his chores. The cost for each activity or privilege will be decided by Jim's Mom. Here is a beginning list of activities that Jim's Mom has developed, with the costs. Jim or his Mom can also add new activities to the list and Jim's Mom will decide on their cost.

Point value	Activity/privilege
2500	Get your own home chemistry set
2000	Go to a professional basketball game
1700	Get your own skateboard
1200	Get a new table game
1000	Get your own soccer ball
900	Go to a movie (theater) with Mom or Dad (movie they approve of)
800	Have a special dinner (something that you like)
600	Rent a movie for VCR (movie that Mom and Dad approve of)
500	Have lunch at fast-food restaurant
400	Get your own fishing pole
250	You get to pick out a shirt or some clothing that you like when shopping with Mom
200	Have friend over to play
200	Visit grandparents on the weekend
200	Get your own Frisbee
100	Make your own ice cream sundae
75	Stop by a fast-food restaurant for a soda
50	Evening snack (cookies, popcorn, soda)
20	"Rent" video game cartridge from Mom for 30 minutes (max. twice per day)
20	Watch TV for 30 minutes (max. twice per day)
10	Spend 15 minutes alone with your Mom or Dad to play a game or do something that you like. You can buy a total of only 1 hour per day, for a total of 40 points

in individual therapy for 2 years. During the 2 years she gradually made substantial improvement. She eventually returned to work, enrolled in and was successful in college, resumed going to church, and developed an extensive network of social supports through contacts made at work, school, and church. Jim continued to do well academically and socially. Occasionally, behavior problems developed in the home setting, particularly during periods when the mother was under stress associated with negotiating issues related to the divorce. At these times the mother generally raised questions or concerns about managing the behavior of Jim and/or his younger brother, and with some suggestions and advice she typically managed these situations effectively. On several occasions the Contingency Management Program was altered to accommodate new circumstances or expectations, and to include new rewards. At the termination of individual therapy Jim and his mother were both doing well. There had been no evidence of significant behavioral problems or oppositional behaviors in over 6 months.

Case Example 2: Michael

Michael attended fourth grade in a public school. His parents and teacher/pupil services personnel initiated the referral, feeling an outside-the-school assessment for suspected hyperactivity would be helpful in gaining information appropriate for classroom management and placement. Previous to the clinical evaluation, Michael's teacher and parents initiated a CAR referral through the school's pupil services department. The school's intervention, as outlined through Michael's Student Educational Plan (SEP), suggested a need for possible exceptional education in the form of a program for the emotionally disturbed. Parents and pupil services staff felt that before such an evaluation took place, a clinical assessment would be appropriate. At the same time, parents were encouraged to seek medical consultation regarding Michael's general health. While Michael's overall health appeared well within the norm, the purpose of this suggestion was to alert his pediatrician to the clinical assessment and the school's concerns, and to seek an opinion as to whether there might be medical factors that had to be considered in managing Michael's behavior. The next step in the SEP called for another meeting subsequent to the medical and psychological evaluation. At that point, a more definitive set of interventions would

TABLE 5.16
Jim's Contingency Management Program—Part IV: Response Cost for Aggressive Behaviors

Jim will not hit, kick, bite, grab, or otherwise hurt his Mom, brother, or anyone else.
If Jim does not know how to stop these behaviors, he can ask the therapist to help him learn.
If he does any of these things he will not be allowed to watch any television for 24 hours. For example, if he hits his Mom at 5 PM on a Friday, he will not be allowed to watch television until after 5 PM on Saturday.
If he does this twice in one day, the 24-hour period will begin again at the time of the second incident. For example, if he hits his brother at 10 AM on a Saturday, he will not be allowed to watch TV until after 10 AM on Sunday. However, if he later hits his Mom at 3 PM, he will not be allowed to watch TV until after 3 PM on Sunday.
If Jim goes from the time that he wakes up until the time that he is scheduled to go to sleep without hurting anyone, he will be allowed to stay up 30 minutes later than his scheduled bedtime.
If Jim goes 7 days in a row without engaging in any of these aggressive behaviors, he will be rewarded with a special treat, such as going out with his Mom to get a soda, an ice-cream cone, etc.

be established. Release-of-information forms were signed, allowing the school to disclose information about Michael's functioning to the physician and psychologist. Parents were asked ensure that physician and psychologist sent their information to the pupil services staff. Parents were quite supportive and willing to pursue all avenues suggested.

The clinical evaluation consisted of an interview with Michael's parents, an interview with Michael, a review of several child behavior questionnaires, and a review of school records. Formal psychometric assessment was not necessary, given information provided through school records.

Evaluation

Parents entered the evaluation in a very pleasant and cooperative manner. They identified many issues of concern to them. Most of these centered around Michael's difficulty in following directions, his high activity level, general disorganization, inattention, and poor impulse control. They also felt that much of the time he chose to be less than compliant with adult directives. Parents felt that Michael's social skills were somewhat immature, in that he had friends and could easily initiate peer interaction but that such interactions were frequently not sustained. Much of this appeared due to his need to control the situation, and also to some degree to inadvertent aggression. Presenting concerns had been chronic, dating back to Michael's preschool years. Parents also indicated that while Michael's behavior could indeed be frustrating, if not embarrassing, he could be a very loving and affectionate child. Fortunately, the parents were in agreement regarding their own inconsistency in managing Michael's behavior. While both generally agreed which behaviors under which conditions were most problematic, parents did not present with a consistent format of behavior management. It was particularly helpful to use R. A. Barkley's Diagram of Noncompliant Interaction (Barkley, 1987) in sorting through not only some of the parent–child interactions but also the dynamics involved with parental expectations for Michael's behavior and their own capacity for follow-through. It became clear that Michael's behavior, along with the parental attitudes, were adversely affecting family dynamics. Parents readily admitted that many times it was much easier to acquiesce to the directive rather than to seek full compliance. The family history for psychopathology was not significant.

Michael's general health appeared normal, with no outstanding previous or current medical complications or anomalies. Michael's pre-, peri-, and post-natal development appeared normal. Developmental milestones occurred within the norm, though language seemed delayed. School attendance has not been a problem. Parents described Michael as being a restless sleeper; he did not require much rest. As noted earlier, Michael presented with significant behavior problems quite early. Parents sought psychiatric consultation while Michael was in the middle of first grade. Over the course of the next year, parents reported that Michael had taken Ritalin, Dexedrine, Cylert, and Ritalin S-R (20 mg). Each new medication was attempted because the previous medicine proved ineffective. Ritalin S-R apparently resulted in the most improved behavior, but caused too much weight loss. Parents then stopped the medicine altogether. General parental frustration with the medication was also a factor. Other than general impressions as to behavior changes, parents could not identify methods of monitoring drug effects at home or school. By the middle of second grade, Michael was completely off medication. Parents reported that since the medicine was terminated, his behavior within school and home had worsened and the overall stress level increased.

Michael's academic history appeared significant. Prior to age 3, he participated in an Infant Stimulation Program. He had been referred for an exceptional education needs assessment during kindergarten due to language delays and behavior problems. The M-Team evaluation resulted in a recommendation for speech and language therapy but not for enrollment into a program for the emotionally disturbed. The M-Team did however note Michael's poor attention span, capacity to comply consistently with directives, poor impulse control, and motor restlessness. General cognitive ability was assessed to be well within the average range. At the time the CAR process began, Michael's academic skills appeared grade-appropriate (B's and C's), with primary concerns relating more to productivity and consistency than deficits in skill acquisition. By this time, language therapy had assisted Michael in developing more appropriate receptive and expressive skills. It was speculated that by the end of the present school year, he might be dismissed from therapy. Other than attempting to structure Michael's activity as much as possible within the confines of regular education and implementing consequences for noncompliance (academic and behavior), not much well-coordinated effort involving home and school was evident.

Table 5.17 presents results of the parent- and teacher-completed child behavior questionnaires. As illustrated, a host of concerns crossing externalizing and internalizing domains were evident within the home and school settings. Results of parent questionnaires appeared fairly consistent with their verbal reports of concern focusing upon behaviors associated with Michael's poor impulse control, poor rule-governed behavior, inattention, noncompliance, needs for attention, and immaturity. The elevated Internalizing factors appear as a result of the many negative interactions with teacher, parents, and peers Michael had experienced. By this point in time, the negative cycle has been well ingrained. Part of the reason for the consistent elevation, in this case, appeared related to the overall frustration of these parents in dealing with Michael and their tendency to "overfocus" upon the less than favorable aspects of his behavior. This is not to suggest that Michael did not present as a difficult child to manage, only that during the interview parents could identify many positive aspects of Michael's behavior that, when considered, would put his behavior profile into perspective. Teacher reports also suggest Michael displayed disruptive behavior within the academic setting, had difficulty with peer interaction, and showed a high degree of impulsivity. She commented that many times Michael behaves without forethought and will frequently deny any wrongdoing. His teacher also commented as to the degree of carelessness across all aspects of school functioning.

Even though there were no significant academic deficits as noted during the interview or in comments by the teacher, parents did ask that some formal measurement of academic skills be made due to the degree of frustration associated with work completion. Consequently, the Kaufman Test of Educational Achievement was administered. While there was some degree of variability between reading, math, and spelling, all standard scores ranged from 92 through 104. Testing academic skills also allowed for observation of behavior. Michael was easily distracted, though easily brought back to task (as long as the examiner was close). Some errors were thought to be related to a lack of concentration. Michael was appropriately verbal and not particularly reticent in his manner. This also fostered an opportunity to discuss with Michael feelings

TABLE 5.17

A 10-Year-Old Boy with a Diagnosis of ADHD and Oppositional Defiant Disorder

CBCL-T		CBCL-P		CPRS-R	
Anxious	55	Schizoid/Anxious	68	Conduct	66
Social Withdrawal	66	Depressed	65	Impulsive–Hyperactive	76
Unpopular	67	Uncommunicative	75	Hyperactivity Index	83
Self-destructive	66	Obsessive–Compulsive	78		
Obsessive–Compulsive	82	Somatic Complaints	57	CTRS-R	
Inattentive	68	Social Withdrawal	88	Conduct	71
Nervous–Overactive	66	Hyperactive	83	Hyperactivity	76
Aggressive	66	Aggressive	73	Inattentive–Passive	71
		Delinquent	78	Hyperactivity Index	75
SSQ		HSQ			
Number of problems	10	Number of problems	10		
Mean severity	6.5	Mean severity	4.9		
Unsupervised setting	6.5	Nonfamily transactions	4.7		
Task performance	6.8	Custodial transactions	1.0		
Special events	2.5	Task-performance transactions	4.7		
		Isolate play	1.0		

about school, his behavior, and friends. Generally speaking, he did a nice job of circumventing certain specific inquiries. He was also rather at odds with parent and teacher comments as to the degrees of the problems. Michael did, however, readily admit he is tired of being yelled at by parents and did not understand why he couldn't be going out for recess more at school. In essence, much of what Michael presented (despite a level of superficial cooperativeness) was to deny the significance of his behavior. Given the chronological age and general immaturity, this was not unexpected.

Summary and Treatment

Given the nature, historical significance, pervasiveness, and current status of Michael's behavior, a diagnosis of Attention-deficit Hyperactivity Disorder with Oppositional Defiant Disorder appeared appropriate. Other diagnoses (e.g., mood/anxiety/adjustment disorders) were considered but ruled out. A report from the physician indicated that Michael was free from significant medical anomaly. In following the models suggested in Table 5.2 and Figure 5.1, it became apparent that the major issue to be resolved was Michael's behavior, as well as parent and teacher management of this behavior. While Michael's social skills and level of self-esteem were poor, they were viewed as a function of his behavior rather than as causes of the behavior problems. Issues not requiring direct attention were academic skill level, family psychopathology, parental/teacher unwillingness to work toward a unified goal of positive behavior from Michael, and a high degree of aggression from the child. The *first* approach was to solidify parent expectations and management skills. This was accomplished by encouraging both parents to attend a parent-training program specifically designed to acquaint them with Disruptive Behavior Disorders and effective behavior management techniques. Both parents were quite willing to follow this recommendation. The parent-training program adopted in this case was the one proposed by Barkley (1987). By chance, they were one of five other sets of parents also beginning this program. The group presentation of this program proved quite helpful to these parents as it gave them exposure to other parents with similar concerns and frustrations. The entire program was implemented and Michael's parents missed but one session. Each week parents would report relevant behavior changes. While Michael's behavior did not change too much until well into the training program, his parents did note they were becoming more consistent in their views of expectations and consequences as well the manner of giving directives to Michael.

The *second* recommendation involved contacting the physician in order to gain her opinion as to the need for a trial dose of medication. The clinician felt that, due to the severity and ramifications of Michael's behavior at home and at school, a more immediate intervention was warranted. In addition, Michael was now more mature than when he last took psychotropic medication. The suggestion was to start him off with 10 mg Ritalin in the morning and at noon. Given the set of circumstances in this case, it did not seem warranted to proceed with a drug–placebo assessment. Rather, parents and teacher agreed to monitor drug side effects weekly using the questionnaires offered in Appendices B and C. These data were coordinated by the school guidance counselor, who then forwarded information to the physician. It was also suggested that, if a positive effect was observed through the first 2 weeks with few adverse side-effects, a late afternoon dose of 5 mg would be given. This was suggested in an effort to assist in "taking the edge off" some of the behaviors that fostered negative parent–child interactions during the evening hours. This pharmacologic intervention was based upon Michael having a positive response to the 10 mg of Ritalin and the fact that neither the 10 mg nor the additional 5 mg altered sleep patterns substantially. Once the late-afternoon dose was given, parents were asked to monitor drug effects for at least 2 weeks. It turned out that Michael had a positive response to the Ritalin. It was not necessary to increase the dose in order to observe more appropriate behavior.

The *third* suggestion was actually a result of the parent training program. The session that involved developing a home behavior management program was expanded to incorporate a home–school model. Two sessions were devoted to this very important intervention. Using the principles discussed in Barkley's manual, parents and teacher developed a relatively brief but specific program designed to reduce three annoying behaviors. The system involved a format very similar to the example found in our earlier case example. Michael seemed to "catch on" to the system nicely. When combined with the medication, this intervention seemed to result in greater success in peer–academic–parent interactions.

Individual sessions with Michael were not deemed necessary as the parent-training program and medication resulted in some degree of positive behavior change, and this was thought to have a positive effect upon Michael's social skills and self-esteem. The only time it was necessary to meet with Michael was to explain the "chip" system, which was done by the school guidance counselor.

The aforementioned suggestions were proposed at the school's follow-up CAR meeting. Parents were informed of these recommendations at the time of the evaluation and felt comfortable with them. It was important to include school personnel in this process as the classroom teacher had an obviously important role in developing and implementing the home–school management program. By involving the CAR process, it was also possible to have all school personnel who might be involved in working with Michael at the meeting. The pupil services staff and Michael's teacher were pleased that the medication would be tried and were quite willing to abandon the EEN referral for suspected emotional disturbance. Parents and teacher were to continue their efforts in managing Michael's behavior and monitoring drug effects periodically throughout the school year. Should Michael's behavior prove resistant to these interventions, those in attendance of the CAR meeting felt that an EEN referral would then be appropriate.

SUMMARY

We opened this chapter by discussing several issues involved in conducting evaluations of children who present with disruptive behavior problems. We then summarized and integrated the information presented in the previous chapters and recommended a relatively standardized protocol that clinicians might follow when conducting these types of evaluations. The protocol we have recommended includes: (1) completion by the parent of the developmental questionnaire presented and discussed in Chapter 2; (2) interviews with the parents, the child, and where appropriate, the teacher; (3) the completion of several parent and teacher behavior rating scales, including the Child Behavior Checklist (CBCL), Revised Conners Parent Rating Scale (CPRS-R), Home Situations Questionnaire (HSQ), Teacher Report Form of the Child Behavior Checklist (TRF), ADD-H Comprehensive Teacher Rating Scale (ACTeRS), and School Situations Questionnaire (SSQ). Each questionnaire was selected because of its adequate psychometric properties and evidence suggesting that it discriminates disruptive-behavior-disordered children from nonclinical and non-disruptive-behavior-disordered clinical samples. We noted that in some situations additional data may also be necessary. We recommended several more specialized questionnaires (e.g., BDI, RADS, PSI, etc.), as well as measures of general intellectual functioning (e.g., WISC-R, KABC) and academic achievement (e.g., WJ-R, PIAT-R).

We then discussed how the data that is produced through this process might be integrated and interpreted in reaching a differential diagnosis. The point was made that the clinician should engage in both a statistical and a functional interpretation of the child behavior questionnaires. It has been our contention that such a comprehensive, standardized assessment protocol would yield sufficient data to allow for meaningful consideration of complex differential diagnostic considerations. In addition, this assessment protocol would yield a baseline against which the effectiveness of subsequent treatment might be assessed. We then presented an overview of the process, moving from the initial presentation, through the assessment process, and into relevant and appropriate treatment interventions.

We noted that comprehensive treatment/management of children identified as having a Disruptive Behavior Disorder often includes pharmacologic, psychotherapeutic, behavioral, and educational interventions. Therefore, we discussed integrating and monitoring these intervention strategies. A detailed, step-by-step method for assessing the effectiveness of medication was outlined. It has been our experience that this protocol is reasonably easy to implement and very useful in helping to determine if medication is beneficial for an individual child. Next, we outlined the steps involved in developing a contingency management program with parents and provided some practical suggestions in working with parents. We then discussed how the contingency management program could be modified for school use, resulting in an integrated home–school program. Finally, two case examples were presented.

CONCLUDING REMARKS

We started this manuscript by noting that outdated and ambiguous assessment methods continue to be utilized by practitioners who assess children presenting with disruptive behavior problems. There has been a notable lack of consistency in assessment practices within the various disciplines typically involved in assessing these children and across the disciplines as well. In short, there is a clear need for a more standardized, systematic, and integrated assessment protocol for use with children who present with disruptive, externalizing behavior problems. Finally, it has been our contention that greater cooperation across the relevant disciplines can only facilitate better assessment and treatment for these children and their families. Thus it would be beneficial if a standardized assessment protocol incorporated perspectives of the various disciplines. This would offer the opportunity for greater interdisciplinary communication and collaboration. The primary goal of this text has been to meet the need for a standardized psychometrically acceptable, treatment-focused assessment protocol for use with these children. A secondary goal has been to develop and articulate the protocol in such a manner that it will be understandable and acceptable from within the various disciplinary perspectives. We hope that we have reached the goals set for the text, and thereby met the need for a systematic yet practical assessment protocol.

APPENDIX A
DEVELOPMENTAL QUESTIONNAIRE

DIRECTIONS: Please read this questionnaire carefully and complete the items that apply to you and your child. This information is necessary to ensure a thorough evaluation of your child. All information is for the confidential use of staff involved in evaluating and treating your child. No information will be released without your prior written permission.

Family Identification

Name of child_____ Sex_____ Date of birth_____
School_____ Grade_____ Teacher_____
Child's physician_____
Child reffered by_____

Father:

    Name_____

    Address_____

    Age_____

    Education_____

    Occupation_____

    Home phone_____

    Work phone_____

Mother:

    Name_____

    Address_____

    Age_____

    Education_____

    Occupation_____

    Home phone_____

    Work phone_____

List all children/significant others in the family. (If more room is needed, please use back of this page.)

Name	Age	Residing in or outside of home

Do your children or your immediate relatives' children have unique medical, physical, learning, or emotional needs? If so, please describe them. (If more room is needed, please use back of this page.)

_____

_____

_____

_____

Insurance Information

Name of insurance carrier_____

Address_____

Insured's name_____ ID/Group #_____

History Of Pregnancy and Delivery

Length of pregnancy_____ Birth weight_____

Did mother take alcohol, other drugs, or prescription medications during pregnancy? If so, please indicate the type of chemical and any implications or complicaitons._____

_____

Were there any unusual factors relating to the pregnancy or birth? If so, please note them._____

_____

Child's Medical History

General health of child: Good_____ Fair_____ Poor_____

Describe any significant medical conditions, illnesses, accidents, or operations your child has experienced._____

_____

_____

Has your child frequently been absent from school?_____

Is your child taking medication prescribed by a physician? If so, indicate type, amount, length of time taking the medication, and any known side effects_____

_____

Please check the following as applied to your child:

	Yes	No		Yes	No
Frequent colds	____	____	Head injury	____	____
Ear infections	____	____	Allergies	____	____
Hearing problems	____	____	Lacks energy	____	____

	Yes	No		Yes	No
Speech problems	___	___	Asthma	___	___
Language problems	___	___	Headaches	___	___
Visual problems	___	___	Eating problems	___	___
Sleeping problems	___	___	Tics/Twitches	___	___
Physical complaints	___	___	Seizures	___	___
Coordination problems	___	___	Lethary	___	___

Development and Behavior

Please indicate the age at which your child began:

Walking alone_____   Using meaningful words_____

Bowel control_____   Bladder control_____

Does your child experience difficulty in conveying his/her thoughts or feelings? If so, please describe._____

_____

Does your child experience academic delays? If so, please describe the areas of delay._____

How does your child interact with

    Mother_____

    Father_____

    Brothers and sisters_____

    Other children_____

    Other adults_____

Does your child display behavior that is particularly stressful for you to manage? If so, please describe._____

_____

Is your child able to initiate and maintain friendships for an expected period of time?_____

Do you suspect your child to be using alcohol or other drugs? If so, please describe._____

_____

What are your child's favorite activities?_____

_____

What are your child's most positive characterestics?_____

_____

_____

Education

Has your child been evaluated by the school or an outside agency for social–emotional, intellectual, or academic delays? If so, please describe._____

_____

_____

Has your child been enrolled in an exceptional education program (learning disabilities, emotional disturbance, mental retardation, speech/language therapy)? If so, please describe the type of program and initial enrollment/dismissal date._____

Do your feel comfortable with your child's current educational program?_____

_____

How does your child relate to his/her teacher?_____

Can your child sustain his/her attention longer for certain activities than others? If so, please describe._____

_____

Under what conditions is your child's behavior least/most tolerable?_____

_____

_____

Please indicate whether the following represent areas of concern you have regarding your child's functioning:

	Yes	No		Yes	No
Following directions	___	___	Reading	___	___
Completing homework	___	___	Math	___	___
Poor concentration	___	___	Spelling	___	___
Excessive daydreaming	___	___	Anger	___	___
Easily distracted	___	___	Impulsiveness	___	___
Verbal aggression	___	___	Fidgety	___	___
Social immaturity	___	___	Seems spacey	___	___
Lying/Stealing	___	___	Defiant behavior	___	___
Temper tantrums	___	___	Withdrawn	___	___
Emotional sensitivity	___	___	Running away	___	___
Physical aggression	___	___	Irritability	___	___
Wetting	___	___	Argumentative	___	___
Soiling	___	___	Shyness	___	___
Sexual behavior	___	___	Low self-esteem	___	___
Preoccupations	___	___	Disorganized	___	___

	Yes	No		Yes	No
Verbal comprehension	____	____	Mood swings	____	____
Remembering things	____	____	Fearful	____	____
Written language	____	____	Social skills	____	____

Reason for referral

What prompted you to seek assistance at this time?_____

_____

Please describe the specific concerns you wish to have addressed._____

_____

_____

What information do you hope to gain as a result of this evaluation?_____

_____

_____

Who in your family appears most and least stressed by the child's behavior? Please describe._____

_____

_____

Name of person completing this form_____

Date_____

Relationship to the child_____

_____

APPENDIX B
QUESTIONNAIRE INFORMATION

For the convenience of the reader, a brief summary of pertinent information for each questionnaire or rating scale reviewed in Chapter 3 is presented below. Included is information concerning the copyright status, current price, if any, availability of computer scoring disks, and where to purchase the materials. Prices and other data were accurate at the time that they were collected but may change over time. They are followed by copies of HSQ, SSQ, and some relevant statistics. These were included because they have been recommended for use in the current assessment protocol. In addition, some have been recently developed and may not yet be familiar to some readers.

PARENT QUESTIONNAIRES

1. Child Behavior Checklist (CBCL)

Number of items: 138   Time to complete: 20–25 minutes
Response format: 0 (not true), 1 (somewhat true), or 2 (very true)

Factors assessed (vary with gender and age): Social withdrawal, depressed, immature, somatic complaints, sex problems, schizoid, aggressive, delinquent, uncommunicative, obsessive–compulsive, hyperactive, hostile withdrawal, obese, cruel

Reliability data available: Yes
Validity data available: Yes
Normative data: Yes ($n = 1,300$)
Ages: 4–16 years

Developer: Thomas M. Achenbach and Craig Edelbrock
Date of publication (most recent revision): 1983
Copyrighted: Yes
Scoring software available: Yes, IBM-PC compatible and Apple II series
Cost: $15.00 for sample packet; $18.00 for manual; $25.00 for 100 forms
Where to obtain: Thomas M. Achenbach, PhD, Department of Psychiatry, University of Vermont, 1 South Prospect, Burlington, VT 05401–3456.
     Phone: 1–802–656–4563

2. Conners Parent Rating Scale (Original) (CPRS)

Number of items: 93   Time to complete: 10–15 minutes
Response format: 0 (not at all) through 3 (very much)

Factors assessed: Conduct disorder, anxious–shy, restless–disorganized, learning
  problem, psychosomatic, obsessive–compulsive, antisocial, hyperactive–immature

Reliability data available: Yes
Validity data available: Yes
Normative data: Yes (*n* = 683)
Ages: 6–14 years

Developer: C. Keith Conners
Date of publication (most recent revision): Originally 1970; manual revised 1989
Copyrighted: Yes
Scoring software available: Yes, IBM-PC compatible only
Cost: $80.00 for complete set of Conners Scales: $16.00 for 25 CPRS forms
Where to obtain: Multi-Health Systems, Inc., 908 Niagara Falls Blvd.,
  North Tonawanda, NY, 14120–2060. Phone: 1–800–666–7007

3. Conners Parent Rating Scale—Revised (CPRS-R)

Number of items: 48   Time to complete: 5–10 minutes
Response format: 0 (not at all) through 3 (very much)

Factors assessed: Conduct problems, learning problems, psychosomatic, impulsive–
  hyperactive, and anxiety.

Reliability data available: Yes
Validity data available: Yes
Normative data: Yes (*n* = 578)
Ages: 3–17 years

Developer: C. Keith Conners (see Goyette, Conners, & Ulrich, 1978)
Date of publication (most recent revision): Originally 1978; manual revised 1989
Copyrighted: Yes
Scoring software available: Yes, IBM-PC compatible only
Cost: $80.00 for complete set of Conners Scales; $16.00 for 25 CPRS-R forms
Where to obtain: Multi-Health Systems, Inc., 908 Niagara Falls Blvd.,
  North Tonawanda, NY, 14120–2060. Phone: 1–800–666–7007

4. Conners Abbreviated Symptom Questionnaire (ASQ)

Number of items: 10 (included in CPRS-R)   Time to complete: 5 minutes or less
Response format: 0 (not at all) through 3 (very much)

Factors assessed: none (not factor analyzed)
Reliability data available: Yes
Validity data available: Yes
Normative data: Yes (n = 578)
Ages: 3–17 years

Developer: C. Keith Conners (see Goyette, Conners, & Ulrich, 1978)
Date of publication (most recent revision): Originally 1978; manual revised 1989
Copyrighted: Yes
Scoring software available: Yes, IBM-PC compatible only
Cost: $80.00 for complete set of Conners Scales; $16.00 for 25 CPRS-R forms
Where to obtain: Multi-Health Systems, Inc., 908 Niagara Falls Blvd.,
    North Tonawanda, NY, 14120–2060. Phone: 1–800–666–7007

5. Revised Behavior Problem Checklist (for use with parents and teachers)

Number of items: 89   Time to complete: 15–20 minutes or less
Response format: 0 (not a problem) through 2 (a severe problem)

Factors assessed: Conduct disordered, socialized aggressive, attention problems—
    immaturity, anxiety-withdrawal, psychotic behavior, and motor excess

Reliability data available: Yes
Validity data available: Yes
Normative data: Yes (n = 578)
Ages: 5–17 years

Developer: Herbert C. Quay and Donald R. Peterson
Date of publication (most recent revision): 1987
Copyrighted: Yes
Scoring software available: No
Cost: $25.00 for kit; $22.00 for 100 additional checklist forms
Where to obtain: Herbert C. Quay, PhD, P. O. Box 248074, University of Miami,
    Coral Gables, FL 33124. Phone: 1–305–284–5208

6. Eyberg Child Behavior Inventory (ECBI)

Number of items: 36   Time to complete: 10 minutes or less
Response format: 1 (never a problem) through 7 (always a problem)

Factors assessed: Conduct problems (unidimensional)
Reliability data available: Yes
Validity data available: Yes
Normative data: No (preliminary comparative data available)
Ages: 2–16 years

Developer: Sheila M. Eyberg
Date of publication (most recent revision): 1980
Copyrighted: Yes
Scoring software available: Yes
Cost: None
Where to obtain: Sheila M. Eyberg, PhD, Department of Clinical and Health
    Psychology, Box J-165, Health Science Center, University of Florida, Gainesville,
    FL 32610–0165. Phone: 1–904–392–4551

7. Home Situations Questionnaire (HSQ)

Number of items: 16   Time to complete: 5 minutes
Response format: 1 (mild problem) through 9 (severe problem)

Factors assessed: Non-family transactions, custodial transactions, task-performance
    transactions, and isolate play

Reliability data available: Yes
Validity data available: Yes
Normative data: Yes (n = 995; see Altepeter & Breen, 1989)
Ages: 4–11 years

Developer: Russell A. Barkley
Date of publication (most recent revision): 1981; norms, 1989
Copyrighted: Yes
Scoring software available: No
Cost: None
Where to obtain: See below, or write Russell A. Barkley, PhD, Department of
    Psychiatry, University of Massachusetts Medical Center, 55 Lake Avenue North,
    Worcester, MA 01605

TEACHER QUESTIONNAIRES

1. Child Behavior Checklist—Teacher Report Form (TRF)

Number of items: 118   Time to complete: 20 minutes
Response format: 0 (not true), 1 (somewhat true), or 2 (very true)

Factors assessed: (vary with gender and age): Anxious, social withdrawal, unpopular, self-destructive, obsessive–compulsive, inattentive, nervous–overactive, aggressive, immature, depressed, delinquent

Reliability data available: Yes
Validity data available: Yes
Normative data: Yes ($n = 1,100$)
Ages: 6–16 years

Developer: Thomas M. Achenbach and Craig Edelbrock
Date of publication (most recent revision): 1984
Copyrighted: Yes
Scoring software available: Yes, IBM-PC compatible and Apple II series
Cost: $15.00 for sample packet; $18.00 for manual; $25.00 for 100 forms
Where to obtain: Thomas M. Achenbach, PhD, Department of Psychiatry, University of Vermont, 1 South Prospect, Burlington, VT 05401–3456. Phone: 1–800–656–4563

2. Conners Teacher Rating Scale (Original) (CTRS)

Number of items: 39   Time to complete: 5–10 minutes
Response format: 0 (not at all) through 3 (very much)

Factors assessed: Hyperactivity, conduct problem, emotional–overindulgent, anxious–passive, asocial, daydream–attention problem

Reliability data available: Yes
Validity data available: Yes
Normative data: Yes ($n = 9583$; see Trites, Blouin, & Laprade, 1982)
Ages: 4–12 years

Developer: C. Keith Conners
Date of publication (most recent revision): Originally 1969; norms, 1982; manual revised 1989
Copyrighted: Yes
Scoring software available: Yes, IBM-PC compatible only
Cost: $80.00 for complete set of Conners Scales; $16.00 for 25 CTRS forms
Where to obtain: Multi-Health Systems, Inc., 908 Niagara Falls Blvd., North Tonawanda, NY, 14120–2060. Phone: 1–800–666–7007

3. Conners Teacher Rating Scale—Revised (CTRS-R)

Number of items: 28   Time to complete: 5 minutes
Response format: 0 (not at all) through 3 (very much)

Factors assessed: Conduct problem, hyperactive, inattentive-passive
Reliability data available: Yes
Validity data available: Yes
Normative data: Yes ($n = 388$)
Ages: 3–17 years

Developer: C. Keith Conners (see Goyette, Conners, & Ulrich, 1978)
Date of publication (most recent revision): Originally 1978; manual revised 1989
Copyrighted: Yes
Scoring software available: Yes, IBM-PC compatible only
Cost: $80.00 for complete set of Conners Scales; $16.00 for 25 CTRS-R forms
Where to obtain: Multi-Health Systems, Inc., 908 Niagara Falls Blvd.,
    North Tonawanda, NY, 14120–2060. Phone: 1–800–666–7007

4. Conners Abbreviated Symptom Questionnaire (ASQ)

Number of items: 10 (included in CTRS-R)   Time to complete: 5 minutes or less
Response format: 0 (not at all) through 3 (very much)

Factors assessed: None (not factor analyzed)
Reliability data available: Yes
Validity data available: Yes
Normative data: Yes ($n = 383$)
Ages: 3–17 years

Developer: C. Keith Conners (see Goyette, Conners, & Ulrich, 1978)
Date of publication (most recent revision): Originally 1978; manual revised 1989
Copyrighted: Yes
Scoring software available: Yes, IBM-PC compatible only
Cost: $80.00 for complete set of Conners Scales; $16.00 for 25 CTRS-R forms
Where to obtain: Multi-Health Systems, Inc., 908 Niagara Falls Blvd.,
    North Tonawanda, NY, 14120–2060. Phone: 1–800–666–7007

5. IOWA Conners Teacher Rating Scale

Number of items: 10 (modified from the original CTRS)
Time to complete: 5 minutes or less
Response format: 0 (not at all) through 3 (very much)

Factors assessed: Hyperactivity and aggression
Reliability data available: No
Validity data available: No
Normative data: No
Ages: 4–12 years

Developer: Jan Loney and Richard Milich
Date of publication (most recent revision): 1981
Copyrighted: No
Scoring software available: No
Cost: None
Where to obtain: Jan Loney, PhD, Department of Psychiatry, State University of
    New York at Stoney Brook, Stony Brook, NY 11794–8790

6. ADD/H Comprehensive Teacher Rating Scale (ACTeRS)

Number of items: 24   Time to complete: 5–10 minutes
Response format: 1 (almost never) through 4 (almost always)

Factors assessed: Attention, hyperactivity, social skills, and oppositional

Reliability data available: Yes
Validity data available: Yes
Normative data: Yes (n = 1,347)
Ages: 5–12 years

Developer: Rina K. Ullmann, Esther K. Sleator, and Robert L. Sprague
Date of publication (most recent revision): 1988
Copyrighted: Yes
Scoring software available: Yes IBM compatible only
Cost: $48.00 for kit; $40.00 for 100 forms
Where to obtain: MetriTech, Inc., 111 North Market Street, Champaign, IL 61820.
    Phone: 1–800–747–4868

7. School Situations Questionnaire (SSQ)

Number of items: 12   Time to complete: 5 minutes
Response format: 1 (mild problem) through 9 (severe problem)

Factors assessed: Unsupervised settings, task performance, and special events

Reliability data available: Yes
Validity data available: Yes
Normative data: Yes ($n = 615$; see Altepeter & Breen, 1989)
Ages: 6–11 years

Developer: Russell A. Barkley
Date of publication (most recent revision): Originally 1981; norms, 1989
Copyrighted: Yes
Scoring software available: No
Cost: None
Where to obtain: See below, or write Russell A. Barkley, PhD, Department of
   Psychiatry, University of Massachusetts Medical Center, 55 Lake Avenue North,
   Worcester, MA 01605

8. The Stony Brook Scale

Number of items: 68   Time to complete: 10–15 minutes
Response format: 0 (not at all) through 3 (very much)

Factors assessed: Aggression, anxiety–depression, hyperactivity, and uncoordination

Reliability data available: No
Validity data available: No
Normative data: No
Ages: 5–11 years

Developer: Susan G. O'Leary and Patricia L. Steen
Date of publication (most recent revision): 1982
Copyrighted: No
Scoring software available: No
Cost: None
Where to obtain: Susan G. O'Leary, PhD, Department of Psychology, State
   University of New York at Stony Brook, Stony Brook, NY 11794–8790

9. Self-Control Rating Scale

Number of items: 33   Time to complete: 5–10 minutes
Response format: 1 (maximum self-control) through 7 (maximum impulsivity)

Factors assessed: Cognitive–behavioral self-control (unidimensional)
Reliability data available: Yes
Validity data available: Yes
Normative data: Yes (ages 8–12, $n = 110$; see Kendall & Wilcox, 1979)
     (ages 9–11, $n = 763$; see Humphrey, 1982)

Ages: 8–12 years

Developer: Phillip C. Kendall and Lance E. Wilcox
Date of publication (most recent revision): Originally 1979; norms, 1982
Copyrighted: No
Scoring software available: No
Cost: None
Where to obtain: Phillip C. Kendall, PhD, Department of Psychology, Temple
 University, Philadelphia, PA 19122

YOUTH SELF-REPORT QUESTIONNAIRES

1. Child Behavior Checklist—Youth Self-Report (YSR)

Number of items: 103   Time to complete: 20 minutes
Response format: 0 (not true), 1 (somewhat true), or 2 (very true)

Factors assessed (vary with gender): Depressed, unpopular, somatic complaints,
 thought disorder, self-destructive, aggressive, delinquent

Reliability data available: Yes
Validity data available: Yes (limited to information in the manual)
Normative data: Yes ($n = 686$)
Ages: 11–18 years

Developer: Thomas M. Achenbach and Craig Edelbrock
Date of publication (most recent revision): 1987
Copyrighted: Yes
Scoring software available: Yes, IBM-PC compatible and Apple II series
Cost: $15.00 for sample packet; $18.00 for manual; $25.00 for 100 forms
Where to obtain: Thomas M. Achenbach, PhD, Department of Psychiatry,
 University of Vermont, 1 South Prospect, Burlington, VT 05401–3456.
 Phone: 1–800–656–4563

2. Child Depression Inventory (CDI)

Number of items: 27   Time to complete: 10–15 minutes
Response format: 0 through 2

Factors assessed: Inconclusive (diverse findings across several studies)
Reliability data available: Yes
Validity data available: Yes
Normative data: Yes ($n = 1,463$; see Finch et al., 1985; other independent norm
   samples are also available)
Ages: 8–13 years

Developer: Maria C. Kovacs
Date of publication (most recent revision): 1981
Copyrighted: Yes
Scoring software available: No
Cost: None
Where to obtain: Maria C. Kovacs, PhD, Western Psychiatric Institute and Clinic,
   3811 O'Hara Street, Pittsburgh, PA 15213

3. Reynolds Adolescent Depression Scale (RADS)

Number of items: 30   Time to complete: 5–10 minutes
Response format: 0–3

Factors assessed: Generalized demoralization, despondency and worry, somatic–
   vegetative symptoms, anhedonia, and lowered self-worth

Reliability data available: Yes
Validity data available: Yes
Normative data: Yes ($n = 2,460$)
Ages: 12–18 years

Developer: William M. Reynolds
Date of publication (most recent revision): 1986
Copyrighted: Yes
Scoring software available: No
Cost: $29.00 for kit; $12.00 for 25 additional forms
Where to obtain: Psychological Assessment Resources, Inc., P. O. Box 998, Odessa,
   FL 33556. Phone: 1–800–331–8378

PARENTAL/FAMILY RATING SCALES

1. Beck Depression Inventory (BDI)

Number of items: 21   Time to complete: 5–10 minutes
Response format: 0–3

Factors assessed: Generalized depression, negative attitudes, performance difficulties, and somatic complaints

Reliability data available: Yes
Validity data available: Yes
Normative data: No; cutoffs based upon comparative data in clinical samples are available
Ages: 18 years and up (requires sixth grade reading level)

Developer: Aaron T. Beck
Date of publication (most recent revision): 1986
Copyrighted: Yes
Scoring software available: No
Cost: $35.00 for kit
Where to obtain: The Psychological Corporation, 555 Academic Court, San Antonio, TX 78204–2498. Phone: 1–800–228–0752

2. Parenting Stress Index (PSI)

Number of items: 120   Time to complete: 15–20 minutes
Response format: 1 (strongly agree) through 5 (strongly disagree)

Factors assessed: Six child domains (adaptability, acceptability, demandingness, mood, distractibility/hyperactivity, and reinforces parent) and seven parent domains (depression, attachment, restriction of role, sense of competence, social isolation, relationship with spouse, and parent health)

Reliability data available: Yes
Validity data available: Yes
Normative data: Yes ($n = 534$)
Ages: parents complete, norms sample includes ages 18–65 (requires fifth grade reading level)

Developer: Richard R. Abidin
Date of publication (most recent revision): 1986
Copyrighted: Yes
Scoring software available: Yes
Cost: $27.50 for kit
Where to obtain: Clinical Psychological Publishing Co., Inc., 4 Conant Square, Brandon, VT 05733. Phone: 1–802–247–6871

3. Conflict Behavior Questionnaire (for use with adolescents and parents)

Number of items: 75 (parent version), 73 (adolescent version)
Time to complete: 10–20 minutes
Response format: true-false

Factors assessed: None (not factor-analyzed)
Reliability data available: Yes
Validity data available: Yes
Normative data: No (comparison data are available)
Ages: Adolescents and parents

Developer: Ronald J. Prinz
Date of publication (most recent revision): 1977
Copyrighted: Yes
Scoring software available: No
Cost: None
Where to obtain: Ronald J. Prinz, PhD, Department of Psychology, University of
South Carolina, Columbia, SC 29208

4. Issues Checklist (for use with adolescents)

Number of items: 44   Time to complete: 15–20 minutes
Response format: Yes-no, frequency of items responded yes, severity (1 to 5) of
items responsed yes

Factors assessed: None (not factor-analyzed)
Reliability data available: Yes
Validity data available: Yes
Normative data: No (comparison data are available)
Ages: Adolescents and parents

Developer: Ronald J. Prinz
Date of publication (most recent revision): 1979
Copyrighted: Yes
Scoring software available: No
Cost: None
Where to obtain: Ronald J. Prinz, PhD, Department of Psychology, University of
South Carolina, Columbia, SC 29208

HOME SITUATIONS QUESTIONNAIRE (HSQ)

Child's name_____ Date_____

Name of person completing this form_____

Instructions: Does your child present any behavior problems in any of these situations? If so, please indicte how severe they are.

	Circle yes or no		If yes, how severe? (Circle one.) Mild → Severe								
1. While playing alone	yes	no	1	2	3	4	5	6	7	8	9
2. While playing with other children	yes	no	1	2	3	4	5	6	7	8	9
3. During mealtime	yes	no	1	2	3	4	5	6	7	8	9
4. While getting dressed	yes	no	1	2	3	4	5	6	7	8	9
5. While washing/bathing	yes	no	1	2	3	4	5	6	7	8	9
6. While you are on the telephone	yes	no	1	2	3	4	5	6	7	8	9
7. While watching TV	yes	no	1	2	3	4	5	6	7	8	9
8. When visitors are in your home	yes	no	1	2	3	4	5	6	7	8	9
9. When you are visiting someone else	yes	no	1	2	3	4	5	6	7	8	9
10. In public places (supermarkets, stores, churches, restaurants, etc.)	yes	no	1	2	3	4	5	6	7	8	9
11. When asked to do chores at home	yes	no	1	2	3	4	5	6	7	8	9
12. At bedtime	yes	no	1	2	3	4	5	6	7	8	9
13. While in the car	yes	no	1	2	3	4	5	6	7	8	9
14. While with a babysitter	yes	no	1	2	3	4	5	6	7	8	9
15. When father is home	yes	no	1	2	3	4	5	6	7	8	9
16. When asked to do school homework	yes	no	1	2	3	4	5	6	7	8	9

Note. From *Hyperactive Children: A Handbook for Diagnosis and Treatment* by R. A. Barkley, 1981, New York: Guilford. Copyright 1981 by The Guilford Press. Adapted by permission.

MEANS, STANDARD DEVIATIONS, AND SIGNIFICANT CUTOFFS FOR THE HOME SITUATIONS QUESTIONNAIRE FACTORIAL DIMENSIONS

Age	N	Non-family transactions			Custodial transactions			Task-performance transactions			Isolate play		
		$\bar{x}$	SD	Cutoff	$\bar{x}$	SD	Cutoff	$\bar{x}$	SD	Cutoff	$\bar{x}$	SD	Cutoff
Boys													
4–5	162	.62	.98	(3)	.45	.83	(2)	.37	.68	(2)	.11	.37	(1)
6–8	203	.78	1.06	(3)	.63	1.06	(3)	.76	.98	(3)	.23	.68	(2)
9–11	139	.65	1.07	(3)	.41	.68	(2)	1.08	1.35	(4)	.21	.58	(1)
Girls													
4–5	146	.39	.67	(2)	.36	.75	(2)	.26	.51	(1)	.18	.87	(2)
6–8	202	.62	1.06	(3)	.51	.93	(2)	.68	1.06	(3)	.16	.53	(1)
9–11	142	.38	.62	(2)	.32	.78	(2)	.83	1.25	(3)	.17	.57	(1)

Note. Factorial dimensions, means, standard deviations, and significant cutoffs taken from "Factor Structure of the Home Situations Questionnaire (HSQ) and the School Situations Questionnaire (SSQ)" by M. Breen, and T. Altepeter, 1990, manuscript under review. Scores for items assigned to each factor were summed and divided by the number of questions assigned to or loading on that factor. Items assigned to each factor are as follows:

Non-family transactions: 2, 6, 8, 9, 10, 13, 14
Custodial transactions: 3, 4, 12, 15
Task-performance transactions: 5, 11, 16
Isolate play: 1, 7

SCHOOL SITUATIONS QUESTIONNAIRE (SSQ)

Child's name_____   Date_____

Name of person completing this form_____

Instructions: Does this child present any behavior problems in any of these situations? If so, please indicte how severe they are.

	Circle yes or no		If yes, how severe? (Circle one.) Mild → Severe								
1. While arriving at school	yes	no	1	2	3	4	5	6	7	8	9
2. During individual deskwork	yes	no	1	2	3	4	5	6	7	8	9
3. During small group activi - ties	yes	no	1	2	3	4	5	6	7	8	9
4. During free play time in class	yes	no	1	2	3	4	5	6	7	8	9
5. During lectures to the class	yes	no	1	2	3	4	5	6	7	8	9
6. During recess	yes	no	1	2	3	4	5	6	7	8	9
7. During lunch	yes	no	1	2	3	4	5	6	7	8	9
8. While in the hallways	yes	no	1	2	3	4	5	6	7	8	9
9. While in the bathroom	yes	no	1	2	3	4	5	6	7	8	9
10. During field trips	yes	no	1	2	3	4	5	6	7	8	9
11. During special assemblies	yes	no	1	2	3	4	5	6	7	8	9
12. While on the bus	yes	no	1	2	3	4	5	6	7	8	9

Note. From *Hyperactive Children: A Handbook for Diagnosis and Treatment* by R. A. Barkley, 1981, New York: Guilford. Copyright 1981 by The Guilford Press. Adapted by permission.

MEANS, STANDARD DEVIATIONS, AND SIGNIFICANT CUTOFFS FOR THE SCHOOL SITUATIONS QUESTIONNAIRE FACTORIAL DIMENSIONS

Age	N	Unsupervised settings			Task performance			Special events		
		$\bar{x}$	SD	Cutoff	$\bar{x}$	SD	Cutoff	$\bar{x}$	SD	Cutoff
Boys										
6–8	169	.69	1.31	(3)	1.06	1.78	(5)	.21	.78	(2)
9–11	124	.99	1.68	(4)	1.23	1.89	(5)	.23	.87	(2)
Girls										
6–8	180	.27	.87	(2)	.44	1.12	(3)	.06	.33	(1)
9–11	142	.25	.56	(1)	.51	1.10	(3)	.03	.21	(1)

Note. Factorial dimensions, means, standard deviations, and significant cutoffs taken from "Factor Structure of the Home Situations Questionnaire (HSQ) and the School Situations Questionnaire (SSQ)" by M. Breen, and T. Altepeter, 1990, Manuscript under review. Scores for items assigned to each factor were summed and divided by the number of questions assigned to or loading on that factor. Items assigned to each factor are as follows:

Unsupervised settings: 1, 4, 6, 7, 8, 9
Task-performance: 2, 3, 5
Special events: 10, 11, 12

MEANS, STANDARD DEVIATIONS, AND SIGNIFICANT CUTOFF POINTS FOR THE NUMBER OF PROBLEM SITUATIONS AND MEAN SEVERITY FOR THE HOME AND SCHOOL SITUATIONS QUESTIONNAIRES

Age	N	Number of problem situations			Mean severity		
		$\bar{x}$	SD	Cutoff	$\bar{x}$	SD	Cutoff
Home Situations Questionnaire							
Boys							
4–5	162	3.15	(2.79)	(9)	1.65	(1.40)	(4)
6–8	203	4.13	(3.36)	(11)	1.98	(1.36)	(5)
9–11	139	3.54	(3.19)	(10)	1.97	(1.54)	(5)
Girls							
4–5	146	2.16	(2.60)	(7)	1.25	(1.42)	(4)
6–8	202	3.40	(3.47)	(10)	1.60	(1.54)	(5)
9–11	142	2.66	(3.24)	(9)	1.55	(1.45)	(5)
School Situations Questionnaire							
Boys							
6–8	169	2.41	(3.25)	(9)	1.51	(1.96)	(5)
9–11	124	2.77	(3.16)	(9)	1.86	(2.09)	(6)
Girls							
6–8	180	.95	(2.00)	(5)	.77	(1.52)	(4)
9–11	126	1.24	(2.11)	(5)	.84	(1.24)	(3)

Note. Normative data are taken from "The Home Situations Questionnaire (SSQ) and the School Situations Questionnaire (SSQ): Normative Data and an Evaluation of Psychometric Properties" by T. Altepeter and M. Breen, 1989, *Journal of Psychoeducational Assessment, 7*, p. 312–322. Copyright 1989 by Grune & Stratton, Inc. Adapted by permission.

APPENDIX C
MEDICATION EVALUATION AND QUESTIONNAIRES

DRUG–PLACEBO EVALUATION

Protocol for Establishing Efficacy of Stimulant Medication

1. Parent-completed questionnaires
   a. Conners Parent Rating Scale
   b. Home Situations Questionnaire
   c. Home Side Effects Questionnaire
2. Teacher-completed questionnaires
   a. Conners Teacher Rating Scale
   b. School Situations Questionnaire
   c. School Side Effects Questionnaire
   d. Child Attention Profile
3. Clinic measures
   a. Matching Familiar Figure Test
   b. Children's Selective Reminding Test
   c. Gordon Diagnostic System
   d. Observations within a Restricted Academic Situation format

Note: For a more extensive protocol, see Barkley et al. (1988,1989).

MEDICATION SIDE EFFECTS QUESTIONNAIRES

Below are two behavior questionnaires we have found useful in monitoring potential side effects of various medications used with disruptive-behavior-disordered children. The first questionnaire, Form A, was adapted from Barkley (1981) for use with stimulant medications (Ritalin, Cylert, and Dexedrine). The second questionnaire, Form B, was designed for use with antidepressant medications (Imipramine and Desipramine). The questionnaires may be completed by any reliable adult informant who has daily contact with the child, including teachers, parents, etc. Obviously, teachers may not have knowledge of some behaviors, such as difficulties with sleep. However, consistent with the assessment approach discussed in this text, we maintain that a more accurate, objective impression is formed if data are gathered from two or more informants across two or more settings. Thus, we attempt to have the questionnaires completed by the

243

primary teacher and at least one parent when possible. We have found that it is best to administer the questionnaire at least once, preferably twice, prior to initiating treatment with any medication. This provides a premedication baseline against which subsequent responses can be assessed. Once medication is initiated, we typically administer the relevant questionnaire on a weekly basis for the first 4–6 weeks, or several weeks after the therapeutic dose has been reached, whichever is longer. Then we typically readminister the questionnaire every 2–3 months while the child remains on the same dosage, or again weekly if the medication being used or the dosage level is changed.

1. Side Effects Questionnaire: Form A (for use with stimulants)

Child's name_____   Date_____

Informant_____

Please rate each behavior from 0 (absent) to 9 (serious). Circle only one number beside each item. A zero means that you have not seen this behavior in your child during the past week. A 9 means that you have noticed it and believe it to be either very serious or occurring very frequently. Thank you.

Trouble sleeping	0	1	2	3	4	5	6	7	8	9
Nightmares	0	1	2	3	4	5	6	7	8	9
Stares a lot or daydreams	0	1	2	3	4	5	6	7	8	9
Talks less with others	0	1	2	3	4	5	6	7	8	9
Disinterested in others	0	1	2	3	4	5	6	7	8	9
Decreased appetite	0	1	2	3	4	5	6	7	8	9
Stomach aches or nausea	0	1	2	3	4	5	6	7	8	9
Headaches	0	1	2	3	4	5	6	7	8	9
Drowsiness or tiredness	0	1	2	3	4	5	6	7	8	9
Sad or unhappy	0	1	2	3	4	5	6	7	8	9
Prone to crying	0	1	2	3	4	5	6	7	8	9
Anxious	0	1	2	3	4	5	6	7	8	9
Bites his nails	0	1	2	3	4	5	6	7	8	9
Unusually happy	0	1	2	3	4	5	6	7	8	9
Dizziness	0	1	2	3	4	5	6	7	8	9
Tics or twitches	0	1	2	3	4	5	6	7	8	9
Nervous movements	0	1	2	3	4	5	6	7	8	9
Skin rash	0	1	2	3	4	5	6	7	8	9
Numbness or tingling in limbs	0	1	2	3	4	5	6	7	8	9

Note. This questionnaire was designed for use with stimulant medications. From *Hyperactive Children: A Handbook for Diagnosis and Treatment* by R. A. Barkley, 1981, New York: Guilford. Copyright 1981 by The Guilford Press. Adapted by permission.

2. Side Effects Questionnaire: Form B (for use with antidepressants)

Child's name_____ Date_____

Informant_____

Please rate each behavior from 0 (absent) to 9 (serious). Circle only one number beside each item. A zero means that you have not seen this behavior in your child during the past week. A 9 means that you have noticed it and believe it to be either very serious or occurring very frequently. Thank you.

Trouble falling sleeping	0	1	2	3	4	5	6	7	8	9
Decreased appetite	0	1	2	3	4	5	6	7	8	9
Has nightmares	0	1	2	3	4	5	6	7	8	9
Has dry mouth	0	1	2	3	4	5	6	7	8	9
Complains of or seems to have blurred vision	0	1	2	3	4	5	6	7	8	9
Motor incoordination	0	1	2	3	4	5	6	7	8	9
Complains of or seems to have weakness or fatigue	0	1	2	3	4	5	6	7	8	9
Nausea	0	1	2	3	4	5	6	7	8	9
Motor tremors	0	1	2	3	4	5	6	7	8	9
Numbness in extremities	0	1	2	3	4	5	6	7	8	9
Irritable or moody	0	1	2	3	4	5	6	7	8	9
Complains of stomach ache	0	1	2	3	4	5	6	7	8	9
Wakes up frequently	0	1	2	3	4	5	6	7	8	9
Complains of headache	0	1	2	3	4	5	6	7	8	9
Drowsiness	0	1	2	3	4	5	6	7	8	9
Skin rash	0	1	2	3	4	5	6	7	8	9
Diarrhea	0	1	2	3	4	5	6	7	8	9
Has convulsions or seizures	0	1	2	3	4	5	6	7	8	9
Seems nervous or anxious	0	1	2	3	4	5	6	7	8	9
Increased urination	0	1	2	3	4	5	6	7	8	9
Complains of or seems dizzy	0	1	2	3	4	5	6	7	8	9
Constipation	0	1	2	3	4	5	6	7	8	9
Increased perspiration	0	1	2	3	4	5	6	7	8	9
Odd or unusual behaviors or nervous mannerisms	0	1	2	3	4	5	6	7	8	9

Note. This questionnaire was designed for use with antidepressant medications. It may be reproduced.

REFERENCES

Abidin, R. R. (1986). *Parenting Stress Index-Manual*. Charlottesville, VA: Pediatric Psychology Press.

Abikoff, H. (1985). Efficacy of cognitive training interventions with hyperactive children: A critical review. *Clinical Psychology Review, 5,* 479–512.

Abikoff, H. (1987). An evaluation of cognitive behavior therapy for hyperactive children. In B. Lahey & A. Kazdin (Eds.), *Advances in clinical child psychology* (Vol. 10, pp. 171–216). New York: Plenum Press.

Abikoff, H., & Gittelman, R. (1984). Does behavior therapy normalize the classroom behavior of hyperactive children? *Archives of General Psychiatry, 41,* 449–454.

Abikoff, H., & Gittelman, R. (1985). Hyperactive children treated with stimulants: Is cognitive training a useful adjunct? *Archives of General Psychiatry, 42,* 953–961.

Abramowitz, A. J., O'Leary, S. G., & Rosen, L. A. (1987). Reducing off-task behavior in the classroom: A comparison of encouragement and reprimands. *Journal of Abnormal Child Psychology, 15,* 153–163.

Achenbach, T. M. (1974). *Developmental psychopathology*. New York: Wiley.

Achenbach, T. M. (1982). *Developmental psychopathology*. New York: Wiley.

Achenbach, T. M., & Edelbrock, C. S. (1978). The classification of child psychopathology: A review and analysis of empirical efforts. *Psychological Bulletin, 55,* 1275–1301.

Achenbach, T. M., & Edelbrock, C. S. (1983). *Manual for the Child Behavior Checklist and Revised Child Behavior Profile*. Burlington, VT: University of Vermont, Department of Psychiatry.

Achenbach, T. M., & Edelbrock, C. S. (1986). *Manual for the Teacher's Report Form and Teacher Version of the Child Behavior Profile*. Burlington, VT: University of Vermont, Department of Psychiatry.

Achenbach, T. M., & Edelbrock, C. (1987). *Manual for the Youth Self-Report and Profile*. Burlington, VT: University of Vermont, Department of Psychiatry.

Acker, M. M., & O'Leary, S. G. (1987). Effects of reprimands and praise on appropriate behavior in the classroom. *Journal of Abnormal Child Psychology, 15*, 549–557.

Ackerman, P. T., Elardo, P. T., & Dykman, R. A. (1979). A psychosocial study of hyperactive and learning disabled boys. *Journal of Abnormal Child Psychology, 7*, 91–99.

Altepeter, T. S., & Breen, M. J. (1989). The Home Situations Questionnaire (HSQ) and the School Situations Questionnaire (SSQ): Normative data and an evaluation of psychometric properties. *Journal of Psychoeducational Assessment, 7*, 312–322.

Aman, M. G., & Werry, J. S. (1984). The Revised Behavior Problem Checklist in clinic attenders and nonattenders: Age and sex effects. *Journal of Clinical Child Psychology, 13*, 237–242.

American Psychiatric Association. (1968). *Diagnostic and statistical manual of mental disorders*. (2nd ed.). Washington, DC: Author.

American Psychiatric Association. (1980). *Diagnostic and statistical manual of mental disorders*. (3rd ed.). Washington, DC: Author.

American Psychiatric Association. (1987). *Diagnostic and statistical manual of mental disorders*. (3rd ed.-rev.). Washington, DC: Author.

Aragona, J. A., & Eyberg, S. M. (1981). Neglected children: Mothers' report of child behavior problems and observed verbal behavior. *Child Development, 52*, 596–602.

Arnold, L. E., Barnebey, N. S., & Smeltzer, D. J. (1981). First-grade norms, factor analysis and cross correlation for Conners, Davids, and Quay-Peterson behavior rating scales. *Journal of Learning Disabilities, 14*, 269–275.

Atkeson, B. M., & Forehand, R. (1979). Home-based reinforcement programs designed to modify classroom behavior: A review and methodological evaluation. *Psychological Bulletin, 86*, 1298–1308.

Atkins, M. C., Pelham, W. E., & Licht, M. H. (1985). A comparison of objective classroom measures and teacher ratings of attention deficit disorder. *Journal of Abnormal Child Psychology, 13*, 155–167.

Ayllon, T., Garber, S., & Pisor, K. (1975). The elimination of discipline problems through a combined school-time motivational system. *Behavior Therapy, 6*, 616–626.

Aylward, G. P., Verhulst, S. J., Bell, S., Kelly, D. P., & Dorry, G. W. (1988). The relationship between the GDS and DSM-III diagnoses: Introduction of the Accuracy Index (AI). *The ADD Hyperactivity Newsletter, 11*, 2–6.

Azrin, N. H., & Besalel, V. A. (1979). *A parent's guide to bedwetting control: A step-by-step method*. New York: Simon & Schuster.

Azrin, N., & Foxx, R. (1976). *Toilet training in less than a day*. New York: Pocket Books.

Baker, L., Cantwell, D. P., & Mattison, R. E. (1980). Behavior problems in children with pure speech disorders and in children with combined speech and language disorders. *Journal of Abnormal Child Psychology, 8,* 245–256.

Bandura, A. (1977). *Social learning theory.* Englewood Cliffs, NJ: Prentice-Hall.

Barkley, R. A. (1977). A review of stimulant drug research with hyperactive children. *Journal of Child Psychology and Psychiatry, 18,* 137–165.

Barkley, R. A. (1981). *Hyperactive children: A handbook for diagnosis and treatment.* New York: Guilford Press.

Barkley, R. A. (1982). Specific guidelines for defining hyperactivity in children (attention deficit disorder with hyperactivity). In B. B. Lahey & A. E. Kazdin (Eds.), *Advances in clinical child psychology* (Vol. 5, pp. 137–180). New York: Plenum Press.

Barkley, R. A. (1983). Hyperactivity. In R. J. Morris & T. R. Kratochwill (Eds.), *The practice of child therapy* (pp. 87–112). New York: Pergamon Press.

Barkley, R. A. (1985a). The social interactions of hyperactive children: Developmental changes, drug effects, and situational variation. In R. McMahon & R. Peters (Eds.), *Childhood disorders: Behavioral-developmental approaches* (pp. 218–243). New York: Brunner/Mazel.

Barkley, R. A. (1985b). Family interaction patterns in hyperactive children: Precursors to aggressive behavior? In M. Wolraich & D. Routh (Eds.), *Advances in behavioral pediatrics* (Vol. 6, pp. 117–150). Greenwich, CT: JAI Press.

Barkley, R. A. (1987). *Defiant children: A clinician's manual for parent training.* New York: Guilford Press.

Barkley, R. A. (1988a). Attention Deficit Disorder with hyperactivity. In E. J. Mash & L. G. Terdal (Eds.), *Behavioral assessment of childhood disorders* (2nd ed., pp. 69–104). New York: Guilford Press.

Barkley, R. A. (1988b). Tic disorders and Gilles de la Tourette syndrome. In E. J. Mash & L. G. Terdal (Eds.), *Behavioral assessment of childhood disorders* (2nd ed., pp. 552–585). New York: Guilford Press.

Barkley, R. A. (1988c). Child behavior rating scales and checklists. In M. Rutter, A. H. Tuma, & I. S. Lann (Eds.), *Assessment and diagnosis in child psychopathology* (pp. 113–155). New York: Guilford Press.

Barkley, R. A. (1988d). The effects of methylphenidate on the interactions of preschool ADHD children with their mothers. *Journal of the American Academy of Child and Adolescent Psychiatry, 27,* 336–341.

Barkley, R. A. (1989a). Attention-deficit Hyperactivity Disorder. In E. J. Mash & R. A. Barkley (Eds.), *Treatment of childhood disorders* (pp. 39–72). New York: Guilford Press.

Barkley, R. A. (1989b). Hyperactive girls and boys: Stimulant drug effects on mother-child interactions. *Journal of Child Psychology and Psychiatry, 3,* 379–390.

Barkley, R. A., & Cunningham, C. E. (1979). Stimulant drugs and activity level in hyperactive children. *American Journal of Orthopsychiatry, 49,* 491–499.

Barkley, R. A., & Edelbrock, C. (1987). Assessing situational variation in children's problem behaviors: The Home and School Situations Questionnaire. In R. Prinz

(Ed.), *Advances in behavioral assessment of children and families* (Vol. 3, pp. 157–176). Greenwich, CT: JAI Press.

Barkley, R. A., Fischer, M., Newby, R., & Breen, M. J. (1988). Development of a multi-method clinical protocol for assessing stimulant drug responses in ADHD children. *Journal of Clinical Child Psychology, 17,* 14–24.

Barkley, R. A., Karlsson, J., & Pollard, S. (1985a). Effects of age on mother-child interactions of hyperactive boys. *Journal of Abnormal Child Psychology, 13,* 631–637.

Barkley, R. A., Karlsson, J., Pollard, S., & Murphy, J. (1985b). Developmental changes in the mother-child interactions of hyperactive boys: Effects of two doses of Ritalin. *Journal of Child Psychology and Psychiatry, 26,* 705–715.

Barkley, R. A., Karlsson, J., Strzelecki, E., & Murphy, J. (1984). Effects of age and Ritalin dosage on the mother-child interactions of hyperactive children. *Journal of Consulting and Clinical Psychology, 52,* 750–758.

Barkley, R. A., McMurray, M. B. Edelbrock, C. S., & Robbins, K. (1989). The response of aggressive and nonaggressive ADHD children to two doses of methylphenidate. *Journal of the American Academy of Child and Adolescent Psychiatry, 28,* 873–881.

Barkley, R. A., Spitzer, R., & Costello, A. (1990). The development of the DSM-III-R criteria for the Disruptive Behavior Disorders. *Manuscript under review.*

Beach, C. F., & Laird, J. D. (1968). Follow-up study of children identified early as emotionally disturbed. *Journal of Consulting and Clinical Psychology, 32,* 369–374.

Beck, A. T. (1976). *Cognitive therapy and the emotional disorders.* New York: International Universities Press.

Beck, A. T., & Beamesderfer, A. (1974). Assessment of depression: The Depression Inventory. In P. Pichot (Ed.), *Modern problems in pharmacopsychiatry* (pp. 151–169). Basel, Switzerland: Karger.

Beck, A. T., & Beck, R. W. (1972). Screening depressed patients in family practice: A rapid technique. *Postgraduate Medicine, 52,* 81–85.

Beck, A. T., Rush, A. J., Shaw, B. F., & Emergy, G. (1979). *Cognitive therapy of depression.* New York: Guilford Press.

Beck, A. T., Steer, R. A., & Garbin, M. G. (1988). Psychometric properties of the Beck Depression Inventory: Twenty-five years of evaluation. *Clinical Psychology Review, 8,* 77–100.

Beck, A. T., Ward, C. H., Mendelson, M., Mock, J., & Erbaugh, J. (1961). An inventory of measuring depression. *Archives of General Psychiatry, 4,* 561–571.

Becker, W. C., Madsen, C. H., Arnold, C. R., & Thomas, D. R. (1967). The contingent use of teacher attention and praising in reducing classroom problems. *Journal of Special Education, 1,* 287–307.

Befera, M., & Barkley, R. A. (1985). Hyperactive and normal girls and boys: Mother–child interactions, parent psychiatric status, and child psychopathology. *Journal of Child Psychology and Psychiatry, 26,* 439–452.

Behar, D., Rapoport, J. L., Adams, A. J., Berg, C. J., & Cornblath, M. (1984). Sugar challenge testing with children considered behaviorally "sugar reactive." *Nutrition and Behavior, 1,* 227–288.

Bemporad, J. R., & Schwab, M. E. (1986). The DSM-III and clinical child psychiatry. In T. Millon & G. L. Lerman (Eds.), *Contemporary directions in psychopathology: Toward the DSM-IV* (pp. 135–150). New York: Guilford Press.

Bender, L. (1942). Post encephalitic behavior disorders in childhood. In L. Bender (Ed.), *Encephalitis: A clinical study*. New York: Grune & Stratton.

Berkowitz, B. P., & Graziano, A. M. (1972). Training parents as behavior therapists: A review. *Behavioral Research and Therapy, 10*, 297–317.

Bernal, M. E. (1984). Consumer issues in parent training. In R. F. Dangel & R. A. Polster (Eds.), *Parent training: Foundations of research and practice* (pp. 477–503). New York: Guilford Press.

Berndt, D. J., Schwartz, S., & Kaiser, C. F. (1983). Readability of self-report depression inventories. *Journal of Consulting and Clinical Psychology, 51*, 627–628.

Biederman, J., Baldessarini, R. J., Wright, V., Knee, D., & Harmatz, J. S. (1989a). A double-blind placebo-controlled study of desipramine in the treatment of ADD: I. Efficacy. *Journal of the American Academy of Child and Adolescent Psychiatry, 28*, 777–784.

Biederman, J., Baldessarini, R. J., Wright, V., Knee, D., Harmatz, J., & Goldblatt, A. (1989b). A double-blind placebo-controlled study of desipramine in the treatment of ADD: II. Serum drug levels and cardiovascular findings. *Journal of the American Academy of Child and Adolescent Psychiatry, 28*, 903–911.

Bierman, K. L. (1983). Cognitive development and clinical interviews with children. In B. B. Lahey & Kazdin, A. E. (Eds.), *Advances in clinical child psychology* (pp. 217–250). New York: Plenum Press.

Bijou, S. W. (1984). Parent training: Actualizing the critical conditions of early childhood development. In R. F. Dangel & R. A. Polster (Eds.), *Parent training: Foundations of research and practice* (pp. 15–26). New York: Guilford Press.

Birmaher, B., Greenhill, L., Cooper, T. B., Fried, J., & Maminski, B. (1989). Sustained release methylphenidate: Pharmacokinetic studies in ADHD males. *Journal of the American Academy of Child and Adolescent Psychiatry, 28*, 768–772.

Blechman, E. A. (1984). Competent parents, competent children: Behavioral goals of parent training. In R. F. Dangel & R. A. Polster (Eds.), *Parent training: Foundations of research and practice* (pp. 34–63). New York: Guilford Press.

Block, J., Block, J. H., & Harrington, D. (1975). Comment on the Kagan-Messer reply. *Developmental Psychology, 11*, 249–252.

Bond, C. R., & McMahon, R. J. (1984). Relationships between marital distress and child behavior problems, maternal personal adjustment, maternal personality, and maternal parenting behavior. *Journal of Abnormal Psychology, 93*, 348–351.

Bornstein, P. H., & Quevillon, R. P. (1976). The effects of a self-instructional package on overactive preschool boys. *Journal of Applied Behavior Analysis, 9*, 179–188.

Brantner, J. P., & Doherty, M. A. (1983). A review of timeout: A conceptual and methodological analysis. In S. Apelrod & J. Apache (Eds.), *The effect of punishment on human behavior*. New York: Academic Press.

Braswell, L., & Kendall, P. C. (1988). Cognitive-behavioral methods with children. In K. S. Dobson (Ed.), *Handbook of cognitive-behavioral therapies* (pp. 167–213). New York: Guilford Press.

Breen, M. J. (1984). Analysis of Wide Range Achievement Test and Woodcock-Johnson achievement grade and standard scores for learning disabled and nonreferred regular education students. *Educational and Psychological Research, 3,* 115–121.

Breen, M. J. (1989). Cognitive and behavioral differences in ADHD boys and girls. *Journal of Child Psychology and Psychiatry, 5,* 711–716.

Breen, M. J. (1990). The consistency in behavior of ADHD children across measures of attention span and impulse control, behavior questionnaires, and within-clinic observations. *Submitted for publication.*

Breen, M. J., & Altepeter, T. S. (1990a). Situational variability in boys and girls identified as ADHD. *Journal of Clinical Psychology.*

Breen, M. J., & Altepeter, T. S. (1990b). Factor structure of the Home Situations Questionnaire (HSQ) and the School Situations Questionnaire (SSQ). *Submitted for publication.*

Breen, M. J., & Barkley, R. A. (1983). The Personality Inventory for Children (PIC): Its clinical utility with hyperactive children. *Journal of Pediatric Psychology, 4,* 359–366.

Breen, M. J. & Barkley, R. A. (1984). Psychological adjustment of learning disabled, hyperactive, and hyperactive/learning disabled children as measured by the Personality Inventory for Children. *Journal of Clinical Child Psychology, 3,* 232–236.

Breen, M. J., & Barkley, R. A. (1988). Child psychopathology and parenting stress in girls and boys having attention deficit disorder with hyperactivity. *Journal of Pediatric Psychology, 2,* 265–280.

Breen, M. J., & Drecktrah, M. (1989). The similarity between common measures of academic achievement: Implications for assessing specific developmental disabilities. *Submitted for publication.*

Breen, M. J., Lehman, J., & Carlson, M. (1984). Achievement correlates of the Woodcock-Johnson Reading and Math Subtests, Keymath, and Woodcock Reading in an elementary aged learning disabled population. *Journal of Learning Disabilities, 5,* 258–261.

Broad, J. C. (1982). Assessing stimulant treatment of hyperkinesis by Bristol Social Adjustment Guides. *Journal of Psychiatric Treatment and Evaluation, 4,* 355–358.

Brody, G. H., & Forehand, R. (1986). Maternal perceptions of child maladjustment as a function of the combined influence of child behavior and maternal depression. *Journal of Consulting and Clinical Psychology, 54,* 237–240.

Brofenbrenner, U. (1977). Toward an experimental ecology of human development. *American Psychologist, 32*(7), 513–531.

Brofenbrenner, U. (1979). *The ecology of human development.* Cambridge, MA: Harvard University Press.

Brown, G., Ebert, M., Mikkelsen, E., & Hunt, R. (1980). Behavior and motor activity response in hyperactive children and plasma amphetamine levels following a sustained release preparation. *Journal of the American Academy of Child Psychiatry, 19,* 225–239.

Brown, R. T., & Borden, K. A. (1986). Hyperactivity at adolescence: Some misconceptions and new directions. *Journal of Clinical Child Psychology, 3*, 194–209.

Brown, R. T., Borden, K. A., Wynne, M. E., Schleser, R., & Clingerman, S. R. (1986). Methylphenidate and cognitive therapy with ADD children: A methodological reconsideration. *Journal of Abnormal Child Psychology, 14*, 481–497.

Brown, R. T., Wynne, M. E., & Medenis, R. (1985). Methylphenidate and cognitive therapy: A comparison of treatment approaches with hyperactive children. *Journal of Abnormal Child Psychology, 13*, 69–87.

Buchanan, W. L. (1987, November). *Structural-strategic family therapy for hyperactive and learning-disabled children*. Paper presented at the annual meeting of American Association for Marital and Family Therapy, Chicago, IL.

Burgess, R. L., & Richardson, R. A. (1984). Coercive interpersonal contingencies as a determinant of child maltreatment: Implications for treatment and prevention. In R. F. Dangel & R. A. Polster (Eds.), *Parent training: Foundations of research and practice* (pp. 239–259). New York: Guilford Press.

Burke, W. T., & Abidin, R. R. (1978, August). *The development of a parenting stress index*. Paper presented at the annual meeting of the American Psychological Association, Toronto, Ontario, Canada.

Busby, K. A., & Broughton, R. J. (1983). Waking ultradian rhythms of performance and motility in hyperkinetic and normal children. *Journal of Abnormal Child Psychology, 11*, 431–442.

Cadoret, R. J. (1978). Psychopathology in adopted-away offspring of biologic parents with antisocial behavior. *Archives of General Psychiatry, 35*, 176–184.

Cairns, E., & Cammock, T. (1978). Development of a more reliable version of the Matching Familiar Figures Test. *Developmental Psychology, 5*, 555–560.

Camp, B. W., & Bash, M. A. S. (1985). *Think aloud: Increasing social and cognitive skills—A problem-solving approach*. Champaign, IL: Research Press.

Campbell, M., Green, W. H., & Deutsch, S. I. (1985). *Child and adolescent psychopharmacology*. Beverly Hills, CA: SAGE.

Campbell, S. B., Douglas, V. I., & Morganstern, G. (1971). Cognitive styles in hyperactive children and the effect of methylphenidate. *Journal of Child Psychology and Psychiatry, 12*, 55–67.

Campbell, M., & Spencer, E. K. (1988). Psychopharmacology in child and adolescent psychiatry: A review of the past five years. *Journal of the American Academy of Child and Adolescent Psychiatry, 27*, 269–279.

Campbell, S. B., & Steinert, Y. (1978). Comparisons of rating scales of child psychopathology in clinic and nonclinic samples. *Journal of Consulting and Clinical Psychology, 46*, 358–359.

Campbell, S. B., & Werry, J. S. (1986). Attention Deficit Disorder (hyperactivity). In H. C. Quay & J. S. Werry (Eds.), *Psychopathological disorders of childhood* (3rd ed., pp. 111–153). New York: Wiley.

Cantwell, D. (1975). *The hyperactive child*. New York: Spectrum.

Cantwell, D. (1980). A clinician's guide to the use of stimulant medication for the psychiatric disorders of children. *Developmental and Behavioral Pediatrics, 3,* 133–140.

Cantwell, D., & Carlson, G. (1978). Stimulants. In J. Werry (Ed.), *Pediatric psychopharmacology* (pp. 171–207). New York: Bruner/Mazel.

Carey, M. P., Faulstich, M. E., Gresham, F. M., Ruggiero, L., & Enyart, P. (1987). Children's Depression Inventory: Construct and discriminative validity across clinical and nonreferred (control) populations. *Journal of Consulting and Clinical Psychology, 55,* 755–761.

Carlson, C. L. (1986). Attention Deficit Disorder without hyperactivity: A review of preliminary experimental evidence. In B. B. Lahey & A. E. Kazdin (Eds.), *Advances in clinical child psychology* (Vol. 9, pp. 153–175). New York: Plenum Press.

Chambers, W. J., Puig-Antich, J., Hirsch, M., Paez, P., Ambrosini, P. J. Tabrizi, M. A., & Davies, M. (1985). The assessment of affective disorders in children and adolescents by semistructured interview: Test-retest reliability of the Schedule for Affective Disorders and Schizophrenia for School Age Children, Present Episode Version. *Archives of General Psychiatry, 42,* 696–702.

Clement, P. W. (1970). Elimination of sleepwalking in a seven-year-old boy. *Journal of Consulting and Clinical Psychology, 34,* 22–26.

Clements, S. D., & Peters, J. E. (1962). Minimal brain dysfunction in the school-aged child. *Archives of General Psychiatry, 6,* 185–197.

Cloninger, C. R., Reich, T., & Guze, S. G. (1978). Genetic environmental interactions and antisocial behavior. In R. D. Hare & D. Schalling (Eds.), *Psychopathic behavior: Approaches to research* (pp. 225–237). New York: Wiley.

Cohen, N. J., Gotlieb, H., Kershner, J., & Wehrspann, W. (1985). Concurrent validity of the internalizing and externalizing profile patterns on the Achenbach Child Behavior Checklist. *Journal of Consulting and Clinical Psychology, 53,* 724–728.

Cohen, N. J., Kershner, J., & Wehrspann, W. (1988). Correlates of competence in a child psychiatric population. *Journal of Consulting and Clinical Psychology, 56,* 97–103.

Comings, D. E., & Comings, B. G. (1984). Tourette's syndrome and Attention Deficit Disorder with hyperactivity: Are they genetically related? *Journal of the American Academy of Child and Adolescent Psychiatry, 23,* 138–146.

Conde, V., Esteban, T., & Useros, E. (1976). Revision critica de la adaptacion castellana del cuestionario de Beck (Critical revision of the Spanish adaptation of the Beck Inventory). *Revista de Psychologia General Aplicada, 31,* 469–497.

Conners, C. K., (1969). A teacher rating scale for use in drug studies of children. *American Journal of Psychiatry, 126,* 884–888.

Conners, C. K. (1970). Symptom patterns in hyperkinetic, neurotic, and normal children. *Child Development, 41,* 667–682.

Conners, C. K. (1973). Rating scales for use in drug studies with children. *Psychopharmacology Bulletin: Special issues, Pharmacotherapy with children,* 24–84.

Conners, C. K. (1980). *Food additives and hyperactive children.* New York: Plenum Press.

Conners, C. K. (1985). *The Conners Rating Scales: Instruments for the assessment of childhood psychopathology.* Unpublished manuscript.

Conners, C. K. (1989). *Conners' Rating Scales Manual*. North Tonawanda, NY: Multi-Health Systems, Inc.

Conners, C. K., & Blouin, A. G. (1980, August). *Hyperkinetic syndrome and psychopathology in children*. Paper presented at the annual meeting of the American Psychological Association, Montreal.

Conners, C. K., & Wells, K. C. (1986). *Hyperkinetic children: Neuropsychological approach*. Beverly Hills, CA: SAGE.

Coons, H. W., Klorman, R., & Borgstedt, A. D. (1987). Effects of methylphenidate on adolescents with a childhood history of attention deficit disorder: II. Information processing. *Journal of the American Academy of Child and Adolescent Psychiatry, 26*, 368–374.

Copeland, A. P., & Weissbrod, C. S. (1978). Behavioral correlates of the Hyperactivity Factor of the Conners Teacher Questionnaire. *Journal of Abnormal Child Psychology, 6*, 339–343.

Copeland, L., Wolraich, M., Lindgren, S., Milich, R., & Woolson, R. (1987). Pediatricians' reported practices in the assessment and treatment of attention deficit disorders. *Developmental and Behavioral Pediatrics, 4*, 191–196.

Costello, A., Edelbrock, C., Kalas, R., Kessler, M., & Klaric, S. (1982). *The NIMH Diagnostic Interview Schedule for Children (DISC)*. Pittsburgh: Author.

Costello, E. J., & Edelbrock, C. S. (1985). Detection of psychiatric disorders in pediatric primary care: A preliminary report. *Journal of the American Academy of Child Psychiatry, 24*, 771–774.

Craighead, W. E. (1983, August). If you think and feel are you still behavioral? Paper presented at the annual meeting of the American Psychological Association, Anaheim, CA.

Craighead, W. E., Meyers, A. W., & Craighead, L. W. (1985). A conceptual model for cognitive-behavior therapy with children. *Journal of Abnormal Child Psychology, 13*, 331–342.

Cunningham, C., & Barkley, R. A. (1978). The effects of Ritalin on the mother–child interactions of hyperkinetic twin boys. *Developmental Medicine and Child Neurology, 20*, 634–642.

Dangel, R. F., & Polster, R. A. (Eds.). (1984). *Parent training: Foundations of research and practice*. New York: Guilford Press.

Davidson, E. M., & Prior, M. R. (1978). Laterality and selective attention in hyperactive children. *Journal of Abnormal Child Psychology, 6*, 475–481.

Davis, W. E. (1989). The regular education initiative debate: Its promises and problems. *Exceptional Children, 5*, 440–446.

deHass, P. A. (1986). Attention styles and peer relationships of hyperactive and normal boys and girls. *Journal of Abnormal Child Psychology, 14*, 457–467.

deHass, P. A., & Young, R. D. (1984). Attention styles of hyperactive and normal boys and girls. *Journal of Abnormal Child Psychology, 12*, 531–546.

Denson, R., Nanson, J. L., & McWatters, M. A. (1975). Hyperkinesis and maternal smoking. *Canadian Psychiatric Association Journal, 20*, 183–187.

Dodge, K. A. (1985). Attributional bias in aggressive children. In P. C. Kendall (Ed.), *Advances in cognitive-behavioral research and therapy* (Vol. 4, pp. 73–110). Orlando, FL: Academic Press.

Doerfler, L. A., Felner, R. D., Rowllison, R. T., Raley, P. A., & Evans, E. (1988). Depression in children and adolescents: A comparative analysis of the utility and construct validity of two assessment measures. *Journal of Consulting and Clinical Psychology, 56,* 769–772.

Donnelly, M., & Rapoport, J. L. (1985). Attention Deficit Disorders. In J. J. Weiner (Ed.), *Diagnosis and psychopharmacology of childhood and adolescent disorders* (pp. 178–197). New York: Wiley.

Douglas, V. I. (1972). Stop, look, and listen: The problem of sustained attention and impulse control in hyperactive and normal children. *Canadian Journal of Behavioral Science, 4,* 259–282.

Douglas, V. I. (1980). Higher mental processes in hyperactive children: Implications for training. In R. Knights & D. Bakker (Eds.), *Treatment of hyperactivity and learning-disordered children* (pp. 65–92). Baltimore: University Park Press.

Douglas, V. I. (1983). Attention and cognitive problems. In M. Rutter (Ed.), *Developmental neuropsychiatry* (pp. 280–329). New York: Guilford Press.

Douglas, V. I., & Peters, K. G. (1979). Toward a clearer definition of the attentional deficit of hyperactive children. In G. A. Hale & M. Lewis (Eds.), *Attention and the development of cognitive skills* (pp. 173–248). New York: Plenum Press.

Douglas, V. I., Barr, R. G., Amin, K., O'Neill, M. E., & Britton, B. G. (1988). Dosage effects and individual responsivity to methylphenidate in attention deficit disorder. *Journal of Child Psychology and Psychiatry, 29,* 453–475.

Douglas, V. I., Barr, R. G., O'Neill, M. E., & Britton, B. G. (1986). Short-term effects of methylphenidate on the cognitive, learning, and academic performance of children with Attention Deficit Disorder in the laboratory and the classroom. *Journal of Child Psychology and Psychiatry, 27,* 191–212.

Draeger, S., Prior, M., & Sanson, A. (1986). Visual and auditory attention performance in hyperactive children: Competence or compliance. *Journal of Abnormal Child Psychology, 14,* 411–424.

Dubey, D. R. (1976). Organic factors in hyperkinesis: A critical review. *American Journal of Orthopsychiatry, 46,* 353–366.

Dumas, J. E. (1986). Parental perception and treatment outcome in families of aggressive children: A causal model. *Behavior Therapy, 17,* 420–432.

D'Zurillia, T. J. (1986). *Problem-solving therapy: A social competence approach to clinical intervention.* New York: Springer Publications.

D'Zurillia, T. J. (1988). *Problem-solving therapies.* In K. S. Dobson (Ed.), *Handbook of cognitive-behavioral therapies* (pp. 85–135). New York: Guilford Press.

D'Zurillia, T. J., & Goldfried, M. R. (1971). Problem solving and behavior modification. *Journal of Abnormal Psychology, 78,* 107–126.

Edelbrock, C. (1988). Informant reports. In E. S. Shapiro & T. R. Kratochwill (Eds.), *Behavioral assessment in schools: Conceptual foundations and practical applications* (pp. 351–383). New York: Guilford Press.

Edelbrock, C., & Costello, A. (1988). Structured psychiatric interviews for children. In M. Rutter, A. H. Tuma, & I. S. Lann (Eds.), *Assessment and diagnosis in child psychopathology* (pp. 87–112). New York: Guilford Press.

Edelbrock, C., Costello, A. J., & Kessler, M. D. (1984). Empirical corroboration of

Attention Deficit Disorder. *Journal of the American Academy of Child Psychiatry, 23,* 285–290.

Edelbrock, C., Greenbaum, R., & Conover, N. C. (1985). Reliability and concurrent relations between the teacher version of the Child Behavior Profile and Conners' Revised Teacher Rating Scale. *Journal of Abnormal Child Psychology, 13,* 295–304.

Edelbrock, C., & Rancurello, M. D. (1985). Childhood hyperactivity: An overview of rating scales and their applications. *Clinical Psychology Review, 5,* 429–445.

Edelbrock, C., & Reed, M. L. (1984). *Reliability and concurrent validity of the teacher version of the Child Behavior Profile.* Unpublished manuscript.

Einbender, A. J., & Friedrich, W. N. (1989). Psychological functioning and behavior of sexually abused girls. *Journal of Consulting and Clinical Psychology, 57,* 155–157.

Endicott, J., & Spitzer, R. L. (1978). A diagnostic interview: The schedule for affective disorders and schizophrenia. *Archives of General Psychiatry, 35,* 837–844.

Enyart, P. (1984). *Behavioral correlates of self-reported parent-adolescent relationship satisfaction.* Unpublished doctoral dissertation, West Virginia University, Morgantown, WV.

Erenberg, G., Cruse, R. P., & Rothner, A. D. (1985). Gilles de la Tourette's syndrome: Effect of stimulant drugs. *Neurology, 35,* 1346–1348.

Eron, L. D., Lefkowitz, M. M., Walder, L. O., & Huesmann, L. R. (1974). Relation of learning in childhood psychopathology and aggression in young children. In A. Davis (Ed.), *Child personality and psychopathology* (Vol. 1). New York: Wiley.

Evans, R. W., Gualtieri, T. C., & Amara, I. (1986). Methylphenidate and memory: Dissociated effects in hyperactive children. *Psychopharmacology, 90,* 211–216.

Evert, T., & Reynolds, W. M. (1986). *Efficacy of a multi-stage screening model for depression in adolescence.* Unpublished manuscript.

Eyberg, S. M. (1980). Eyberg Child Behavior Inventory. *Journal of Clinical Child Psychology, 9,* 22–28.

Eyberg, S. M. (1985). Behavioral assessment: Advancing methodology in pediatric psychology. *Journal of Pediatric Psychology, 10,* 123–139.

Eyberg, S. M. (1986, August). *Parent-child interaction therapy: Integration of traditional and behavioral concerns.* Paper presented at the annual meeting of the American Psychological Association, Washington, DC.

Eyberg, S. M., & Matarazzo, R. G. (1980). Training parents as therapists: A comparison between individual parent-child interaction training and parent group didactic training. *Journal of Clinical Psychology, 36,* 492–499.

Eyberg, S. M., & Robinson, E. A. (1982). Parent-child interaction training: Effects on family functioning. *Journal of Clinical Child Psychology, 11,* 130–137.

Eyberg, S. M., & Robinson, E. A. (1983). Conduct problem behavior: Standardization of a behavior rating scale with adolescents. *Journal of Clinical Child Psychology, 12,* 347–356.

Eyberg, S. M., & Ross, E. A. (1978). Assessment of child behavior problems: The validation of a new inventory. *Journal of Clinical Child Psychology, 7,* 113–116.

Feldman, R. A., Caplinger, T. E., & Wodarski, J. S. (1983). *The St. Louis conundrum: The effective treatment of antisocial youths.* Englewood Cliffs, NJ: Prentice-Hall.

Feingold, B. (1975). *Why your child is hyperactive.* New York: Random House.

Finch, A. J., Saylor, C. F., & Edwards, G. L. (1985). Children's Depression Inventory: Sex and grade norms for normal children. *Journal of Consulting and Clinical Psychology, 53*, 424–425.

Fischer, M., Barkley, R. A., Edelbrock, C. S., & Smallish, L. (1989). *The adolescent outcome of hyperactive children diagnosed by research criteria: Academic, attentional, and neuropsychological measures.* Manuscript under review.

Forehand, R., & Atkeson, B. M. (1977). Generality of treatment effects with parents as therapists: A review of assessment and implementation procedures. *Behavior Therapy, 8*, 575–593.

Forehand, R., Brody, G., Slotkin, J., Fauber, R., McCombs, A., & Long, N. (1988). Young adolescent and maternal depression: Assessment, interrelations, and family predictors. *Journal of Consulting and Clinical Psychology, 56*, 422–426.

Forehand, R., Long, N., Faust, J., Brody, G. H., Burke, M., & Fauber, R. (1987). Physical and psychological health of young adolescents: The relationship to gender and marital conflict. *Journal of Pediatric Psychology, 12*, 191–201.

Forehand, R., McCombs, A., Long, N., Brody, G., & Fauber, R. (1988). Early adolescent adjustment to recent parental divorce: The role of interparental conflict and adolescent sex as mediating variables. *Journal of Consulting and Clinical Psychology, 56*, 624–627.

Forehand, R. L., & McMahon, R. J. (1981). *Helping the noncompliant child: A clinician's guide to parent training.* New York: Guilford Press.

Foreyt, J. P., & McGavin, J. K. (1988). Anorexia nervosa and bulimia. In E. J. Mash & L. G. Terdal (Eds.), *Behavioral assessment of childhood disorders* (2nd ed., pp. 776–805). New York: Guilford Press.

Foster, S. L., Bell-Dolan, S. J., & Burge, D. A. (1988). Behavioral observation. In A. S. Bellack & M. Herson (Eds.), *Behavioral assessment: A practical handbook* (3rd ed., pp. 119–160). New York: Pergamon Press.

Foster, S. L., Prinz, R. J., & O'Leary, K. D. (1983). Impact of problem-solving communication training and generalization procedures on family conflict. *Child and Family Behavior Therapy, 5*, 1–23.

Foster, S. L., & Robin, A. L. (1988). Family conflict and communication in adolescence. In E. J. Mash & L. G. Terdal (Eds.), *Behavioral assessment of childhood disorders* (2nd ed., pp. 69–104). New York: Guilford Press.

Friedrich, W. N., Urquiza, A. J., & Beilke, R. L. (1986). Behavior problems in sexually abused young children. *Journal of Pediatric Psychology, 11*, 47–57.

Furguson, H. B., Stoddart, C., & Simeon, J. G. (1986). Double-blind challenge studies of behavioral and cognitive effects of sucrose-aspartame ingestion in normal children. *Nutrition Reviews, 44*, 144–150.

Gilbert, G. M. (1957). A survey of "referral problems" in metropolitan child guidance centers. *Journal of Clinical Psychology, 13*, 37–42.

Gillbert, I. C., & Gillberg, M. D. (1988). Generalized hyperkinesis: Follow-up study from age 7–13. *Journal of the American Academy of Child and Adolescent Psychiatry, 1*, 55–59.

Glow, R. A. (1979). Cross-validity and normative data on the Conners Parent Teacher Rating scales. In K. Gadnow & J. Loney (Eds.), *Psychosocial aspects of drug treatment for hyperactivity.* Boulder, CO: Westview Press.

Glow, R. A., Glow, P. H., & Rump, E. E. (1982). The stability of child behavior disorders: A one-year test-retest study of Adelaide versions of the Conners Teacher and Parent Rating scales. *Journal of Abnormal Child Psychology, 10*, 33–60.

Golden, G. S. (1988). The relationship between stimulant medication and tics. *Pediatric Annals, 117*, 405.

Goldman, J. A., Lerman, R. H., Contois, J. H., & Udall, J. N. (1986). Behavioral effects of sucrose on preschool children. *Journal of Abnormal Child Psychology, 14*, 565–577.

Goldstein, A. P., & Keller, H. (1987). *Aggressive behavior: Assessment and intervention.* New York: Pergamon Press.

Goldstein, K. (1936). Modification of behavior consequent to cerebral lesion. *Psychiatric Quarterly, 10*, 539–610.

Goodwin, S., & Mahoney, M. J. (1975). Modification of aggressive behavior through modeling: An experimental probe. *Journal of Behavior Therapy and Experimental Psychiatry, 6*, 200–202.

Gordon, M. (1979). The assessment of impulsivity and mediating behaviors in hyperactive and non-hyperactive children. *Journal of Abnormal Child Psychology, 7*, 317–326.

Gordon, M. (1982). *The Gordon Diagnostic System.* DeWitt, NY: Gordon Systems.

Gordon, M. (1987). How is a computerized attention test used in the diagnosis of Attention Deficit Disorder? In J. Loney (Ed.), *The young hyperactive child: Answers to questions about diagnosis, prognosis, and treatment.* New York: Haworth Press.

Gordon, M., & Mettelman, B. B. (1988). The assessment of attention: 1. standardization and reliability of a behavior-based machine. *Journal of Clinical Psychology, 5*, 682–690.

Gordon, M., DiNiro, D., Mettelman, B. B., & Tallmadge, J. (1989). Observations of test behavior, quantitative scores, and teacher ratings. *Journal of Psychoeducational Assessment, 7*, 141–147.

Gordon, M., Mettelman, B. B., & DiNiro, D. (1989, August). *Are continuous performance tests valid in the diagnosis of ADHD/Hyperactivity?* Paper presented at the meeting of the American Psychological Association, New Orleans, LA.

Gordon, M., Thomason, D., & Cooper, S. (1989, August). *To what extent do IQ tests measure attentiveness?* Paper presented at the meeting of the American Psychological Association, New Orleans, LA.

Gordon, S. B., & Davidson, N. (1981). Behavioral parent training. In A. S. Gurman & D. P. Kniskern (Eds.), *Handbook of family therapy.* New York: Brunner/Mazel.

Gould, M. S., Shaffer, D., Rutter, M., & Sturge, C. (1984). *UK/WHO Study of ICD-9: Issues of classification.* Paper presented at research workshop on psychopathology. Washington, DC: Center for Studies of Child and Adolescent Psychopathology, Clinical Research Branch, NIMH.

Gouze, K. R. (1987). Attention and social problem solving as correlates of aggression in preschool males. *Journal of Abnormal Child Psychology, 15*, 181–197.

Goyette, C. H., Conners, C. K., & Ulrich, R. F. (1978). Normative data for Revised Conners Parent and Teacher Rating Scales. *Journal of Abnormal Child Psychology, 6*, 221–236.

Graziano, A. M. (1977). Parents as behavior therapists. In M. Hersen, R. M. Eisler, & P. M. Miller (Eds.), *Progress in behavior modification* (Vol. 4). New York: Academic Press.

Griest, D. L., & Wells, K. C. (1983). Behavioral family therapy with conduct disorders in children. *Behavior Therapy, 14*, 37–53.

Gross, A. M., & Wixted, J. T. (1988). Assessment of child behavior problems. In A. S. Bellack & M. Hersen (Eds.), *Behavioral assessment: A practical handbook* (3rd ed., pp. 578–608). New York: Pergamon Press.

Gross, M. D. (1984). Effects of sucrose on hyperkinetic children. *Pediatrics, 74*, 876–878.

Gurman, A. S., & Kniskern, D. P. (1978). Research on marital and family therapy: Progress, perspective, and prospect. In S. L. Garfield & A. E. Bergin (Eds.), *Handbook of psychotherapy and behavior change: An empirical analysis* (2nd ed.). New York: Wiley.

Hall, C. W., & Marks, H. (1988). Assessment of subcategories of hyperactivity. *The ADD/Hyperactivity Newsletter, 11*, 4–6.

Hallahan, D. P., Keller, C. E., McKinney, J. D., Lloyd, J. W., & Bryan, T. (1988). Examining the research base of the regular education initiative: Efficacy studies and the adaptive learning environments model. *Journal of Learning Disabilities, 1*, 29–35.

Halperin, J. M., Gittelman, R., Katz, S., & Struve, F. A. (1986). Relationship between stimulant effect, electroencephalogram, and clinical neurological findings in hyperactive children. *Journal of the American Academy of Child and Adolescent Psychiatry, 25*, 820–825.

Halperin, J. M., Gittelman, R., Klein, D. F., & Rudel, R. G. (1984). Reading-disabled hyperactive children: A distinct subgroup of Attention Deficit Disorder with Hyperactivity? *Journal of Abnormal Child Psychology, 12*, 1–14.

Hanf, C. (1969). *A two-stage program for modifying maternal controlling during mother child (M–C) interaction.* Paper presented at the annual meeting of the Western Psychological Association, Vancouver, BC, Canada.

Harley, J. P., Ray, R. S., Tomasi, L., Eichman, P. L., Mathews, C. G., Chun, R., Cleelund, C. S., & Traisman, E. (1981). Hyperkinesis and food additives: Testing the Feingold hypothesis. *Pediatrics, 61*, 818–828.

Harris, J. C., King, S. L., Reifler, J. P., & Rosenberg, L. A. (1984). Emotional and learning disorders in 6–12-year-old boys attending special schools. *Journal of the American Academy of Child Psychiatry, 23*, 431–437.

Harris, K. R., Wong, B. Y., & Keogh, B. K. (Eds.). (1985). Cognitive-behavioral modification with children: A critical review of the state-of-the-art. *Journal of Abnormal Child Psychology, 13*, entire issue.

Hartsough, C. S., & Lambert, N. M. (1985). Medical factors in hyperactive and normal children: Prenatal, developmental, and health history findings. *American Journal of Orthopsychiatry, 55*, 190–201.

Hauenstein, E., Scarr, S., & Abidin, R. R. (1986). *Measurement of parental stress across cultures: Validation of the parenting Stress Index with American and Bermudian parents.* Unpublished manuscript.

Henker, B., & Whalen, C. K. (1989). Hyperactivity and attention deficits. *American*

Psychologist, 2, 216–223.

Herbert, M. (1978). *Conduct disorders of childhood and adolescence: A behavioral approach to assessment and treatment*. New York: Wiley.

Herbert, M. (1982). Conduct disorders. In B. B. Lahey & A. E. Kazdin (Eds.), *Advances in clinical child psychology* (Vol. 5, pp. 95–136). New York: Plenum Press.

Herjanic, B., Brown, F., & Wheatt, T. (1975). Are children reliable reporters? *Journal of Abnormal Child Psychology, 3*, 41–48.

Hersen, M., & Van Hasselt, V. B. (Eds.). (1987). *Behavior therapy with children and adolescents*. New York: Wiley.

Hinshaw, S. P. (1987). On the distinction between attentional deficits/hyperactivity and conduct problems/aggression in child psychopathology. *Psychological Bulletin, 101*, 443–463.

Hinshaw, S. P., Buhrmester, D., & Heller, T. (1989). Anger control in response to verbal provocation: Effects of stimulant medication for boys with ADHD. *Journal of Abnormal Child Psychology, 17*, 393–407.

Hinshaw, S. P., Henker, B., & Whalen, C. K. (1984a). Self-control in hyperactive boys in anger-inducing situations: Effect of cognitive-behavioral training and methylphenidate. *Journal of Abnormal Child Psychology, 12*, 55–77.

Hinshaw, S. P., Henker, B., & Whalen, C. K. (1984b). Cognitive-behavioral and pharmacological interventions for hyperactive boys: Comparative and combined effects. *Journal of Consulting and Clinical Psychology, 52*, 739–749.

Hodges, K. (1987). Assessing children with a clinical research interview: The Child Assessment Schedule. In R. J. Prinz (Ed.), *Advances in behavioral assessment of children and families* (pp. 203–233). Greenwich, CT: JAI Press.

Hodges, K., Kline, J., Stern, L., Cytryn, L., & McKnew, D. (1982a). The development of a child assessment interview for research and clinical use. *Journal of Abnormal Child Psychology, 10*, 173–189.

Hodges, K., McKnew, D., Cytryn, L., Stern, L., & Kline, J. (1982b). The Child Assessment Schedule (CAS) diagnostic interview: A report on reliability and validity. *Journal of the Academy of Child Psychiatry, 21*, 468–473.

Hodges, K., Siegel, L. J., Mullins, L., & Griffin, N. (1983). Factor analysis of the Children's Depression Inventory. *Psychological Reports, 53*, 759–763.

Hogan, A. E., Quay, H. C., Vaughn, S., & Shapiro, K. (1989). Revised Behavior Problem Checklist: Stability, prevalence, and incidence of behavior problems in kindergarten and first-trade children. *Psychological Assessment: A Journal of Consulting and Clinical Psychology, 1*, 103–111.

Hohman, L. B. (1922). Post encephalitic behavior disorders in children. *Johns Hopkins Hospital Bulletin, 380*, 372–375.

Holborow, P., & Berry, P. S. (1986). Hyperactivity and learning difficulties. *Journal of Learning Disabilities, 19*, 426–431.

Holden, E. W., Willis, D. J., & Foltz, L. (1989). Child abuse potential and parenting stress: Relationships in maltreating parents. *Psychological Assessment: A Journal of Consulting and Clinical Psychology, 1*, 64–67.

Horn, W. F., Chatoor, I., & Conners, C. K. (1983). Additive effects of dexedrine and self-control training. *Behavior Modification, 7*, 383–402.

Horn, W. F., Ialongo, N., Popovich, S., & Peradotto, D. (1984, August). *An evaluation of a multi-method treatment approach with hyperactive children*. Paper presented at the annual meeting of the American Psychological Association, Toronto, Ontario, Canada.

Horn, W. F., Ialongo, N. Popovich, S., & Peradotto, D. (1987). Behavioral parent training and cognitive-behavioral self-control therapy with ADD-H children: Comparative and combined effects. *Journal of Clinical Child Psychology, 16*, 57–68.

Horn, W. F., Wagner, A. E., & Ialongo, N. (1989). Sex differences in school-aged children with pervasive Attention-deficit Hyperactivity Disorder. *Journal of Abnormal Child Psychology, 17*, 109–125.

Huesman, L. R., Eron, L. D., Lefkowitz, M. M., & Walder, L. O. (1984). Stability of aggression over time and generations. *Developmental Psychology, 20*, 1120–1134.

Humphrey, L. L. (1982). Children's and teacher's perspectives on children's self-control: The development of two rating scales. *Journal of Consulting and Clinical Psychology, 50*, 624–633.

Hunt, R. (1988). Attention Deficit Disorder and hyperactivity. In C. J. Kestenbaum & D. T. Williams (Eds.), *Handbook of clinical assessment of children and adolescents* (pp. 519–561). New York: New York University Press.

Hurtig, A. L., Koepke, D., & Park, K. B. (1989). Relation between severity of chronic illness and adjustment in children and adolescents with sickle cell disease. *Journal of Pediatric Psychology, 14*, 117–132.

Jary, M. L., & Stewart, M. A. (1985). Psychiatric disorder in the parents of adopted children with aggressive conduct disorder. *Neuropsychobiology, 13*, 7–11.

Jensen, P. S., Bloedau, L., Degroot, J., Ussery, T., & Davis, H. (1990). Children at risk: I. Risk factors and child symptomatology. *Journal of the Academy of Child and Adolescent Psychiatry, 18*, 51–59.

Johnson, C., Pelham, W. E., & Murphy, H. A. (1985). Peer relationships in ADDH and normal children: A developmental analysis of peer and teacher ratings. *Journal of Abnormal Child Psychology, 13*, 89–100.

Johnson, J. H., & Fennell, E. B. (1983). Aggressive and delinquent behavior in childhood and adolescence. In C. E. Walker & M. C. Roberts (Eds.), *Handbook of clinical child psychology* (pp. 475–497). New York: Wiley.

Johnson, J. H., Floyd, B. J., & Isleib, R. (1983). *Parent stress, empathy and dimensions of adult temperament as predictors of child abuse and neglect*. Unpublished manuscript, University of Florida, Gainesville.

Jones, R. N., Latkowski, M. E., Kircher, J. C., & McMahon, W. M. (1988). The Child Behavior Checklist: Normative information for inpatients. *Journal of the American Academy of Child and Adolescent Psychiatry, 27*, 632–635.

Jones, R. T., & Kazdin, A. E. (1981). Childhood behavior problems in the school. In S. M. Turner, & K. S. Calhoun (Eds.), *Handbook of clinical behavior therapy* (pp. 568–606). New York: Wiley.

Kagan, J., & Messer, S. B. (1975). A reply to "Some misgivings about the Matching Familiar Figures Test as a measure of reflection-impulsivity. *Developmental Psychology, 11*, 244–248.

Kagan, J., Rosman, B. L., Day, D., Albert, J., & Phillips, W. (1964). Information processing in the child: Significance of analytic and reflective attitudes. *Psychological Monographs, 78* (578).

Kaplan, W. H. (1988). Conduct disorder. In C. J. Kestenbaum & D. T. Williams (Eds.), *Handbook of clinical assessment of children and adolescents* (pp. 562–582). New York: New York University Press.

Kashani, J. H., Sherman, D. D., Parker, D. R., & Reid, J. C. (1990). Utility of the Beck Depression Inventory with clinic-referred adolescents. *Journal of the Academy of Child and Adolescent Psychiatry, 18*, 278–282.

Kaufman, A. S., & Kaufman, N. L. (1983). *K-ABC: Kaufman Assessment Battery for Children*. Circle Pines, MN: American Guidance Service.

Kaufman, A. S., & Kaufman, N. L. (1985). *Kaufman Test of Educational Achievement*. Circle Pines, MN: American Guidance Service.

Kauffman, J. M., Gerber, M. M., & Semmel, M. I. (1988). Arguable assumptions underlying the regular education initiative. *Journal of Learning Disabilities, 21*, 6–11.

Kazdin, A. E. (1981). Assessment techniques for childhood depression. *Journal of the American Academy of Child Psychiatry, 20*, 358–375.

Kazdin, A. E. (1985). *Treatment of antisocial behavior in children and adolescents*. Homewood, IL: Dorsey Press.

Kazdin, A. E. (1987). Treatment of antisocial behavior in children: Current status and future directions. *Psychological Bulletin, 102*, 187–203.

Kazdin, A. E. (1988). Childhood depression. In E. J. Mash & L. G. Terdal (Eds.), *Behavioral assessment of childhood disorders* (2nd ed., pp. 157–195). New York: Guilford Press.

Kazdin, A. E., Bass, D., Siegel, T., & Thomas, C. (1989). Cognitive behavioral therapy and relationship therapy in the treatment of children referred for antisocial behavior. *Journal of Consulting and Clinical Psychology, 57*, 522–535.

Kazdin, A. E., Colbus, D., & Rodgers, A. (1986). Assessment of depression and diagnosis of depressive disorder among psychiatrically disturbed children. *Journal of Abnormal Child Psychology, 14*, 499–515.

Kazdin, A. E., Esveldt-Dawson, K. & Loar, L. L. (1983). Correspondence of teacher ratings and direct observations of classroom behavior of psychiatric inpatient children. *Journal of Abnormal Child Psychology, 11*, 549–564.

Kazdin, A. E., & Heidish, I. E. (1984). Convergence of clinically derived diagnoses and parent checklists among inpatient children. *Journal of Abnormal Child Psychology, 12*, 421–436.

Kendall, P. C. (1985). Toward a cognitive-behavioral model of child psychopathology and a critique of related interventions. *Journal of Abnormal Child Psychology, 13*, 357–372.

Kendall, P. C., & Braswell, L. (1982). Cognitive-behavioral self-control therapy for children: A component analysis. *Journal of Consulting and Clinical Psychology, 50*, 672–689.

Kendall, P. C., & Braswell, L. (1985). *Cognitive-behavioral therapy for impulsive children*. New York: Guilford Press.

Kendall, P. C., & Finch, A. J. (1978). A cognitive-behavioral treatment for impulsivity: A group comparison study. *Journal of Consulting and Clinical Psychology, 46*, 110–118.

Kendall, P. C., & Urbain, E. S. (1981). Cognitive-behavioral interventions with a hyperactive girl: Evaluation via behavioral observations and cognitive performance. *Behavioral Assessment, 3*, 345–357.

Kendall, P. C., & Wilcox, L. E. (1979). Self-control in children: Development of a rating scale. *Journal of Consulting and Clinical Psychology, 47*, 1020–1029.

Kendall, P. C., & Wilcox, L. E. (1980). Cognitive-behavioral treatment for impulsivity: Concrete versus conceptual training in non-self-controlled problem children. *Journal of Consulting and Clinical Psychology, 48*, 80–91.

Kendall, P.C. & Zupan, B.A. (1981). Individual versus group application of cognitive-behavioral self-control procedures with children. *Behavior Therapy, 12*, 344–359.

Kendall, P. C., Zupan, B. A., & Braswell, L. (1981). Self-control in children: Further analysis of the Self-Control Rating Scale. *Behavior Therapy, 12*, 667–681.

Kerasotes, D., & Walker, C. E. (1983). Hyperactive behavior in children. In C. E. Walker & M. C. Roberts (Eds.). *Handbook of clinical child psychology* (pp. 498–523). New York: Wiley.

Kindlon, D., Solle, N., & Yando, R. (1988). Specificity of behavior problems among children with neurological dysfunctions. *Journal of Pediatric Psychology, 13*, 39–47.

King, C., & Young, D. (1982). Attention deficits with and without hyperactivity: Teacher and peer perceptions. *Journal of Abnormal Child Psychology, 10*, 483–496.

Kirk, S. A., & Bateman, B. (1962). Diagnosis and remediation of learning disabilities. *Exceptional Children, 29*, 73–78.

Klein, R. G., & Abikoff, H. (1989). The role of psychostimulants and psychosocial treatments in hyperkinesis. In T. Sagvolden & T. Archer (Eds.). *Attention Deficit Disorder: Clinical and basic research* (pp. 167–180). Hillsdale, NJ: Erlbaum.

Klein, R. G., & Mannuzza, S. (1989). The long-term outcome of the Attention Deficit Disorder/Hyperkinetic syndrome. In T. Sagvolden & T. Archer (Eds.). *Attention Deficit Disorder: Clinical and basic research* (pp. 71–91). Hillsdale, NJ: Erlbaum.

Klorman, R., Coons, H. W., & Borgestedt, A. D. (1987). Effects of methylphenidate on adolescents with a childhood history of attention deficit disorder. I. Clinical findings. *Journal of the American Academy of Child and Adolescent Psychiatry, 3*, 363–367.

Knight, D., Hensley, V. R., & Waters, B. (1988). Validation of Children's Depression Scale and Children's Depression Inventory in a prepubertal sample. *Journal of Child Psychology and Psychiatry, 29*, 853–863.

Kolvin, I., Nicol, A. R., Garside, R. F., Day, K. A., & Tweedle, E. G. (1982). Temperamental patterns in aggressive boys. In R. Porter & G. M. Collins (Eds.), *Temperamental differences in infants and young children.* (CIBA Foundation Symposium No. 89) (pp. 252–255). London: Pitman.

Kopp, C. B., & Kaler, S. R. (1989). Risk in infancy. *American Psychologist, 2*, 24–236.

Kovacs, M. (1981). Rating scales to assess depression in school-aged children. *Acta Paedopsychiatry, 46*, 305–315.

Kovacs, M. (1983). *The Children's Depression Inventory: A self-rated depression scale for school-aged youngsters*. Unpublished manuscript, University of Pittsburgh.

Kovacs, M. (1985). The Children's Depression Inventory. *Psychopharmacology Bulletin, 21*, 995–998.

Kupietz, S. S., Bialer, I., & Winsberg, B. G. (1972). A behavior rating scale for assessing improvement in behaviorally deviant children: A preliminary investigation. *American Journal of Psychiatry, 128*, 1432–1436.

Lahey, B. B., Gendrich, J. G., Gendrich, S. I., Schnelle, J. F., Gant, D. S., & McNees, M. P. (1977). An evaluation of daily report cards with minimal teacher and parent contacts as an efficient method of classroom intervention. *Behavior Modification, 1*, 381–394.

Lahey, B. B., Russo, M. F., Walker, J. L., & Piacentini, J. C. (1989). Personality characteristics of the mothers and children with Disruptive Behavior Disorders. *Journal of Consulting and Clinical Psychology, 57*, 512–515.

Lahey, B. B., Shaughency, E. A., Frame, C. L., & Strauss, C. C. (1985). Teacher ratings of attention problems in children experimentally classified as exhibiting Attention Deficit Disorders with and without hyperactivity. *Journal of the American Academy of Child Psychiatry, 24*, 613–616.

Lahey, B. B., Shaughency, E. A., Strauss, C. C., & Frame, C. L. (1984). Are Attention Deficit Disorders with and without hyperactivity similar or dissimilar disorders? *Journal of the American Academy of Child Psychiatry, 23*, 302–309.

Laufer, M., & Denhoff, E. (1957). Hyperkinetic behavior syndrome in children. *Journal of Pediatrics, 50*, 463–474.

Lavinge, J. V., Nolan, D., & McLone, D. G. (1988). Temperament, coding, and psychological adjustment in young children with myelomeningocele. *Journal of Pediatric Psychology, 13*, 363–378.

Leon, G. R., Kendall, P. C., & Garber, J. (1980). Depression in children: Parent, teacher, and child perspectives. *Journal of Abnormal Child Psychology, 8*, 221–235.

Lieberman, J. M. (1984). *Preventing special education...for those who don't need it*. Newton, MA: Gloworm.

Lobovits, D. A., & Handal, P. J. (1985). Childhood depression: Prevalence among DSM-III criteria and validity of parent and child depression scales. *Journal of Pediatric Psychology, 10*, 45–54.

Lochman, J. E., Burch, P. R., Curry, J. F., & Lampron, L. B. (1984). Treatment and generalization effects of cognitive-behavioral and goal-setting interventions with aggressive boys. *Journal of Consulting and Clinical Psychology, 52*, 915–916.

Lochman, J. E., & Lampron, L. B. (1986). Situational social problem-solving skills and self-esteem of aggressive and nonaggressive boys. *Journal of Abnormal Child Psychology, 14*, 605–617.

Loeber, R. (1982). The stability of antisocial and delinquent child behavior: A review. *Child Development, 53*, 1431–1446.

Loeber, R. (1988). Natural histories of conduct problems, delinquency, and associated substance use: Evidence for developmental progressions. In B. B. Lahey & Kazdin, A. E. (Eds.), *Advances in clinical child psychology* (Vol. 11, pp. 73–125). New York: Plenum Press.

Loeber, R., & Schmaling, K. B. (1985). Empirical evidence for overt and covert patterns of antisocial conduct problems: A meta-analysis. *Journal of Abnormal Child Psychology, 13,* 337–352.

Loney, J., Langhorne, J. E., & Paternite, C. E. (1978). An empirical basis for subgrouping the hyperkinetic/minimal brain dysfunction syndrome. *Journal of Abnormal Psychology, 87,* 431–441.

Loney, J., & Milich, R. S. (1982). Hyperactivity, inattention, and aggression in clinical practice. In M. Wolraich & D. Routh (Eds.). *Advances in Developmental and Behavioral Pediatrics* (Vol. 2, pp. 113–147). Greenwich, CT: JAI Press.

Long, N., Slater, E., Forehand, R., & Fauber, R. (1978). Continued high or reduced interparental conflict following divorce: Relation to young adolescent adjustment. *Journal of Consulting and Clinical Psychology, 56,* 467–469.

Lowe, T. L., Cohen, D. J., Detlor, J., Kremenitzer, M. W., & Shaywitz, B. A. (1982). Stimulant medication precipitates Tourette's syndrome. *Journal of the American Medical Association, 247,* 1729–1731.

Loyd, B. H., & Abidin, R. R. (1985). Revision of the Parenting Stress Index. *Journal of Pediatric Psychology, 10,* 169–177.

Markwardt, F. C. (1989). *Peabody Individual Achievement Test-R.* Circle Pines, MN: American Guidance Service.

Mash, E. J., & Johnston, C. (1982). A comparison of the mother–child interactions of younger and older hyperactive and normal children. *Child Development, 53,* 1371–1381.

Mash, E. J., & Johnston, C. (1983a). The prediction of mother's behavior with their hyperactive children during play and task situations. *Child and Family Behavior Therapy, 5,* 1–14.

Mash, E. J., & Johnston, C. (1983b). Parental perceptions of child behavior problems, parenting self-esteem, and mother's reported stress in younger and older hyperactive and normal children. *Journal of Consulting and Clinical Psychology, 51,* 86–99.

Mash, E. J., Johnston, C., & Kovitz, K. (1983). A comparison of the mother–child interactions of physically abused and non-abused children during play and task situations. *Journal of Clinical Child Psychology, 12,* 337–346.

Mash, E. J., & Terdal, L. G. (1988). Behavioral assessment of child and family disturbance. In E. J. Mash & L. G. Terdal (Eds.), *Behavioral assessment of childhood disorders* (2nd ed., pp. 3–65). New York: Guilford Press.

Mattes, J. A., & Gittelman, R. (1981). Effects of artificial food colorings in children with hyperactive symptoms. *Archives of General Psychiatry, 38,* 714–718.

Maurer, R. G., & Stewart, M. A. (1980). Attention Deficit Disorder without hyperactivity in a child psychiatry clinic. *Journal of Clinical Psychiatry, 41,* 232–233.

Mayer, J. M. (1977). Assessment of depression. In P. McReynolds (Ed.), *Advances in psychological assessment* (Vol. 4, pp. 358–425). San Francisco, CA: Jossey-Bass.

McCauley, E., Mitchell, J. R., Burke, P., & Moss, S. (1988). Cognitive attributes of depression in children and adolescents. *Journal of Consulting and Clinical Psychology, 56,* 903–908.

McClure, F. D., & Gordon, M. (1984). Performance of disturbed hyperactive and nonhyperactive children of an objective measure of hyperactivity. *Journal of Abnormal Child Psychology, 12,* 561–572.

McMahon, R. J., & Forehand, R. (1984). Parent training for the noncompliant child: Treatment outcome, generalization, and adjunctive therapy procedures. In R. F. Dangel & R. A. Polster (Eds.), *Parent training: Foundations of research and practice* (pp. 298–328). New York: Guilford Press.

McMahon, R. J., & Forehand, R. (1988). Conduct disorders. In E. J. Mash & L. G. Terdal (Eds.), *Behavioral assessment of childhood disorders* (2nd ed., pp. 105–153). New York: Guilford Press.

McMahon, R. J., & Wells, K. C. (1989). Conduct disorders. In E. J. Mash & R. A. Barkley (Eds.), *Treatment of childhood disorders* (pp. 73–132). New York: Guilford Press.

Meichenbaum, D. (1977). *Cognitive behavior modification: An integrative approach*. New York: Plenum Press.

Messer, S. B., & Brodzinsky, D. M. (1981). Three-year stability of reflection-impulsivity in young adolescents. *Developmental Psychology, 6*, 848–850.

Meyer, A. (1904). The anatomical facts and clinical variables of traumatic insanity. *American Journal of Insanity, 60*, 373–441.

Meyers, A. W., & Craighead, W. E. (Eds.). (1984). *Cognitive behavioral therapy with children*. New York: Plenum Press.

Milich, R., & Kramer, J. (1984). Reflections on impulsivity: An empirical investigation of impulsivity as a construct. In K. Gadow & I. Bialer (Eds.), *Advances in learning and behavioral disabilities* (Vol. 3, pp. 57–94). Greenwich, CT: JAI Press.

Milich, R., Landau, S., & Loney, J. (1981, August). *The inter-relationships among hyperactivity, aggression, and impulsivity*. Paper presented at the meeting of the American Psychological Association, Los Angeles, CA.

Milich, R., Wolraich, M., & Lindgren, S. (1986). Sugar and hyperactivity: A critical review of empirical findings. *Clinical Psychology Review, 6*, 493–513.

Mitchell, E., Matthews, K. L. (1980). Gilles de la Tourette's disorder associated with Pemoline. *American Journal of Psychiatry, 137*, 1618–1619.

Moreland, J. R., Schwebel, S. B., Beck, S., & Wells, R. (1982). Parents as therapists: A review of the behavior therapy parent training literature—1975–1981. *Behavior Modification, 2*, 250–276.

Morgan, S. A., & Jackson, J. (1986). Psychological and social concomitants of sickle cell anemia in adolescents. *Journal of Pediatric Psychology, 11*, 429–440.

Morrison, J. R., & Stewart, M. A. (1971). A family study of the hyperactive child syndrome. *Biological Psychiatry, 3*, 189–195.

Morrison, J. R., & Stewart, M. A. (1973). Evidence for a polygenetic inheritance in the hyperactive child syndrome. *American Journal of Psychiatry, 130*, 791–792.

Morrison, R. L. (1988). Structured interviews and rating scales. In A. S. Bellack & M. Hersen (Eds.), *Behavioral assessment: A practical handbook* (3rd ed., pp. 252–277). New York: Pergamon Press.

Nichols, P. (1980). Early antecedents of hyperactivity. *Neurology, 30*, 4–9.

O'Connor, M., Foch, T., Sherry, R., & Plomin, R. (1980). A twin study of specific behavioral problems of socialization as viewed by parents. *Journal of Abnormal Child Psychology, 8*, 189–199.

O'Dell, S. (1974). Training parents in behavior modification: A review. *Psychological Bulletin, 81*, 418–433.

O'Dell, S. L. (1985). Progress in parent training. In M. Hersen, R. M. Eisler, & P. M. Miller (Eds.), *Process in behavior modification* (Vol. 19, pp. 57–108). New York: Academic Press.

O'Donnell, D. J. (1985). Conduct disorders. In J. M. Weiner (Ed.), *Diagnosis and psychopharmacology of childhood and adolescent disorders* (pp. 249–287). New York: Wiley.

O'Leary, K. D., & Emery, R. E. (1984). Marital discord and child behavioral problems. In M. D. Levine & P. Satz (Eds.), *Middle childhood: Development and dysfunction* (pp. 345–364). Baltimore: University Park Press.

O'Leary, K. D., Vivian, D., & Nisi, A. (1985). Hyperactivity in Italy. *Journal of Abnormal Child Psychology, 13*, 485–500.

O'Leary, S. G., & Pelham, W. E. (1978). Behavior therapy and withdrawal of stimulant medication in hyperactive children. *Pediatrics, 61*, 211–217.

O'Leary, S. G., & Steen, P. L. (1982). Subcategorizing hyperactivity: The Stony Brook Scale. *Journal of Consulting and Clinical Psychology, 50*, 426–432.

Oliver, J. M., & Simmons, M. E. (1984). Depression as measured by the DSM-III and the Beck Depression Inventory in an unselected adult population. *Journal of Consulting and Clinical Psychology, 52*, 892–898.

Oliver, J. M., & Simmons, M. E. (1985). Affective disorders and depression as measured by the Diagnostic Interview Schedule and the Beck Depression Inventory in an unselected adult population. *Journal of Clinical Psychology, 41*, 469–477.

Ollendick, T. H., & Hersen, M. (1989). *Handbook of child psychopathology* (2nd ed.). New York: Plenum Press.

Olweus, D. (1979). Stability of aggressive reaction patterns in males: A review. *Psychological Bulletin, 86*, 852–857.

Olweus, D. (1980). Familial and temperamental determinants of aggressive behavior in adolescent boys: A causal analysis. *Developmental Psychology, 16*, 644–660.

Orvaschel, H. (1988). Structured and semistructured psychiatric interviews for children. In C. J. Kestenbaum & D. T. Williams (Eds.), *Handbook of clinical assessment of children and adolescents* (pp. 31–42). New York: New York University Press.

Othmer, E., & Othmer, S. C. (1989). *The clinical interview using DSM-III-R.* Washington, DC: American Psychiatric Press.

Packard, T., Robinson, E. A., & Grove, D. C. (1983). The effect of training procedures on the maintenance of parental relationship building skills. *Journal of Clinical Child Psychology, 12*, 181–186.

Panaccione, V. F., & Wahler, R. G. (1986). Child behavior, maternal depression, and social coercion as factors in the quality of child care. *Journal of Abnormal Child Psychology, 14*, 263–278.

Parsons, O. A. (1987). Neuropsychological consequences of alcohol abuse: Many questions—some answers. In O. A. Parsons, N. Butters, & P. E. Nathan (Eds.), *Neuropsychology of alcoholism: Implications for diagnosis and treatment* (pp. 153–175). New York: Guilford Press.

Patterson, G. R. (1982). *Coercive family process.* Eugene, OR: Castalia.

Patterson, G. R. (1986). Performance models for antisocial boys. *American Psychologist, 41*, 432–444.

Patterson, G. R., & Blank, L. (1986). Bootstrapping your way into the nomological thicket. *Behavioral Assessment, 8*, 49–73.

Patterson, G. R., & Dishioin, T. J. (1985). Contributions of families and peers to delinquency. *Criminology, 23*, 63–79.

Patterson, G. R., & Stouthamer-Loeber, M. (1984). The correlation of family management practices and delinquency. *Child Development, 55*, 1299–1307.

Pelham, W. E., Atkins, M. S., Murphy, H. A., & White, K. J., (1981, November). *Operationalization and validity of attention deficit disorders.* Paper presented at the meeting of the Association for the Advancement of Behavioral Therapy, Toronto, Ont. Canada.

Pelham, W. E., Atkins, M. S., Murphy, H. A., & Swanson, J. (1984). *A teacher rating scale for the diagnosis of Attention Deficit Disorder: Teacher norms, factor analysis, and reliability.* Unpublished manuscript.

Pelham, W. E., Bender, M. E., Caddell, J., Booth, S., & Moorer, S. H. (1985). Methylphenidate and children with Attention Deficit Disorder. *Archives of General Psychiatry, 42*, 948–952.

Pelham, W. E., & Hoza, J. (1987). Behavioral assessment of psychostimulant effects on ADD children in a summer day treatment program. In R. J. Prinz (Ed.). *Advances in behavioral assessment of children and families* (pp. 3–34). Greenwich, CT: JAI Press.

Pelham, W. E., Milich, R., & Walker, J. L. (1986). Effects of continuous and partial reinforcement and methylphenidate on learning in children with Attention Deficit Disorder. *Journal of Abnormal Child Psychology, 14*, 319–325.

Pelham, W. E., Schnedler, R. W., Nender, M. E., Nilsson, D. E., Miller L., Budrow, M. S., Ronnei, M., Paluchowski, C., & Marks, D. A. (1988). The combination of behavior therapy and methylphenidate in the treatment of Attention Deficit Disorders: A therapy outcome study. In L. M. Bloomingdale (Ed.). *Attention Deficit Disorder. Vol. 3: New research in attention, treatment, and psychopharmacology* (pp. 29–48). New York: Pergamon Press.

Pelham, W. E., Walker, J. L., Sturges, J., & Hoza, J. (1989). Comparative effects of methylphenidate on ADD girls and ADD boys. *Journal of the American Academy of Child and Adolescent Psychiatry, 5*, 773–776.

Peterson, D. R. (1961). Behavior problems of middle childhood. *Journal of Consulting Psychology, 25*, 205–209.

Phares, V., Compas, B. E., & Howell, D. C. (1989). Perspectives on child behavior problems: Comparisons of children's self-reports with parent and teacher reports. *Psychological Assessment: A Journal of Consulting and Clinical Psychology, 1*, 68–71.

Piotrwoski, C., Sherry, D., & Keller, J. W. (1985). Psychodiagnostic test usage: A survey of the Society of Personality Assessment. *Journal of Personality Assessment, 49*, 115–119.

Pliszka, S. R. (1987). Tricyclic antidepressants in the treatment of children with Attention Deficit Disorder. *Journal of the American Academy of Child and Adolescent Psychiatry, 2*, 127–132.

Pollard, S., Ward, E. M., & Barkley, R. A. (1983). The effects of parent training and Ritalin on the parent-child interactions of hyperactive boys. *Child and Family Therapy, 5*, 51–69.

Price, R. A., Leckman, J. F., Pauls, D. L., Cohen, D. J., & Kidd, K. (1986). Gilles de la Tourette's syndrome. *Neurology, 36,* 232–237.

Prinz, R. J. (1977). *The assessment of parent-adolescent relations: Discriminating distressed and non-distressed dyads.* Unpublished doctoral dissertation, SUNY, Stony Brook, NY.

Prinz, R. J., Connor, P., & Wilson, C. (1981). Hyperactive and aggressive behaviors in childhood: Intertwined dimensions. *Journal of Abnormal Child Psychology, 9,* 191–202.

Prinz, R. J., Foster, S. L., Kent, R. N., & O'Leary, K. D. (1979). Multivariate assessment of conflict in distressed and nondistressed mother–adolescent dyads. *Journal of Applied Behavioral Analysis, 12,* 691–700.

Prinz, R. J., Moore, P. A., & Roberts, W. A. (1986). Measurement of childhood hyperactivity. In R. J. Prinz (Ed.), *Advances in behavioral assessment of children and families* (Vol. 2, pp. 99–119). Greenwich, CT: JAI Press.

Prinz, R. J., Roberts, W. A., & Hantman, E. (1980). Dietary correlates of hyperactive behavior in children. *Journal of Consulting and Clinical Psychology, 48,* 760–769.

Puig-Antich, J., & Chambers, W. (1978). *The Schedule for Affective Disorders and Schizophrenia for School-Aged Children.* New York: New York State Psychiatric Institute.

Puig-Antich, J., Orvaschel, H., Tabrizi, M. A., & Chambers, W. (1980). *The schedule for affective disorders and schizophrenia for school-aged children—epidemiologic version (Kiddle-SADS-E)* (3rd. ed.). New York: New York State Psychiatric Institute.

Quay, H. C. (1964). Dimensions of personality in delinquent boys as inferred from factor analysis of case history data. *Child Development, 35,* 470–484.

Quay, H. C. (1977). Measuring dimensions of deviant behavior: The Behavior Problem Checklist. *Journal of Abnormal Child Psychology, 5,* 277–287.

Quay, H. C. (1979). Classification. In H. C. Quay & J. S. Werry (Eds.), *Psychopathological disorders of childhood* (2nd ed., pp. 1–42). New York: Wiley.

Quay, H. C. (1983). A dimensional approach to behavior disorder: The Revised Behavior Problem Checklist. *School Psychology Review, 12,* 244–249.

Quay, H. C. (1986). A critical analysis of DSM-III as a taxonomy of psychopathology in childhood and adolescence. In T. Millon & G. L. Klerman (Eds.), *Contemporary directions in psychopathology: Toward the DSM-IV* (pp. 151–165). New York: Guilford Press.

Quay, H. C., & Peterson, D. R. (1975). *Manual for the Behavior Problem Checklist.* Unpublished manuscript, University of Miami.

Quay, H. C., & Peterson, D. R. (1983). *Interim manual for the Revised Behavior Problem Checklist.* Unpublished manuscript. University of Miami.

Quay, H. C., & Peterson, D. R. (1984). *Appendix I to the interim manual for the Revised Behavior Problem Checklist.* Unpublished manuscript, University of Miami.

Quay, H. C., & Peterson, D. R. (1987). *Manual for the Revised Behavior Problem Checklist.* Unpublished manuscript, University of Miami.

Quay, H. C., & Werry, J. S. (1986). *Psychopathological disorders of childhood* (3rd ed.). New York: Wiley.

Rapoport, J. L. (1983). The use of drugs: Trends in research. In M. Rutter (Ed.), *Developmental Neuropsychiatry* (pp. 385–403). New York: Guilford Press.

Rapport, M. D. (1987). Attention Deficit Disorder with hyperactivity. In M. Hersen & V. B. Van Hasselt (Eds.), *Behavior therapy with children and adolescents: A clinical appraoch* (pp. 325–361). New York: Wiley.

Rapport, M. D., Murphy, A., & Bailey, J. S. (1982). Ritalin versus response cost in the control of hyperactive children: A within-subject comparison. *Journal of Applied Behavior Analysis, 15,* 205–216.

Rapport, M. D., Jones, J. T., DuPaul, G. J., Kelly, K. L., Gardner, M. J., Tucker, S. B., & Shea, M. S. (1987). Attention deficit disorder and methylphenidate: Group and single-subject analyses of dose effects on attention in clinic and classroom settings. *Journal of Clinical Child Psychology, 4,* 329–338.

Rapport, M. D., Stoner, G., DuPaul, G. J., Birmingham, B. K., & Tucker, S. (1985). Methylphenidate in hyperactive children: Differential effects of dose on academic, learning, and social behavior. *Journal of Abnormal Child Psychology, 13,* 227–243.

Rapport, M. D., Stoner, G., DuPaul, G. J., Kelly, K. L., Tucker, S. B., & Schoeler, T. (1988). Attention Deficit Disorder and methylphenidate: A multilevel analysis of dose-response effects on children's impulsivity across settings. *Journal of the American Academy of Child and Adolescent Psychiatry, 1,* 60–69.

Reatig, N. (1984). Attention Deficit Disorder: A bibliography. *Psychopharmacology Bulletin, 20,* 693–718.

Reed, M. L., & Edelbrock, C. S. (1983). Reliability and validity of the Direct Observation Form of the Child Behavior Checklist. *Journal of Abnormal Child Psychology, 11,* 521–530.

Reid, J. B., Baldwin, D. V., Patterson, G. R., & Dishion, T. J. (1988). Observations in the assessment of childhood disorders. In M. Rutter, A. Tuma, & I. Lann (Eds.), *Assessment and diagnosis in child psychopathology* (pp. 156–195). New York: Guilford Press.

Reid, W. J., & Crisafulli, A. (1990). Marital discord and child behavior: A meta-analysis. *Journal of Abnormal Child Psychology, 19,* 105–117.

Remschmidt, H. (1984). *Multiaxial classification in child psychiatry: Results of some empirical studies.* Paper presented at research workshop on Assessment, Diagnosis, and Classification in child and adolescent psychopathology. Washington, DC: Center for Studies of Child and Adolescent Psychopathology, Clinical Research Branch, NIMH.

Reynolds, M. C., Wang, C., & Walberg, H. J. (1987). The necessary restructuring of special and regular education. *Exceptional Children, 53,* 391–398.

Reynolds, W. M. (1986). A model for the screening and identification of depressed children and adolescents in school settings. *Professional School Psychology, 1,* 117–129.

Reynolds, W. M. (1987). *Reynolds Adolescent Depression Scale: Professional Manual.* Odessa, FL: Psychological Assessment Resources.

Reynolds, W. M., & Anderson, G. (1986). Unpublished data reported in W. M. Reynolds (1987). *Reynolds Adolescent Depression Scale: Professional manual.* Odessa, FL: Psychological Assessment Resources.

Reynolds, W. M., & Coats, K. I. (1986). A comparison of cognitive-behavioral therapy and relaxation training for the treatment of depression in adolescents. *Journal of Consulting and Clinical Psychology, 54*, 653–660.

Richardson, E., Kupietz, S. S., Winsberg, B. G., Maitinsky, S., & Mendell, N. (1988). Effects of methylphenidate dosage in hyperactive reading-disabled children: II: Reading achievement. *Journal of the American Academy of Child and Adolescent Psychiatry, 1*, 78–87.

Riddle, M. A., Hardin, M. T., Cho, S. C., Woolston, J. L., & Leckman, J. F. (1988). Desipramine treatment of boys with Attention-deficit Hyperactivity Disorder and tics: Preliminary clinical experience. *Journal of the American Academy of Child and Adolescent Psychiatry, 6*, 811–814.

Rincover, A., Koegel, R. L., & Russo, D. C. (1978). Some recent behavioral research on the education of autistic children. *Education and Treatment of Children, 1*, 31–45.

Robin, A. L. (1981). A controlled evaluation of problem-solving communication training with parent-adolescent conflict. *Behavior Therapy, 12*, 593–609.

Robin, A. L., Fischel, J. E., & Brown, K. E. (1984). The measurement of self-control in children: Validation of the Self-Control Rating Scale. *Journal of Pediatric Psychology, 9*, 165–175.

Robin, A. L., & Foster, S. L. (1984). Problem-solving communication training: A behavioral-family systems approach to parent-adolescent conflict. In P. Karoly & J. J. Steffen (Eds.), *Adolescent behavior disorders: Foundations and contemporary concerns* (pp. 195–240). Lexington, MA: D. C. Heath.

Robin, A. L., & Foster, S. L. (1989). *Negotiating parent-adolescent conflict: A behavioral-family systems approach*. New York: Guilford Press.

Robin, A. L., & Weiss, G. (1980). Criterion-related validity of behavioral and self-report measures of problem-solving communication skills in distressed and non-distressed parent-adolescent dyads. *Behavioral Assessment, 2*, 339–352.

Robins, L. N. (1966). *Deviant children grown up: A sociological and psychiatric study of sociopathic personality*. Baltimore: Williams & Wilkins.

Robins, L. N. (1978). Sturdy childhood predictors of adult antisocial behavior: Replications from longitudinal studies. *Psychological Medicine, 8*, 611–622.

Robins, L. N. (1981). Epidemiological approaches to natural history research: Antisocial disorders in children. *Journal of the American Academy of Child Psychiatry, 20*, 566–680.

Robinson, E. A., & Anderson, L. L. (1983). Family adjustment, parental attitudes, and social desirability. *Journal of Abnormal Child Psychology, 11*, 247–256.

Robinson, E. A., & Eyberg, S. M. (1981). The dyadic parent–child interaction coding system: Standardization and validation. *Journal of Consulting and Clinical Psychology, 49*, 245–250.

Robinson, E. A., Eyberg, S. M., & Ross, E. A. (1980). The standardization of an inventory of child conduct problem behaviors. *Journal of Clinical Child Psychology, 9*, 22–29.

Rogers, T. R., Forehand, R., & Griest, D. L. (1981). The conduct disordered child: An analysis of family problems. *Clinical Psychology Review, 1*, 139–147.

Romano, B. A., & Nelson, R. O. (1988). Discriminative and concurrent validity of measures of children's depression. *Journal of Clinical Child Psychology, 17,* 255–259.

Rosen, L. A., Booth, S. R., Bender, M. E., McGrath, M. L. Sorrell, S., & Drabman, R. S. (1988). Effects of sugar (sucrose) on children's behavior. *Journal of Consulting and Clinical Psychology, 56,* 583–589.

Rosenberg, R. P., & Beck, S. (1986). Preferred assessment methods and treatment modalities for hyperactive children among clinical child and school psychologists. *Journal of Clinical Child Psychology, 15,* 142–147.

Ross, D. M., & Ross, S. A. (1982). *Hyperactivity* (2nd ed.). New York: Wiley.

Rutter, M. (1977). Brain damage syndromes in childhood: Concepts and findings. *Journal of Child Psychology and Psychiatry, 18,* 1–21.

Rutter, M. (1983). Introduction: Concepts of brain dysfunction syndromes. In M. Rutter (Ed.), *Developmental neuropsychiatry* (pp. 1–11). New York: Guilford Press.

Rutter, M. (1989). Attention Deficit Disorder/Hyperkinetic Syndrome: Conceptual and research issues regarding diagnosis and classification. In T. Sagvolden & T. Archer (Eds.), *Attention Deficit Disorder: Clinical and basic research* (pp. 1–24). Hillsdale, NJ: Erlbaum.

Rutter, M., Chadwick, O., & Shaffer, D. (1983). Head injury. In M. Rutter (Ed.), *Developmental neuropsychiatry* (pp. 83–111). New York: Guilford Press.

Rutter, M., Tizard, J., Yule, W., Graham, P., & Whitmore, K. (1976). Research report: Isle of Wight studies, 1964–1974. *Psychological Medicine, 6,* 313–332.

Safer, D. J. (1984). Subgrouping conduct disordered adolescents by early risk factors. *American Journal of Orthopsychiatry, 54,* 603–612.

Safer, D. J., & Allen, D. (1976). *Hyperactive children.* Baltimore: University Park Press.

Salkind, N. J. (1978). Development of norms for the Matching Familiar Figures Test. *JSAS Catalog of Selected Documents in Psychology, 8* (1718).

Sanders, M. R., & James, J. E. (1983). The modification of parent behavior: A review of generalization and maintenance. *Behavior Therapy, 7,* 3–27.

Sandoval, J. (1977). The measurement of hyperactive syndrome in children. *Review of Educational Research, 47,* 293–318.

Sandoval, J., & Lambert, N. M. (1985). Hyperactive and learning disabled children: Who gets help? *The Journal of Special Education, 18,* 495–503.

Satterfield, J. H., Hoppe, C. M., & Schell, A. M. (1982). A prospective study of delinquency in 110 adolescent boys with attention deficit disorder and 88 normal adolescent boys. *American Journal of Psychiatry, 139,* 795–798.

Sattler, J. (1988). *Assessment of children's intelligence and special abilities* (3rd ed.). Boston: Allyn and Bacon.

Saylor, C. F., Finch, A. J., Spirito, A., & Bennet, B. (1984). The Children's Depression Inventory: A systematic evaluation of psychometric properties. *Journal of Consulting and Clinical Psychology, 52,* 955–967.

Schachar, R., Taylor, E., Wieselberg, M., Thorley, G., & Rutter, M. (1987). Changes in family function and relationships in children who respond to methylphenidate. *Journal of the American Academy of Child and Adolescent Psychiatry, 26,* 728–732.

Schaefer, C. E., & Briesmeister, J. M. (1989). *Handbook of parent training: Parents as co-therapists for children's behavior problems.* New York: Wiley.

Schatzberg, A. F., & Cole, J. O. (1986). *Manual of clinical psychopharmacology*. Washington, DC: American Psychiatric Press.

Schinka, J. A. (1985). *Personal Problems Checklist For Adolescents* Odessa, FL: Psychological Assessment Resources.

Schmitt, B. (1977). Guidelines for living with a hyperactive child. *Pediatrics, 60,* 387.

Schroeder, J. S., Mullin, A. V., Elliott, G. R., Steiner, H., Nichols, M., Gordon, A., & Paulos, M. (1989). Cardiovascular effects of desipramine in children. *Journal of the American Academy of Child and Adolescent Psychiatry, 28,* 376–379.

Seagull, E. A., & Weinshank, A. B. (1984). Childhood depression in a selected group of low-achieving seventh graders. *Journal of Clinical Child Psychology, 13,* 134–140.

Sergeant, J. A., & Scholten, C. A. (1985a). On resource strategy limitations in hyperactivity: Cognitive impulsivity reconsidered. *Journal of Child Psychology and Psychiatry, 26,* 97–109.

Sergeant, J. A., & Scholten, C. A. (1985b). On data limitations in hyperactivity. *Journal of Child Psychology and Psychiatry, 26,* 111–124.

Shaffer, D., Schonfeld, I., O'Conner, P. A., Stockman, C., Trautman, P., Shafer, S., & Ng, S. (1985). Neurological soft signs: Their relationship to psychiatric disorders and intelligence in childhood and adolescence. *Archives of General Psychiatry, 42,* 342–351.

Shapiro, B. A., & Garfinkel, B. D. (1986). The occurrence of behavior disorders in children: The interdependence of Attention Deficit Disorder and Conduct Disorder. *Journal of the American Academy of Child Psychiatry, 6,* 809–819.

Shaywitz, B. A., Cohen, D. J., & Bowers, M. B. (1977). CSF monoamine metabolites in children with minimal brain dysfunction—evidence for alteration of brain dopamine. *Journal of Pediatrics, 90,* 67–71.

Shaywitz, S. E., Cohen, D. J., & Shaywitz, B. A. (1978). The biochemical basis of minimal brain dysfunction. *Journal of Pediatrics, 92,* 179–187.

Shaywitz, S. E., Cohen, D. J., & Shaywitz, B. A. (1980). Behavior and learning difficulties in children of normal intelligence born to alcoholic mothers. *Journal of Pediatrics, 96,* 978–982.

Shaywitz, S. E., & Shaywitz, B. A. (1989). Critical issues in Attention Deficit Disorder. In T. Sagvolden & T. Archer (Eds.), *Attention Deficit Disorder: Clinical and basic research* (pp. 53–69). Hillsdale, NJ: Erlbaum.

Shaywitz, S. E., Shaywitz, B. A., Cohen, D. J., & Young, D. J. (1983). Monoaminergic mechanisms in hyperactivity. In M. Rutter (Ed.), *Developmental neuropsychiatry* (pp. 330–347). New York: Guilford Press.

Skinner, B. F. (1969). *Contingencies of reinforcement: A theoretical analysis*. New York: Appleton-Century-Crofts.

Sleator, E. K., & Ullmann, R. K. (1981). Can the physician diagnose hyperactivity in the office? *Pediatrics, 67,* 13–17.

Slotkin, J., Forehand, R., Fauber, R., McCombs, A., & Long, N. (1988). Parent-completed and adolescent-completed CDIs: Relationship to adolescent social and cognitive functioning. *Journal of Abnormal Child Psychology, 16,* 207–217.

Smith, M. T., Smith, M. P., & L'Abate, L. (1985). Systems interventions with hyperactive children: An interdisciplinary perspective. In L. L'Abate (Ed.)., *Hand-*

book of family psychology and therapy (pp. 1152–1178). Homewood, IL: Dorsey Press.

Smucker, M. R., Craighead, W. E., Craighead, L. W., & Green, B. J. (1986). Normative and reliability data for the Children's Depression Inventory. *Journal of Abnormal Child Psychology, 14*, 25–39.

Speltz, M. L., Varley, C. K., Peterson, K., & Beilke, R. L. (1988). Effects of dextroamphetamine and contingency management on a preschooler with ADHD and Oppositional Defiant Disorder. *Journal of the American Academy of Child and Adolescent Psychiatry, 27*, 175–178.

Spirito, A., Stark, L., Fristad, M., Hart, K., & Owens-Stively, J. (1987). Adolescent suicide attempters hospitalized on a pediatric unit. *Journal of Pediatric Psychology, 12*, 171–189.

Spitzer, R. L., Davies, M. & Barkley, R. A. (1990). The DSM-III-R field trial of the Disruptive Behavior Disorders. *American Journal of Child and Adolescent Psychiatry.*.

Spivack, G., Platt, J. J., & Shure, M. B. (1976). *The problem-solving approach to adjustment.* San Francisco: Jossey-Bass.

Sprague, R. L., Cohen, M. N., & Eichlseder, W. (1977, August). *Are there hyperactive children in Europe and the South Pacific?* Paper presented at the annual meeting of the American Psychological Association. San Francisco, CA.

Sprague, R. L., & Sleator, E. K. (1977). Methylphenidate in hyperkinetic children: Differences in dose effects on learning and social behavior. *Science, 198*, 1274–1276.

Steer, R. A., Beck, A. T., & Garrison, B. (1986). Application of the Beck Depression Inventory. In N. Sartorious & T. A. Ban (Eds.), *Assessment of depression* (pp. 121–142). Geneva, Switzerland: World Health Organization.

Stephens, R., Pelham, W. E., & Skinner, R. (1984). The state-dependent and main effects of pemoline and methylphenidate on paired-associate learning and spelling in hyperactive children. *Journal of Consulting and Clinical Psychology, 52*, 104–113.

Stevenson, R. D., & Wolraich, M. L. (1989). Stimulant medication therapy in the treatment of children with Attention-deficit Hyperactive Disorder. *Pediatric Clinics of North America, 36*, 1183–1197.

Stewart, M. A., Cummings, C., Singer, S., & deBlois, C. S. (1981). The overlap between hyperactive and unsocialized aggressive children. *Journal of Child Psychology and Psychiatry, 22*, 23–45.

Stewart, J. T., Myers, W. C., Burket, R. C., & Lyles, W. B. (1990). A review of the pharmacotherapy of aggression in children and adolescents. *Journal of the Academy of Child and Adolescent Psychiatry, 18*, 269–277.

Strauss, A. A., & Lehtinen, L. E. (1947). *Psychopathology and education of the brain-injured child.* New York: Grune & Stratton.

Sturge, C. (1982). Reading retardation and antisocial behavior. *Journal of Child Psychology and Psychiatry, 23*, 21–31.

Sullivan, W. (1985). Unpublished data reported in Reynolds, W. M. (1987). *Reynolds Adolescent Depression Scale: Professional manual* Odessa, FL: Psychological Assessment Resources.

Sverd, J., Curley, A., Jandorf, L., & Volkersz, L. (1988). Behavior disorder and attention deficits in boys with Tourette Syndrome. *Journal of the American Academy of Child and Adolescent Psychiatry, 27*, 413–417.

Sverd, J., Gadow, K. D., & Paolicelli, L. M. (1989). Methylphenidate treatment of Attention-Deficit Disorder in boys with Tourette's Syndrome. *Journal of the American Academy of Child and Adolescent Psychiatry, 28*, 574–579.

Szatmari, P., Boyle, M., & Offord, D. R. (1989). ADDH and conduct disorder: Degree of diagnostic overlap and differences among correlates. *Journal of the American Academy of Child and Adolescent Psychiatry, 28*, 865–872.

Tannock, R., Schachar, R. J., Carr, R. P., Chajczyk, D., & Logan, G. D. (1989). Effects of methylphenidate on inhibitory control in hyperactive children. *Journal of Abnormal Child Psychology, 17*, 473–491.

Taylor, E., & Sandberg, S. (1984). Hyperactive behavior in English schoolchildren: A questionnaire survey. *Journal of Abnormal Child Psychology, 12*, 143–156.

Taylor, H. G. (1988). Learning disabilities. In E. J. Mash & L. G. Terdal (Eds.), *Behavioral assessment of childhood disorders* (2nd ed., pp. 402–450). New York: Guilford Press.

Taylor, H. G. (1989). Learning disabilities. In E. J. Mash & R. A. Barkley (Eds.), *Treatment of childhood disorders* (pp. 347–380). New York: Guilford Press.

Taylor, V. L., Cornwell, D. D., & Riley, M. T. (1984). Home-based contingency management programs that teachers can use. *Psychology In The Schools, 3*, 368–374.

Thorley, G. (1983). Data on Conners' Teacher Rating Scale on a British population. *Journal of Behavioral Assessment, 5*, 1–10.

Tramontana, M. G., Hooper, S. R., Curley, A. D., & Nardolillo, E. M. (1990). Determinants of academic achievement in children with psychiatric disorders. *Journal of the Academy of Child and Adolescent Psychiatry, 18*, 265–268.

Trites, R. L., Blouin, A. G., Ferguson, H. B., & Lynch, G. W. (1981). Conners Teacher Rating Scale: An epidemiological inter-rater reliability and follow-up investigation. In K. Gadow & J. Loney (Eds.), *Psychosocial aspects of drug treatment for hyperactivity*. Boulder, CO: Westview Press.

Trites, R. L., Blouin, A. G., & Laprade, K. (1982). Factor analysis of the Conners Teacher Rating Scale based upon a large normative sample. *Journal of Consulting and Clinical Psychology, 50*, 615–623.

Trites, R. L., Dugas, E., Lynch, G., & Ferguson, H. B. (1979). Prevalence of hyperactivity. *Journal of Pediatric Psychology, 4*, 179–188.

Trites, R. L., & Laprade, K. (1984). *Traduction et normes pour une version francaise du Conners Teacher Rating Scale*. Unpublished manuscript. Royal Ottawa Hospital, Ottawa, Ont., Canada.

Twardosz, S., & Norquist, V. M. (1987). Parent training. In M. Hersen & V. B. Van Hasselt Routh (Eds.), *Behavior therapy with children and adolescents: A clinical approach* (pp. 75–105). New York: Wiley.

Ullmann, R. K. (1985). ACTeRS useful in screening learning disabled from Attention Deficit Disorder (ADD-H) children. *Psychopharmacology Bulletin, 21*, 547–551.

Ullmann, R. K., & Sleator, E. K. (1985). Attention Deficit Disorder children with and without hyperactivity: Which behaviors are helped by stimulants. *Clinical Pediatrics, 24*, 547–551.

Ullmann, R. K., & Sleator, E. K. (1986). Responders, nonresponders, and placebo responders among children with Attention Deficit Disorder: Importance of a blinded placebo evaluation. *Clinical Pediatrics, 25*, 594–599.

Ullmann, R. K., Sleator, E. K., & Sprague, R. L. (1984a). A new rating scale for diagnosis and monitoring of ADD children. *Psychopharmacology Bulletin, 20*, 160–164.

Ullmann, R. K., Sleator, E. K., & Sprague, R. L. (1984b). ADD children: Who is referred from the school? *Psychopharmacology Bulletin, 20*, 308–312.

Ullmann, R. K., Sleator, E. K., & Sprague, R. L. (1985). A change of mind: Conners' Abbreviated Rating Scales reconsidered. *Journal of Abnormal Child Psychology, 13*, 553–566.

Ullmann, R. K., Sleator, E. K., & Sprague, R. L. (1988). *Manual for the ADD-H Comprehensive Teacher's Rating Scale*. Champaign, IL: MeriTech, Inc.

United States Public Law 94-142 (learning disability and emotional disturbance federal guidelines). (1984, July 1). *Federal Register* Parts 300–399, pp. 700–701.

van der Meere, J., & Sergeant, J. (1988). Controlled processing and vigilance in hyperactivity: Time will tell. *Journal of Abnormal Child Psychology, 16*, 641–655.

Varni, J. W., & Henker, B. (1979). A self-regulation approach to the treatment of three hyperactive boys. *Child Behavior Therapy, 1*, 171–192.

Vincent, J. P., Williams, B. J., Harris, G. E., & Duvall, G. (1977, August). *Classroom observations of hyperactive children: A multiple validation study*. Paper presented at the annual meeting of the American Psychological Association. San Francisco, CA.

Voelker, S. L., Carter, R. A., Sprague, D. J., Gdowski, C. L., & Lachar, D. (1989). Developmental trends in memory and metamemory in children with Attention Deficit Disorder. *Journal of Pediatric Psychology, 14*, 75–88.

Wahler, R. G. (1980). The insular mother: Her problems in parent–child treatment. *Journal of of Applied Behavior Analysis, 13*, 207–219.

Walker, C. E. (1978). Toilet training, enuresis, encopresis. In P. Magrab (Ed.), *Psychological management of pediatric problems: Vol. 1, Early life conditions*. Baltimore: University Park Press.

Walker, C. E., Milling, L., & Bonner, B. (1988). Incontinence disorders: Enuresis and encopresis. In D. Routh (Ed.), *Handbook of pediatric psychology* (pp. 363–397). New York: Guilford Press.

Walker, C. E., & Roberts, M. C. (Eds.). (1983). *Handbook of clinical child psychology*. New York: Wiley.

Walker, J. L., Lahey, B. B., Hynd, G. W., & Frame, C. L. (1987). Comparison of specific patterns of antisocial behavior in children with Conduct Disorder with or without coexisting hyperactivity. *Journal of Consulting and Clinical Psychology, 55*, 910–913.

Walker, J. L., & Green, J. W. (1989). Children with recurrent abdominal pain and their parents: More somatic complaints, anxiety, and depression than other patient families? *Journal of Pediatric Psychology, 14*, 231–243.

Wallander, J. L., & Hubert, N. C. (1985). Long-term prognosis for children with Attention Deficit Disorder with hyperactivity (ADD/H). In B. B. Lahey & A. E.

Kazdin (Eds.), *Advances in clinical child psychology* (Vol. 8, pp. 113–147). New York: Plenum Press.

Wallander, J. L., Feldman, W. S., & Varni, J. W. (1989). Physical status and psychosocial adjustment in children with spina bifida. *Journal of Pediatric Psychology, 14*, 89–102.

Wallander, J. L., Varni, J. W., Babani, L., Banis, H. T., & Wilcox, K. T. (1988). Children with chronic physical disorders: Maternal reports of their psychological adjustment. *Journal of Pediatric Psychology, 13*, 197–212.

Watter, N., & Dreifuss, F. E. (1973). Modification of hyperkinetic behavior by nortriptyline. *The Virginia Medical Monthly, 2*, 123–126.

Webster-Stratton, C. (1981a). Modification of mothers' behaviors and attitudes through a videotape modeling and group discussion program. *Behavior Therapy, 12*, 634–642.

Webster-Stratton, C. (1981b). Videotape modeling: A method of parent education. *Journal of Clinical Child Psychology, 10*, 93–98.

Webster-Stratton, C. (1982a). Teaching mothers through videotaped modeling to change their children's behavior. *Journal of Pediatric Psychology, 7*, 279–294.

Webster-Stratton, C. (1982b). Long-term effects of a videotape modeling parent training program: Comparison of immediate and 1-year follow-up results. *Behavior Therapy, 13*, 702–714.

Webster-Stratton, C. (1984a). Randomized trial of two parent training programs for families with conduct-disordered children. *Journal of Consulting and Clinical Psychology, 52*, 666–678.

Webster-Stratton, C. (1984b). Mothers' and fathers' perceptions of child deviance: Roles of parent and child behaviors and parent adjustment. *Journal of Consulting and Clinical Psychology, 56*, 909–915.

Webster-Stratton, C. (1987). *The parents and children series*. Eugene, OR: Castalia.

Webster-Stratton, C., & Eyberg, S. M. (1982). Child temperament: Relationship with child behavior problems and parent-child interactions. *Journal of Clinical Child Psychology, 11*, 123–129.

Webster-Stratton, C., Hollingsworth, T., & Kolpacoff, M. (1989). The long-term effectiveness and clinical significance of three cost-effective training programs for families with conduct problem children. *Journal of Consulting and Clinical Psychology, 57*, 550–553.

Webster-Stratton, C., Kolpacoff, M., & Hollingsworth, T. (1988). Self-administered videotape therapy for families with conduct problem children: Comparison of two cost-effective treatments and a control group. *Journal of Consulting and Clinical Psychology, 56*, 558–566.

Wechsler, D. (1974). *Manual for the Wechsler Intelligence Scale for Children-Revised*. San Antonio, TX: The Psychological Corporation.

Weiss, B. (1984). Food additive safety evaluation: The link to behavioral disorders in children. In B. B. Lahey & A. E. Kazdin (Eds.), *Advances in clinical child psychology* (Vol. 7, pp. 221–259). New York: Plenum Press.

Weiss, G., & Hechtman, L. (1986). *Hyperactive children grown up*. New York: Guilford Press.

Weiss, G., Hechtman, L., Milroy, T., & Perlman, T. (1985). Psychiatric status of hyperactives as adults: A controlled prospective 15-year follow-up of 63 hyperactive children. *Journal of the American Academy of Child Psychiatry, 24*, 211–220.

Weiss, G., Hechtman, L., & Perlman, T. (1978). Hyperactives as young adults: School, employer, and self-rating scales obtained during a ten-year follow-up evaluation. *American Journal of Orthopsychiatry, 48*, 438–445.

Wells, K. C., & Forehand, R. (1985). Conduct and oppositional disorders. In P. H. Bornstein & A.E. Kazdin (Eds.), *Handbook of clinical behavior therapy with children* (pp. 218–265). Homewood, IL: Dorsey.

Welsh, R. (1968). *Stimulus satiation as a technique for the elimination of juvenile firesetting behavior*. Washington, DC: Eastern Psychological Association.

Wender, P. H. (1971). *Minimal brain dysfunction in children*. New York: Wiley.

Werner, H., & Strauss, A. A. (1941). Pathology of the figure-background relation in the child. *Journal of Abnormal and Social Psychology, 36*, 236–248.

Werry, J. S. (1982). Pharmacotherapy. In B. B. Lahey & A. E. Kazdin (Eds.), *Advances in clinical child psychology* (Vol. 5, pp. 283–321). New York: Plenum Press.

Werry, J. S., & Hawthorne, D. (1976). Conners Teacher Questionnaire: Norms and validity. *Australian and New Zealand Journal of Psychiatry, 10*, 257–262.

Werry, J. S., Methven, R. J., Fitzpatrick, J., & Dixon, H. (1983). The interrater reliability of DSM-III in children. *Journal of Abnormal Child Psychology, 11*, 341–354.

Werry, J. S., Sprague, R. L., & Cohen, M. N. (1975). Conners Teacher Rating Scale for use in drug studies with children: Am empirical study. *Journal of Abnormal Child Psychology, 3*, 217–229.

Whalen, C. K. (1983). Hyperactivity, learning problems, and the Attention Deficit Disorders. In T. H. Ollendick & M. Hersen (Eds.), *Handbook of child psychopathology* (pp. 151–199). New York: Plenum Press.

Whalen, C. K., Henker, B., & Dotemoto, S. (1981). Teacher response to the methylphenidate (Ritalin) versus placebo status of hyperactive boys in the classroom. *Child Development, 52*, 1005–1014.

Whalen, C. K., Henker, B., & Hinshaw, S. P. (1985). Cognitive-behavioral therapies for hyperactive children: Premises, problems and prospects. *Journal of Abnormal Child Psychology, 13*, 391–410.

Whalen, C. K., Henker, B., Swanson, J. M., Granger, D., Kliewer, W., & Spencer, J. (1987). Natural social behaviors in hyperactive children: Dose effects of methylphenidate. *Journal of Consulting and Clinical Psychology, 55*, 187–193.

White, J. H. (1977). *Pediatric psychopharmacology*. Baltimore: William & Wilkins.

Will, M. C. (1986). Educating children with learning problems: A shared responsibility. *Exceptional Children, 52*, 411–415.

Williams, J. R., & Gold, M. (1972). From delinquent behavior to official delinquency. *Social Problems, 20*, 209–229.

Wilson, G. T., Franks, C. M., Brownell, K. D., & Kendall, P. C. (1984). *Annual review of behavior therapy: Theory and practice* (Vol. 9). New York: Guilford Press.

Wirt, R., Lachar, D., Klinedinst, J., & Seat, P. (1984). *Multidimensional description of child personality; A manual for the Personality Inventory for Children*. (2nd ed., rev. by D. Lachar). Los Angeles, CA: Western Psychological Services.

Wisconsin Statutes. (1983). Rules implementing subchapter V of chapter 115. *Wisconsin Department of Public Instruction*, 125.

Wolfe, D. A., Sandler, J., & Kaufman, K. (1981). A competency-based parent training program for child abusers. *Journal of Consulting and Clinical Psychology, 49*, 633–640.

Wolraich, M., Milich, R., Stumbo, P., & Schultz, F. (1985). The effects of sucrose ingestion on the behavior of hyperactive boys. *Journal of Pediatrics, 106*, 675–682.

Worchel, F. F., Nolan, B. F., Wilson, V. L., Purser, J. S., Copeland, D. R., & Pfefferbaum, B. (1988). Assessment of depression in children with cancer. *Journal of Pediatric Psychology, 13*, 101–112.

Zentall, S. S., & Barack, R. S. (1979). Rating scales for hyperactivity: Concurrent validity, reliability, and decisions to label for the Conners and Davids abbreviated scales. *Journal of Abnormal Child Psychology, 7*, 179–190.

Zentall, S. S., & Meyer, M. J. (1987). Self-regulation of stimulation for ADD-H children during reading and vigilance task performance. *Journal of Abnormal Child Psychology, 15*, 519–536.

INDEX